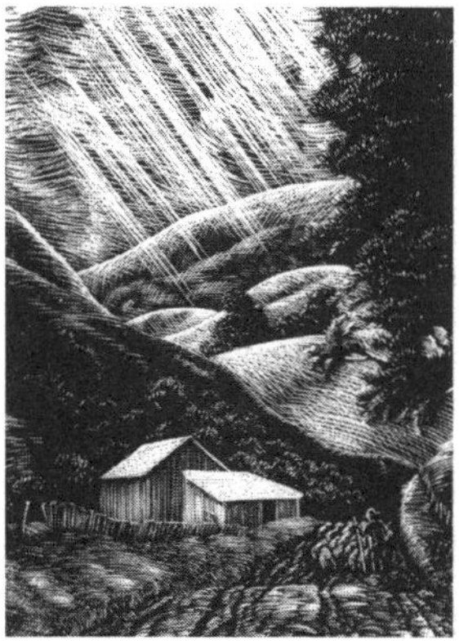

Old Black Cloud

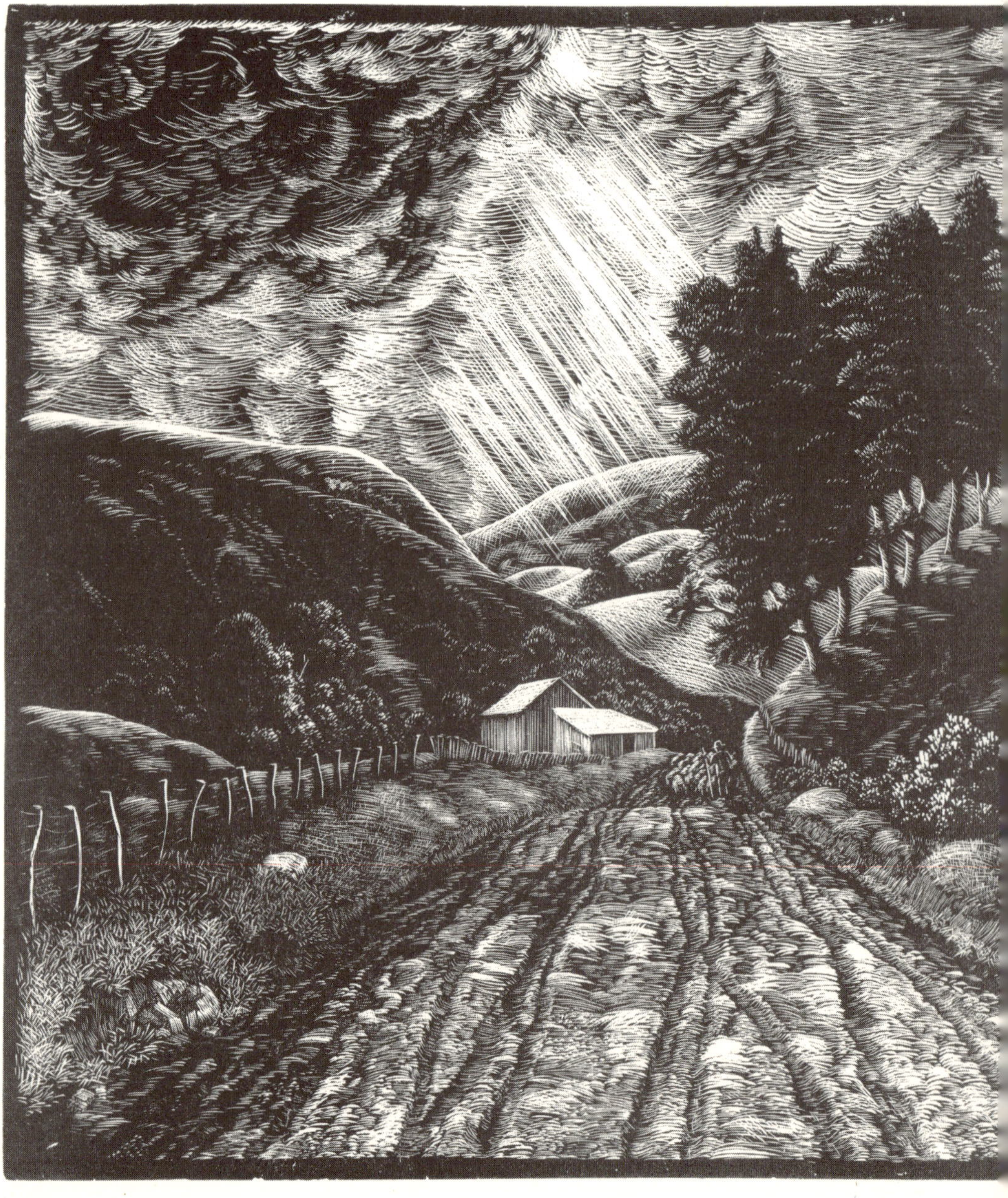

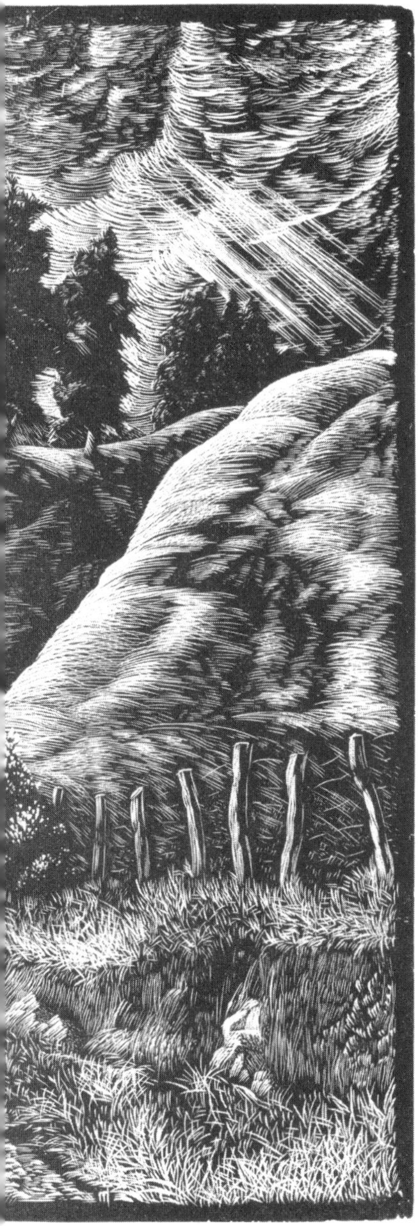

Old Black Cloud

A cultural history of mental depression in Aotearoa New Zealand

Jacqueline Leckie

MASSEY
UNIVERSITY
PRESS

Previous page: E. Mervyn Taylor,
Dark Valley, 1937

Contents

Introduction

When, in the 1990s, my family doctor put it to me that I was depressed, the biochemical model of brain chemistry was ascendant in the understanding and treatment of depression.[1] This science emphasised an imbalance of neurotransmitters — chemical messengers — whereby depression is linked to a lack of serotonin receptors in the brain, serotonin being responsible for many key body functions, such as mood modulation, feelings of reward, sleep, digestion and healing, among many others. The implication was that my depression was due to a biochemical imbalance instead of, or perhaps in combination with, my grief over my mother's recent death.

At times during my life I have been prescribed medications and encountered therapists who have pushed different approaches to coping with depression that seemed to relate to major loss. In 1979, after my former husband's sudden disappearance to live with another woman, an expensive therapy session involved facing a large circle of coloured cushions that I was meant to beat or embrace. I couldn't inflict such actions on those bits of fluff. This was a version of the Gestalt therapy that I had learned about in a first-year university psychology paper, but even so my imagination fell short. Fortunately — thanks to the excellent public health system of the time — I was treated by an empathetic psychiatrist at Auckland Hospital. We explored my family history and dynamics, my economically poor background, politics and, yes, my relationship with my mother. The sessions were structured loosely within psychoanalysis.

That psychiatrist saved my life and encouraged me to complete my PhD and pursue a career.[2] I still recall walking along the Devonport waterfront in 1980, and seeing the sun setting, smelling the sea, hearing the waves and the seagulls and feeling the warmth of the day. For at least the previous year I had felt absolutely nothing except pain.

Depression still lurked in my background and could become unbearable when I experienced intimate or professional stress, or profound loneliness. But like so many people living with depression, I pressed on with hard work, a demanding but rewarding career, and immersed myself in social activism through concern for the suffering of others. My sense of loneliness did not preclude a vibrant social life and wonderful friendships.

My closest bond was with my wonderful mum, Violet, who was born in 1922. She was prone to deep sadness; probably today this would bring a diagnosis of depression. She was also very ill throughout her life with cardiovascular and kidney illness. Her own mother had died when she was only nine years old. Her family was poor, and there could have been abuse.

One of Mum's sisters, who was also my godmother, shot herself in the head in 1961.[3] She had been a patient at Seacliff Psychiatric Hospital, at Karitane, north of Dunedin, and her mental turmoil included suffering from depression. Mum was devastated by her sister's death, and Mum's unhappy marriage and financial hardship also contributed to her own despondency. Her mood disturbance may have been accelerated by the side effects of the drugs she was taking for her heart condition, such as Serpasil (reserpine). Nevertheless, Mum was full of fun and spontaneity, and taught me the exuberance and power of trying and enduring, despite living under a 'black cloud'.

My depression returned after Mum's sudden death on 4 September 1994. The grief was prolonged and numbing, so my doctor prescribed the new wonder drug Prozac, which worked for me, and I began to feel better. After I gave birth to my daughter, Tara, in 1998, I felt very low but I never reached the depths of postnatal depression that many women in Aotearoa have experienced.[4]

My mental descent resumed when redundancy faced several staff in the Division of Humanities at Otago University in 2016. When I lost my academic position of 26 years, my decline into depression was rapid, and I knew how serious this could be if not dealt with. So, even amid the chaos of Christmas, I managed to see my fantastic family doctor. Meanwhile the wonderful support of family, friends and colleagues kept me going. As did the memory of my late mother's love and words of advice to keep trying.

Mine is just one perspective of how the black cloud can cast its shadow over people's lives, but also how they may reflect upon this experience. The book explores the much greater variation of how depression is expressed and experienced over time and place, and across cultures in Aotearoa, with individuals having a range of outcomes. It also traces how the language and treatments for depression have changed.

During the twenty-first century there has been a backlash, both globally and in Aotearoa, against the medicalisation of depression, and a view has emerged that depression is just part of life's woes.[5] After all, our ancestors went through economic depression and wars, raised families and endured difficult marriages, and yet took such adversity in their stride. Given my personal experience with mental health, and interactions with health professionals, alongside academic research in the history of mental health, including within different cultures, I am aware of the way attitudes, diagnoses and treatments change over time. I would suggest that many people in the past, as today, did *not* cope with life's upheavals, often with disastrous consequences.

Depression, far from being new, hangs over humanity. And although those who are prone to depression may endure several years of relief, the dark cloud is always on the horizon. The New Zealand writer Alistair Te Ariki Campbell wrote to his wife, Meg Campbell, in 1963:

> As you know, when you start improving, you don't as a rule climb steadily to the surface. You still have ups and downs, but the troughs get steadily shallower. So keep your pecker up, my sweet.[6]

In 2019 Wendy Parkins, an academic at the University of Otago and later a professor of English in the United Kingdom, wrote an insightful memoir about living with depression, anxiety and obsessive-compulsive disorder in which she described the slow, but hardly dramatic, path to some kind of acceptance and recovery.

> Think of what makes you feel alive, what gives you vitality, and then think of the absence of all those qualities. You're not dead — you get up each day and drag yourself around the daily routines, or as many of them as you can still manage — but it's not much of a life. You're un-alive . . . When I did not have the energy to work I somehow always had the energy for plenty of self-reviling . . .
>
> It's like living underwater or inside a tunnel — life is going on elsewhere, where people are managing to have fun and also pay their bills on time. You can catch a glimpse of them and their world, you may even vaguely recall living there yourself, but you can't get to it. A numbing inertia robs you of the capacity to be either convivial or responsible. And the desire for recovery becomes simply a wish to live a quiet life without desperation.[7]

This book is a history of depression and its forebear, melancholia, in Aotearoa New Zealand. It is not a memoir, even less a therapy book. Rather it aims to show how diverse cultures and ethnicities have experienced and lived with mental depression in our past.

Today there is rightful concern, globally and in Aotearoa, about a contemporary and unprecedented epidemic of depression, but this book reveals that depression has long plagued people within all cultures, across wide-ranging environments and circumstances. What we now recognise as depression may have once been called melancholia, nervous disease or simply part of life's woes. Over the years people who live with depression have endured and tried to overcome it in a range of ways, from confinement in mental asylums and hospitals and care within the community to spirituality, drugs and technologies, or talking and other therapies.

The language and stories in this book can be confronting and disturbing. Depression can lead some people into extreme black holes, but most people who have encountered depression — whether their own or that of loved ones — press on; like mine, their lives are not constantly consumed by it.

The dark outcomes for some that are described in this book are neither inevitable nor unavoidable.

Mental health hospital records, mostly of asylums and hospitals, are key to researching the early history of depression in Aotearoa. These archives may contain patient registers, case notes and admission papers. Under the 1846 Lunatics Ordinance a mentally ill person who threatened public safety or themselves, or who was unable to care for themselves or had no one else to do so, could be certified by two doctors and a magistrate and compulsorily held in either in a gaol, a hospital or an asylum.[8]

The ordinance was replaced by the Lunatics Act in 1868, with revisions in 1882 and 1908. Its successor, the 1911 Mental Defectives Act, enabled people to admit themselves voluntarily. The current Mental Health Act was passed in 1969 and remains in force, with subsequent revisions and the lengthening of its title to the Mental Health (Compulsory Assessment and Treatment) Act in 1992.

Asylum and hospital records can provide only a partial history of depression, however, because most sufferers of the condition were never certified as insane or of unsound mind, and so did not fall within the medical system's ambit. Although there are records for those who were admitted, access to these mental health records remains hugely restricted, usually for 100 years following admission. Even then, their notes may appear in case books that extend beyond that date and so are out of bounds, meaning that only part of the story is available.

For example, I tried to research the early mental health records of Jane Dick from Scotland — whose story is told in chapter 3, and who was admitted to Seacliff Mental Hospital in 1923 — but her case notes are likely to be in volumes that extend beyond that date given that she lived for many years after her first admission. Because of the privacy restrictions on New Zealand's mental health records, I could not consult most public mental hospital records after about 1916.[9]

Within those parameters I have sampled accessible records at the mental asylums and hospitals in Auckland, Dunedin, Hokitika and Christchurch. In 1911 the official term 'asylum' was nationally replaced by that of 'mental

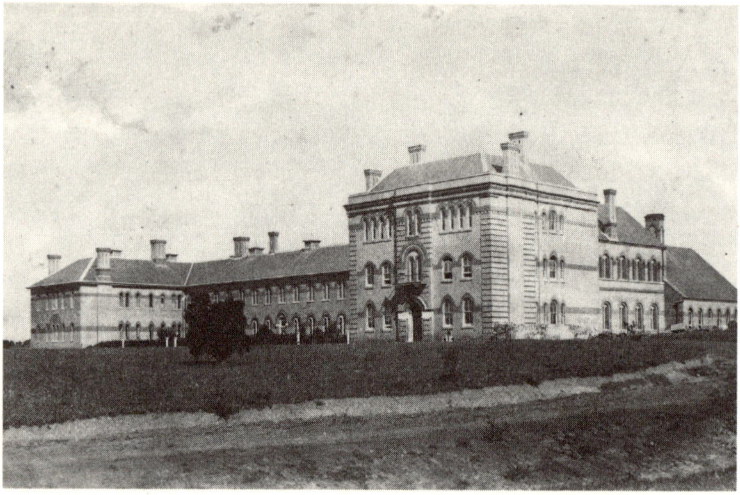

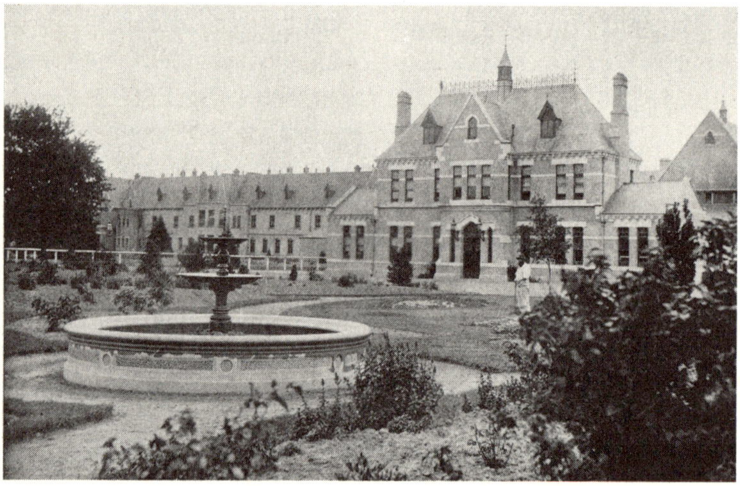

Clockwise from top left:
Auckland Lunatic Asylum, Point Chevalier, 1870s; Seacliff Mental Hospital, north of Dunedin, c. 1917; Seaview Lunatic Asylum, Hokitika, c. 1904; Porirua Lunatic Asylum, Wellington, 1903; Sunnyside Lunatic Asylum, Christchurch, 1906.

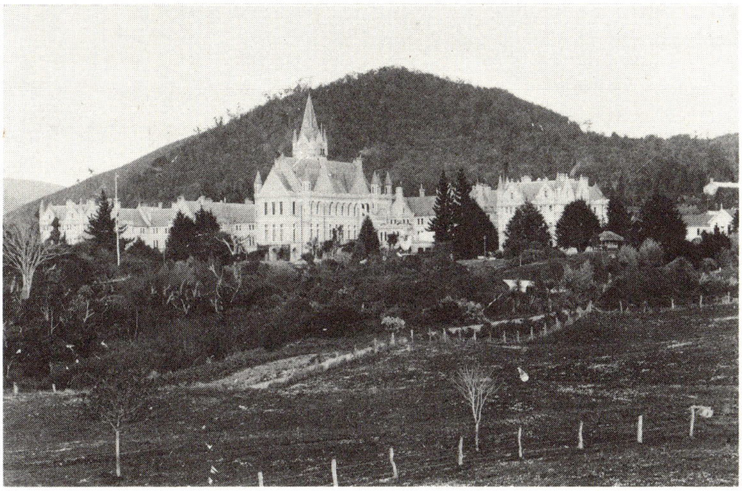

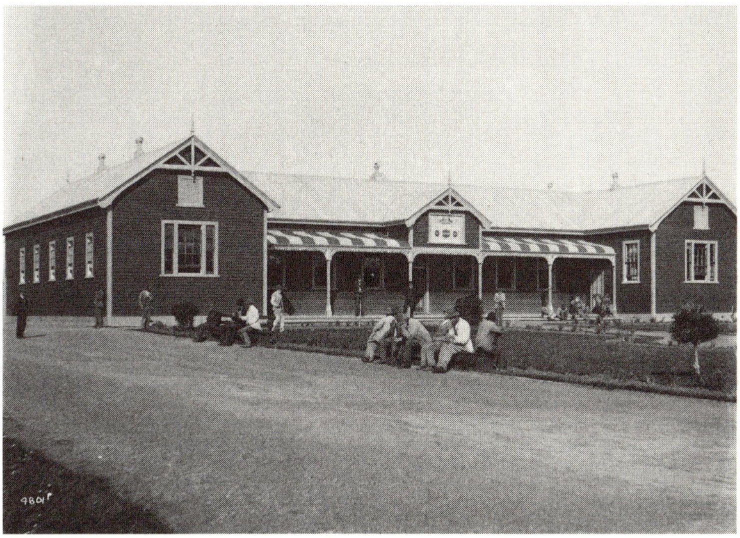

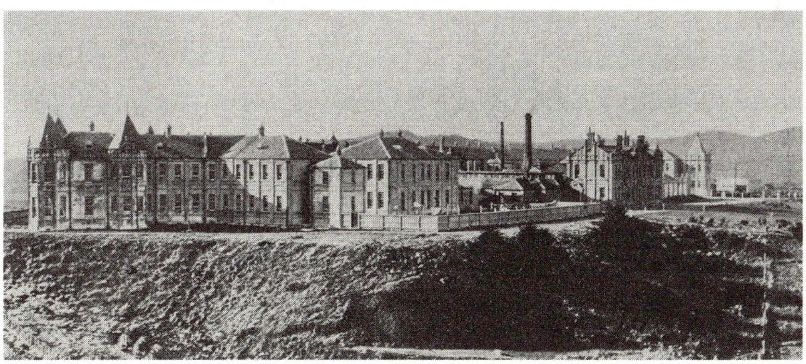

hospital'. Auckland's first asylum was the Whau Lunatic Asylum, later named the Auckland Provincial Lunatic Asylum and then the Auckland Mental Hospital.[10] I consulted its records dating from 1853 to 1916. Otago was served between 1863 and 1878 by the Dunedin Lunatic Asylum, which from 1879 shifted further up the coast to the Seacliff Lunatic Asylum, later renamed the Seacliff Mental Hospital. Its records were available from 1879 to 1916.

Mentally ill patients on the West Coast were initially admitted to the lunatic ward at South Spit Hospital in Hokitika, then to the Seaview Lunatic Asylum, later renamed the Seaview Psychiatric Hospital. I researched its records dating from 1869 to 1916. For Canterbury patients I was able to access the records of Sunnyside Lunatic Asylum and Sunnyside Psychiatric Hospital dating from 1863 to 1917.

For public hospitals I selected records within the date ranges of the earliest available, 1900, and latest available (usually in the years before 1916). With Ashburn Hall, a private psychiatric hospital in Dunedin, I sampled records at five-yearly intervals to identify cases of melancholia and depression from 1885 until October 1945 (51 cases: 18 males and 33 females). I also examined the first 100 cases for melancholia, and checked admissions for 1948 at Ashburn. But because of access restrictions to the individuals' actual mental health records, we often do not know what happened to these patients after they were admitted to a psychiatric institution.

Record-keeping procedures also varied between asylums and hospitals, meaning that a quantitative analysis of melancholia and depression across asylums is not possible. During the early colonial years, diagnoses were not always recorded, making it difficult to identify patients who were possibly admitted with depression. For example, early records at Sunnyside Lunatic Asylum in Christchurch often only recorded terms such as 'mentally insane'. Mental health diagnoses have been and remain subjective, being heavily dependent on experts' training, knowledge and experience.[11] Doctors' assessment of patients relied on testimony provided by family, whānau, friends, police, employers and others. Patient records for Ashburn Hall often contained elaborate family trees (genealogical charts) to show how insanity could be hereditary. This early medical 'science' provides only limited insight into the history of depression in Aotearoa.

Although I draw heavily on mental hospital records before 1920 for primary data, as I emphasise throughout the book, and elaborate on in chapter 7, in Aotearoa most people with depression either soldiered on — often denying their pain, perhaps diverting it through hard work, care for others, their faith or substance abuse — or had the support of whānau, family and friends. Family doctors might be turned to but, until antidepressants became available from the late 1950s, the medication that general practitioners could offer was limited. It is not surprising, therefore, that many people self-medicated through over-the-counter medicines or turned to alternative practitioners, known as quacks.

The asylum records I had access to provided only sparse, if any, details of the treatments patients received within the asylum or mental hospital. Before the 1950s, there was certainly very little drug therapy available for the treatment of melancholia or depression apart from the sedatives described in chapter 7. Generally, hospital regimens stressed the importance of routines such as regular meals, maintaining personal cleanliness, sleep, and working within the hospital or its grounds. At some asylums, such as Seaview in Hokitika, capable patients could work outside the asylum during the day, and some asylums had farms. In most asylums wholesome recreational and social activities — such as exercise, sports, games, needlework (for the ladies), dances and Christian worship — were encouraged for those patients able to participate. Melancholic patients were not usually restrained unless they became unruly.

Clearly, then, patient records can form only part of this history of depression in Aotearoa. In any event, as American historian Jonathan Sadowsky has pointed out, archives are not always the best source for unearthing histories of depression: 'The strength of asylums and hospitals for historical research is also their weakness: they are document factories, and historians need documents . . . Depression is often a "quiet" condition, with a lot of pain directed inward, and less "acting out".'[12]

Few public records speak to a mental state such as depression because most sufferers did not ever encounter a psychiatric professional. So how did those who were not institutionalised experience depression? And how did communities deal with melancholia and depression, and what is unique within Aotearoa?

Sadowsky has also found the use of oral history in histories of mental illness challenging because of privacy concerns. I, too, faced this ethical issue, but in reverse: it was access to the archival evidence the historian craves that was made difficult due to privacy issues. Jane Dick's story is one example of the complexity and frustration of unearthing oral and archival histories of depression. Her grandchildren supported her narrative being retold in this book, and much of her story has been verified through non-medical public records and family memories, but persistent requests to the Southern District Health Board to access Jane's records as a patient at Seacliff Mental Hospital, Orokonui Hospital and Cherry Farm Psychiatric Hospital from 1923 to 1975 were denied. I was informed that Jane Dick was not identifiable in any of the Otago records, yet when I consulted the national index of patients at the archives in Wellington, her admission as a patient was recorded.[13]

To enrich this history, I have used sources from the media, coronial inquiries, military records, and genealogy sites and collections, many available online.[14] These sources often enable investigation of individuals well after access to asylum records is closed. Other sources for non-asylum records were memoirs, creative outputs, student dissertations, and manuscripts and oral histories deposited in the Alexander Turnbull Library and in the Hocken Collections.

There are now many governmental and non-governmental online documents and websites on mental health and depression in Aotearoa, some of which contain case studies and provide insight into diverse cultures. The epilogue makes considerable use of material available through the internet.

Citing historical data related to mental health is also contentious and complicated. Privacy guidelines and legislation must be followed. Some historians, survivors and descendants of those with mental illness consider that keeping names hidden perpetuates an unhealthy silence and stigma. Where feasible, I have followed the convention of referring to a mental health patient by their first name, followed by the initial of their surname. This style does not always apply to people with different cultural and naming practices. It is difficult to keep private earlier patients' names that are now accessible through archives. Sometimes, when a name has been published, I disclose this. In a few sensitive cases I have used pseudonyms.

Coronial inquests up until around 1970 are openly available through New Zealand's national archives. Again, I have used first names when referring to these records. Although I was given access to some later coronial inquests, I am not allowed to publish this material — a situation very different to that faced by historian John Weaver, whose 2014 book *Sorrows of the Century* analysed data from twentieth-century coronial records that could be published.[15]

Citation from theses or secondary sources usually follows the styles those authors have used. Dissertations written by medical school students within the fifth-year programme of preventative medicine at the University of Otago from the 1920s until the 1970s provide a good insight into mental and public health in Aotearoa. However, strict conditions are imposed by the Hocken Collections on reading these dissertations to ensure the privacy of both the participants and the students. The coursework of the latter was never intended to be in the public domain, and it is also a matter of sensitivity to the authors' ages and career stages at the time of their writing.

Old Black Cloud traces a history of mental depression in Aotearoa through various themes that span the nineteenth century through to the late twentieth century, and with an epilogue that reaches into the twenty-first century. The title is a twist on Aotearoa as the 'land of the long white cloud', derived from the title of a book written in 1898 by the politician, writer and poet William Pember Reeves.[16]

This book digs into our past, long before depression was regarded as an epidemic in Aotearoa. Between 2011 and 2021 the recorded rates of depression in New Zealand increased from 14 per cent to 17 per cent; rates among Māori rose from 15 per cent to 21 per cent.[17] The 2017/18 New Zealand Mental Health Survey found that Māori and Pasifika, along with women and the poor, were most at risk of being diagnosed with depression.

Here, Sadowsky's questioning of whether there is a global and contemporary epidemic of depression seems pertinent.[18] Certainly, depression is being diagnosed more than ever, but why is this so? Is it a genuine increase in incidence, or might the burgeoning statistics indicate that feelings of depression have become more medicalised, and therefore more prone to diagnosis, perhaps partly because of the global reach and power of the pharmaceutical industry? And as more people become unafraid to seek support for the symptoms of depression, the medical statistics will likely increase accordingly. Again, we must ask whether the actual incidence of depression has increased, or whether it is rather a matter of depression having become more visible, as more of us who experience depression 'come out' and share our experience of living with it.

This book also considers depression within New Zealand's Indigenous and immigrant societies, cultures and environments. Historical and global literature have overlooked depression in Aotearoa and the South Pacific. Can depression be considered cross-culturally? And how do we avoid cultural stereotyping while acknowledging the different ways depression is recognised and treated within cultures and is clinically diagnosed?

The exploration of historical and cultural evidence again raises the question of whether depression is a modern 'disease'. What are the links with melancholia? How have depressive conditions and moods been medicalised? Interwoven throughout the chapters are the stories of how many people have lived with melancholia and depression. Only a small percentage were ever sent to mental institutions, and far fewer committed suicide. Many New Zealanders have silently lived with depression, or indeed have regarded their 'black cloud' as part of the human experience of sadness and life's woes rather than a medical illness. New Zealanders living with depression will often laugh at themselves; humour can mask depression, but it can also bring relief.

Mental depression is a serious issue within contemporary Aotearoa, and especially affects Māori, Pasifika, women and the poor, a radically different pattern compared to the colonial era, when depression was considered predominately the curse of 'civilised' men. To date there has been no history of mental depression in Aotearoa, in part because New Zealand has been somewhat peripheral in international medical history, and also because depression has been hidden under the long black cloud of Kiwi denial that we have not always lived up to the New Zealand ideal of being pragmatic and getting on with things. Mental depression may be universal, but how it has been experienced, understood, treated and lived with varies hugely. It is timely to offer this story from Aotearoa New Zealand.

1.

Discourse and diagnosis

At the end of 1930, when Aotearoa was beset by economic depression, unemployment and suffering, the director general of mental hospitals, Dr Theodore Gray, made an extraordinary speech at the launch of new radio equipment at Porirua Mental Hospital.

> I have no hesitation in asserting that the depression itself is of less moment to this country than is the manner in which the people of the country rise to meet their difficulties. Mass psychology is not a negligible factor in time of national stress, whether of war or of peace, and when times are hard our Cassandras, our prophetesses and prophets of woe, our defeatists, have their opportunity. Depression and gloomy foreboding . . . are highly contagious in a community and are liable to end disastrously to it in the same way as fear in an individual soldier may cause panic and stampede in a company or even an army in war.
>
> Appropriate remedies have to be taken for national as well as bodily disorders, but sheer funk pessimism and alarm should not be allowed to replace or be mistaken for prudence, for they will get us nowhere except into deeper waters. The spirit of a nation is the snip of the qualities possessed by its individual

> citizens, and it is in fostering a prudent, restrained optimism, a philosophic readiness to meet reverses with a smile and a community spirit of helpfulness.[1]

Gray's use of the discourse of mental depression to refer to the economic and social wellbeing of the nation was remarkable, as was his view that an optimistic spirit could lift the nation out of its doldrums. More than many, Gray would have known that there was no simple cure for depression. His speech also indicates how the discourse of depression has been a catch-all way of referring to individual and collective depression, in both a human and a material sense; the 'Great Depression' comes to mind. Other examples conflated the discourses of mental and economic depression; the New Zealand Women's Christian Temperance Movement, for example, recommended in 1931 that a 'smile' could lift sufferers from this fog:

> How we hate to read in our weather reports that a depression is approaching us over the Tasman Sea. But we sit calmly down and wait for that depression, and endure it until it passes on, fortunately not a long endurance. But a mental depression has overtaken our country, and we are wrapped in a fog of doubt, debt, uncertainty, and unemployment. Now, Christian women should rise above this mist and fog and dwell in the radiant sunshine of God's love and the clear atmosphere of faith in His promises.
>
> Were I an absolute ruler, I would enact a law that anybody talking about depression and [b]lack should be shut away by themselves. Let White Ribboners meet everybody with a smile, and like Pippa, tell it out 'God's In His Heaven, all's right with the world.'
>
> Fear has laid its deadly grip even on our churches; they dread for the future. Let fear give place to faith.[2]

The Congregational Church in Dunedin offered pragmatic suggestions for fighting the mental depression that so often accompanied economic depression for unemployed men. In the 1930s it operated a rest room 'to assist men to fight mental depression and to keep in a happy state of mind. We deem it important to keep unemployed men from becoming disgruntled with life by filling their time with interests.'[3] This noble initiative echoed the New Zealand attitude that activity could stave off the 'blues', even if in 1932 being busy failed to relieve starvation.

During the second half of the twentieth century, mental depression became more tightly defined in a clinical sense, but since colonial times both medical and lay observers in Aotearoa have intertwined the terms 'depression' and 'melancholia'. The latter was a common medical diagnosis until 'mental depression' became a diagnostic category in the twentieth century. As the historian Jonathan Sadowsky has noted, the term 'depression' came into use in Europe during the eighteenth century to refer to a mood, while the terms 'melancholia' and 'melancholy' were descriptions of a sickness.[4]

Melancholia embraced mania, as well as a range of conditions including psychosis, anxiety, irrationality, neurasthenia, delusions, nostalgia, suicidal attempts and ideation, and acute and chronic depression.[5] Depression could be subsumed under the terms of melancholia, neurasthenia, mental or nervous breakdowns. For example, one man admitted to Seaview for seven months during 1884–1885 was diagnosed with melancholia, although his notes described him as 'depressed'.[6]

Elizabeth S.'s case notes for 1916–1919 at Sunnyside also show how melancholia and depression were used interchangeably.[7] On admission, her doctor described her as depressed, and worrying over everything. She could not provide any reason for jumping through a window or going out in the middle of the night. Her daughter stated that no one could live with her owing to her constant depression. She was diagnosed with melancholia. In 1917 Elizabeth was allowed to leave on probation, but later returned, depressed, to Sunnyside.

In 1947 a patient admitted to hospital in Gisborne suffered from melancholia and depression. He was to be sent to a mental hospital, but he disappeared from his bed after midnight and hanged himself.[8]

Global historiography has divergent and complex views on the relationship between melancholia and depression.[9] Most of this literature has concerned Western Europe and North America. In 1892 Daniel Tuke, an alienist (a former term for psychiatrist), recorded mental depression in the *Dictionary of Psychological Medicine* as a synonym for melancholia. Nervous depression was defined as 'a term applied sometimes to a morbid fancy or melancholy of temporary duration'.[10] Janet Oppenheim, who wrote one of the first histories of depression in Victorian and Edwardian Britain, linked depression with nervous disease and neurasthenia, and emphasised the similarity between melancholia and depression.[11]

> Nervous breakdown, a popular name for incapacitating depression, is not a specific disease that can be traced to a single cause. It is an abstract concept, encompassing many symptoms that vary from one patient to another, with invariably devastating effect. The characteristic sense of overwhelming hopelessness, emptiness, impotence, and uselessness, the incapacity to focus attention or reach decisions, the obsessive thoughts and fears, the diminished self-esteem, the extreme lethargy, and the inability to take interest or pleasure in any aspect of life make existence scarcely tolerable.[12]

In 1984 the American psychiatrist Nancy Andreasen also stressed the link between melancholia and depression through taking a biological and organic — rather than a moral or social approach — to mental illness.[13] Psychiatrist and medical historian Stanley Jackson offered an inclusive view of the relationship between melancholia and depression in a survey of medical writings from over 2000 years in the Western and Islamic worlds:

> At any particular time during these many centuries the term that was in common use might have denoted a disease or a troublesome condition of sufficient severity and duration to be conceived of as a clinical entity; or it might have referred to a symptom within a cluster of symptoms that were thought to constitute a disease; or it might have been used to indicate a mood or emotional state of some duration, perhaps troublesome, certainly unusual, and yet not pathological, not a disease; or it might have referred to a temperament or type of character, involving a certain emotional tone and disposition, and yet not pathological; or it might have meant merely a feeling

> state of relatively short duration, unhappy in tone, but hardly a disease. These states were unusual mental states but covered a much wider spectrum than that covered by the term 'disease'.[14]

In Aotearoa, terms such as 'depression', 'melancholia' and 'melancholy' were used in both medical and popular discourse by the late nineteenth century. Elsewhere, 'depression' was often included in 'descriptive accounts of melancholic disorders to denote affect or mood, rather than having yet acquired any sort of formal status' as a diagnostic term.[15] Sadowsky includes 'melancholy in the history of depression because certain features, notably sadness that appears to others out of proportion to events, or gloomy expectation that a terrible fate await, are frequently if not always present . . . Some descriptions of melancholia look very similar to modern descriptions of depression, some less so.'[16]

Many historians pinpoint the shift in recognising depression as a diagnosis to European psychiatrists Emil Kraepelin and Adolf Meyer.[17] Kraepelin used the term 'depressive insanity' during the 1880s, but still referred to forms of 'melancholia'. Depression was commonly described as affect or mood, but the melancholias were considered to be types of mental depression. Manic-depressive insanity as a disease entity was introduced by Kraepelin in 1899. In 1904 Meyer advocated renaming melancholia as 'depression'. Although 'depression' became more widespread in medical discourse, 'melancholia' as a descriptor and diagnosis continued, including in Aotearoa.

Sadowsky's synthesis of melancholia and depression diagnoses stresses that the rising rates of depression reflected a drift; those who would once have been diagnosed with nerves or nervous breakdowns have since been diagnosed as depressed.[18] The word 'depression' retained reference as a mood, but by the 1960s (and I would suggest much earlier) increasingly had meaning as a disease. The historian Åsa Jansson, who teaches at Durham University, has also argued that melancholia as understood in the nineteenth century was different from clinical depression as understood today, suggesting the historical coexistence of two types of depression:

> One is a mild to moderate form of mood disorder, what is usually meant by the term 'clinical depression' today: low mood and sadness, often accompanied by sleeplessness, appetite

> disruption, and anxiety. The other is an endogenous form that is more than a mental disorder, it is an illness where the entire system is, in effect, 'pressed down', resulting in retarded speech and slow bodily movement. This illness often manifests with delusions (psychosis) and can in its most severe forms leave sufferers in a catatonic stupor. This condition is usually referred to as psychotic or melancholic depression.[19]

The American psychologist Gary Greenberg's take on the rise of depression in the twentieth century is evident in the title of his 2011 book *Manufacturing Depression: The Secret History of a Modern Disease*,[20] in which he asks whether the disease was promoted and marketed by drug companies to sell antidepressants. This was a critique of the biomedical model of depression, whereby unhappiness was increasingly considered an illness. A similar perspective had earlier been given by American professor of psychiatry Dan Blazer, whose 2005 book *The Age of Melancholy* placed depression within society and culture and the pressures of modern life (mainly in the United States), but argued that depression was reified as a disease, obscuring our emotionally toxic world.[21]

By the late nineteenth century, the concept of melancholia had been subdivided into various definitions by European and American psychiatrists, employing a disease classification process known as 'nosology'. This resulting nosology was transferred to Aotearoa by doctors who had trained in Britain, most in Scotland. They remained in touch with the global circulation of medical knowledge through medical journals and conferences, or when overseas experts visited. These were crucial ways of keeping up to date with the changing nature of psychiatry, especially when postgraduate qualifications in psychiatry were not available in Aotearoa until the second half of the twentieth century.

Although the Otago Medical School opened in 1875, for decades it offered only limited courses in what was termed 'mental pathology' and later 'mental disease'. Truby King, medical superintendent of the Seacliff asylum from 1889 to 1921 and who had a progressive approach to the treatment of mentally ill patients, taught the first of these courses in the late 1880s, and provided clinical instruction. In 1910 Ashburn Hall established a neuro-pathological laboratory at Dunedin Hospital to train local doctors in mental pathology.[22] However, more specialised psychiatry was not taught in Aotearoa until 1953, when Dr Wallace Ironside from Leeds University was appointed at the medical school. In 1962 he became the first professor of psychological medicine when a separate department was established at Otago.[23] The Auckland Medical School did not open until 1968. John Werry, a New Zealander, was appointed from the University of Illinois as the first professor of psychiatry at Auckland.[24]

Meanwhile, during these slow decades in Aotearoa when medical students had very little exposure to the latest advances in psychiatry, and even less to the nuances of melancholia and depression, the public might be kept informed about these conditions through newspapers that reported on local and visiting medical experts, or when mental illness was implicated in murders or suicides. After the 1951 Coroners Act came into force, only limited details of deaths due to suicide could be published, and the names of these persons could not be disclosed.

The term 'simple melancholia' was coined by the British psychiatrists John Charles Bucknill, Daniel Tuke and Henry Maudsley to denote melancholia without delusions.[25] In 1898, *The Auckland Star* reported a lecture by Dr Burnet, from Kansas City Medical College: 'The first important symptom of simple melancholia is sleeplessness. Another symptom of the greatest importance, is a dull pain in the back of the neck, extending to the back of the head . . . The third symptom is depression of spirits, accompanied by slower mental movements and retarded speech and actions.'[26]

Some doctors were reluctant to equate simple melancholia with insanity — a precursor of the way in which depression has long been regarded as a mental condition that does not always require hospitalisation or legal certification as insane. But not so for Ernest C., a patient at Mount View Asylum in Wellington in 1897, who was diagnosed with simple melancholia. Even though Ernest ultimately committed suicide, the asylum's medical superintendent, Dr Gray Hassell, testified that he should not have been sent to the asylum because he was not insane.[27]

This tragedy drew attention to overcrowding, understaffing and the need for separate facilities in mental hospitals for patients with different mental disorders. As early as 1870, John King, New Zealand's inspector of asylums, asked in his annual report whether nervous cases and those with melancholia should be treated separately within an asylum from long-term or severely mentally ill patients.[28]

A Wellington solicitor who was admitted to Ashburn Hall for 10 weeks in 1900 was diagnosed with simple melancholia. The medical superintendent doubted his insanity, despite a family tree revealing that nervousness ran in the family.[29] He had been working too hard, and it seems that 'time out' in a supportive environment was beneficial. A month after his admission he was cheerful and attending church and the theatre in Dunedin.

When Frederick W., a 53-year-old teacher at a native school, was admitted to Auckland Mental Hospital in 1915 he had simple melancholia, attributed to stress, overwork and dyspepsia (indigestion).[30] His case notes recorded his frightened appearance and his declaration that he had made a mess of his life and thought best to end it. 'He has lost confidence in his ability to teach and dreads returning to scholastic duties and the nearer he gets to this the more he becomes depressed,' his notes stated. He was afraid to be alone, and he told a doctor that he had experienced attacks of 'great depression' over many years 'during which he quite loses control of himself and screams and yells and is seized with the desire to end his life'. Frederick was discharged after four months, but his depression continued and he was readmitted.[31]

Despite the qualifier 'simple', this form of melancholia could be associated with violence. In 1912 a 29-year-old patient was admitted to Auckland Mental Hospital after striking her mother in the throat and saying that she wished that her parents were dead.[32] She had spent several months at Porirua Mental Hospital, and remained in the Auckland Mental Hospital for eight years. A man from Waihi, with at least three admissions to Auckland Mental Hospital between 1912 and 1917, threatened self-violence and violence against others; contrary to the usual definition of simple melancholia, he heard voices telling him to commit suicide, saying 'you are going mad'.[33] His case notes recorded both the terms 'melancholy' and 'depressed'.

When returned soldier Jack Oldfield murdered his wife, Christine, only four weeks after they had married, in 1930 at Seadown near Tīmaru, doctors Thomas Beale and F. F. A. Ulrich, and medical superintendents

Alexander McKillop of Sunnyside Mental Hospital and T. W. J. Charles of Seacliff Mental Hospital, gave conflicting expert opinions at his trial as to whether he was insane or rational at the time of the act. They agreed that he had intended to kill himself, and that he was suffering from severe depression. Ulrich qualified this as simple melancholia brought on by the plummeting value of Oldfield's farm and probably also from the ongoing effects of war wounds, which compromised his ability to work. (Chapter 4 further discusses how depression and suicide could be consequences of the lingering effects of injuries sustained in the First World War, combined with economic worries during the Great Depression.) Did these pressures and Oldfield's mental state induce him to commit murder?[34] The jury found him not guilty on the grounds of insanity, and he was sent to Sunnyside for an indefinite period.

Simple melancholia sometimes embraced what doctors once called 'neurasthenia', and which may have been anxiety and/or depression.[35] At age 23, in 1915, Margaret A. tried to drown herself in a water race at Reefton on the West Coast.[36] Her husband said she had become melancholic two years earlier, and had tried to break and burn items. Margaret said that she hated her child. Yet the case notes from her time at Sunnyside described her melancholia as mild. 'She is the typical neurasthenic who swings back and forward over the borderland. She complained of the usual subject of sensations in the head, she is emotional and self centred,' her notes state.

Acute melancholia was another subtype. In 1898 Annie B., in her thirties and with two children, had 'an attack of melancholia' some months after nursing her elderly and infirm father.[37] She was brought to Hokitika, where she lived in a lodging house for six weeks and was treated by Dr Ebenezer Teichelmann, Westland's medical superintendent. She appeared to become 'almost well' and returned to her home. Annie was still suicidal, and her brother (presumably playing the devil's advocate) 'led her to the water and told her to jump in but she declined'.

Annie was subsequently admitted to Seaview Asylum in Hokitika in March 1899 in a state of acute melancholia, 'with its usual symptoms. Her face is expressive and of intense mental suffering, her attention is difficult

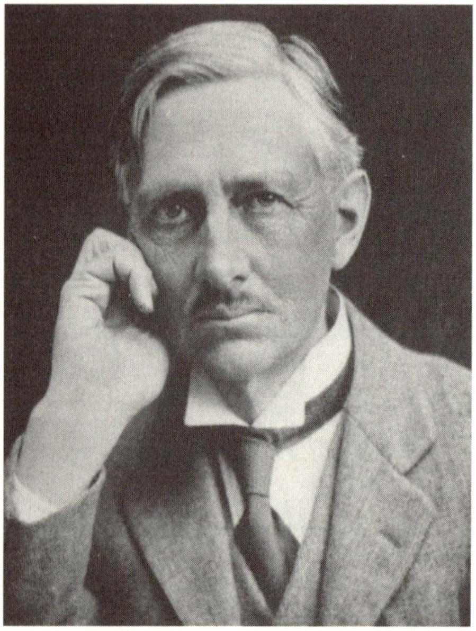

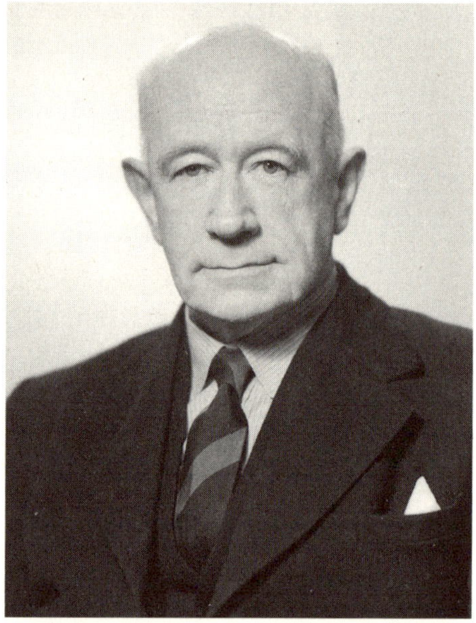

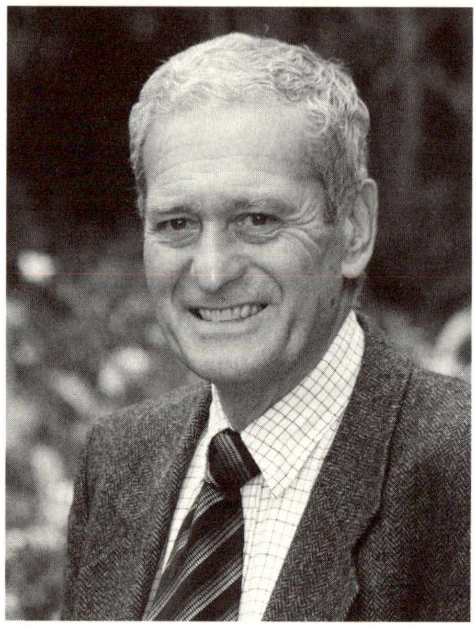

Some prominent doctors in Aotearoa New Zealand's history of the treatment of depression. *Clockwise from top left:* Dr Truby King; Dr Theodore Gray; Professor Mason Durie.

Ashburn Hall

(near Dunedin)

Licensed Hospital for Mental Diseases

Special Features

COMPLETE classification for the mentally unsound of both sexes, and for patients labouring under the lesser neuroses. The latter, and cases of incipient or uncertifiable mental disorder, are received as voluntary boarders.

EVERY patient is encouraged to work and join in active recreations. The farm (100 acres) and gardens afford healthy channels for misplaced energies, and tennis, croquet and bowls form the principal out-door recreations.

PATIENTS are taken to the theatre and other outside entertainments. For the evenings and during inclement weather, music and a variety of indoor occupations and amusements are provided.

INDIVIDUAL tastes are studied and indulgently considered and patients receive individual medical treatment, each patient having a separate room.

The last Annual Report of the Director-General of Mental Hospitals says in regard to Ashburn Hall: "It continues to fulfil a most useful function, and to do it well. This is a homelike retreat in beautiful surroundings, and its administration is personal and kindly."

For further information apply to

THE MEDICAL SUPERINTENDENT

Private Bag 934, DUNEDIN.

A 1921 advertisement for the private psychiatric hospital Ashburn Hall, near Dunedin.

to arrest, and when spoken to she will answer in monosyllables only, and in a voice little above a whisper. Appears to be troubled by delusions of impending evil,' her notes record. In Seaview she started to recover, doing some needlework and laundry, and attending a hospital dance. In September 1901 Annie was discharged to her husband's care, on a bond under the 1882 Lunatics Act for which he had applied, as he was relocating to the North Island.[38]

By the early twentieth century, some women with acute melancholia were described as 'self-centred and depressed' or having 'acute melancholia with self absorption', such as a 24-year-old music teacher admitted, 'morose and depressed', to Seacliff in 1915.[39] Her younger brother found her with a rope around her neck, talking about 'going out to meet her fate'. She was discharged within five months, continued to teach music, and lived until 1979, a happier outcome than another patient who, in 1913, tidied the nurses' mess room at the Auckland Mental Hospital after breakfast and then jumped to her death from a window. She had also been diagnosed with acute melancholia.[40] While men were diagnosed with acute melancholia, they were seldom described as being 'self-absorbed' or in other similar terms that tended to be given to women.

Diagnoses of sub-acute melancholia — a state between acute and chronic melancholia — were also given to patients. Twenty-two-year-old Ethel H. was admitted to Seacliff in 1914, probably with post-partum depression.[41] Her husband said that 'she has become listless and inattentive to work whereas she was [normally] bright and cheerful'. Ethel had delusions in which she saw angels and was violent, threatening to kill her husband's mother. Seacliff's medical superintendent, Frederick Truby King, observed that Ethel was 'markedly depressed' and 'her thoughts are seated on herself and her morbid fancies'.

Emil Kraepelin introduced the term 'involutional melancholia' to refer to serious depression presenting later in life — at about age 45.[42] For women this was also associated with the 'climacteric', an old term referring to women experiencing menopause. In 1935, only six among approximately 1230 patients at Seacliff were diagnosed with involutional melancholia, and at Porirua Hospital during the mid-1940s there were only three such cases among about 1000 resident patients.[43] Some research in New Zealand reported that involutional melancholics tended to 'bewail' that 'the future had nothing in store. The mind was preoccupied with the "might have been" and in consequence doubt, indecision, anxiety readily showed itself.'[44]

New Zealand doctor Gordon Short described a 56-year-old gardener with involutional melancholia (and mental depression) who became down-hearted and despondent, had no ambition and had lost interest in everything.[45] He complained of physical pain, but Short could not find any cause for this except the patient's mental state.

Similar thoughts by a farmer in his fifties led to suicide in 1942. The patient's doctor said he was 'a morose unsmiling man, over-concerned with his own small troubles. During the past six months, he has developed a definite mental illness "involutional melancholia". He has been very depressed . . . not certifiably insane, but would have become so, had he lived, within the next year.'[46]

By the 1960s, admission statistics for psychiatric hospitals in Aotearoa combined manic-depressive reaction and involutional melancholia,[47] but outside of official statistics the concept of involutional melancholia persisted. Chapter 5 recounts the story of Ivan Sutherland, whose tragic ending followed treatment for involutional melancholia that had arisen from professional, personal and physical stress. As a successful philosophy and psychology academic, Sutherland hardly conformed to the stereotype offered by one student researcher of involutional melancholia: those who 'may have performed a dull, uninteresting job in a methodical fashion'.[48]

Severe cases of depression or melancholia were qualified as 'resistive melancholia', 'stuporous melancholia' or 'melancholia attonita'. A patient at Auckland Mental Hospital in 1913 with 'resistive melancholia . . . had an expression that denotes depression and anxiety', requiring artificial feeding.[49] A 27-year-old farmer from Hāwea who refused to eat, stayed in bed, asked to be left alone and tried to swallow matchheads was admitted to Ashburn Hall in a stuporous condition as a voluntary boarder by his father in February 1905.[50] The following month he was committed as a patient.

A few months later he had improved and returned to an active life on the family farm. He married in 1911, had five children, and lived until 1945.

Other diagnoses of melancholia during the early twentieth century in Aotearoa included 'delusional melancholia', 'excited melancholia', 'agitated melancholia', 'confusional melancholia', 'impulsive melancholia' and 'hypochondriacal melancholia'. Case notes suggest that the terms were fluid. For example, a 30-year-old farmer admitted to Ashburn Hall and then to Seacliff had various diagnoses of melancholia (hypochondriacal), adolescent insanity (presumably from when younger) and melancholia (excited), and alcoholic melancholia.[51]

The term that appeared on an individual's mental health records depended on the medical superintendent of the facility to which they were admitted; their use of the various terms was influenced by their training, which for psychiatry until the mid-1950s was overseas, usually in England or Scotland. Psychiatric knowledge was also acquired from attending conferences and from medical literature, including *The New Zealand Medical Journal*, which was first published in 1887 (and is still going).

Classification often depended on whether delusions or hallucinations were present. Dr Burnet, whose lecture on different melancholias was reported in Aotearoa in 1898, described 'agitated melancholia': 'There are generally terrifying hallucinations, an utter indifference to one's self and one's surroundings, aversion to food and inability to sleep except under the influence of drugs. The propensity to take life may come on suddenly, or be gradually developed.'[52]

It is not clear when depression replaced melancholia as a diagnosis in medical assessments in Aotearoa. Many people with symptoms of depression were never considered as such by police, doctors, whānau or families. Melancholia and depression were interchangeably used terms in medical and lay discourse, but depression was usually regarded as distinct from insanity, whereas melancholia could be (but was often not) implicated with madness. For example, boarding-housekeeper Gina Martin described a resident's mental state to a coroner in 1912: 'I do not consider that he was insane but severely depressed.'[53]

In 1862 William Murray, a private in the police force at Coromandel, committed suicide by cutting his own throat. He had been drinking heavily and had submitted his resignation to the commissioner of police. Murray was a former soldier in the 58th Regiment, which came to New Zealand during the New Zealand Wars. After he was discharged from military duty, he took up bush work and later joined the police, where, according to Constable Patrick Cahill, he 'seemed always out of his place'. James Spinks, a miner, stated at the inquest into Murray's death that he had lately 'seemed much depressed in his spirits', and the coroner's verdict was that he had committed suicide 'whilst labouring under a state of great mental depression'.[54]

This or similar expressions — 'suffering from mental depression',[55] 'owing to the depression of mind',[56] for example — were frequently used in the coronial verdicts of suicides, and sometimes implicated among the causes of murder, or in subsequent remorse for a crime. On 22 September 1863 Richard Harper, who operated a butchery business on Queen Street in Auckland, was hanged at the Mount Eden Stockade after stabbing his wife, Jane Alice Harper, to death. A reporter from *The Daily Southern Cross* acquired details (possibly from visiting clergy) of Richard Harper's state of mind during the 18 days since the death sentence was passed — he alternated between being 'somewhat cheerful, and at other times suffering under great mental depression'.[57]

When Reverend William Shirriffs, originally from Aberdeen, Scotland, a minister at Waipukurau and chief clerk in the New Zealand Assembly of the Presbyterian Church, hanged himself in Wellington in 1883 at the age of 42, the jury at his inquest returned a verdict of 'suicide while not in a sound state of mind'.[58] An obituary published in *The Auckland Star* provided further details of his mental state leading up to his death.[59] He had been reluctant to accept the position of chief clerk because of the extra labour and responsibility that the position entailed, but was promised by the church that he would be supported in the role. The 'responsibility was too much for him. Deeply anxious for the prosperity of the Church, he was easily depressed when things did not go on as smoothly as he desired.' His peers had noticed that since the church's last assembly Shirriffs had not been his usual cheerful self, and despaired at the lack of 'vital Godliness in the Church' and the lack of progress in advancing temperance in Aotearoa.

About six weeks before his suicide, his wife, concerned about her husband's mental and physical decline, had asked William's friend John McLean to visit them. Soon after, Shirriffs was sent to a local 'asylum', diagnosed by two doctors with melancholia and committed by the magistrate to the Mount View Asylum in Wellington.[60] But the documentation required for his admission was delayed, and so his friends decided to closely watch him while he was in the care of a nursing attendant. This appeared to be a good plan; about three weeks later, he was a guest in McLean's home, participating in family worship, attending church, singing hymns, gardening, and assisting in the examination of a student. But on 23 September, when Shirriffs did not come to breakfast, McLean had to force open a window to his room, where he found his friend dead.

At Christchurch's Sunnyside hospital in 1915, Dr A. F. Mickle observed that James A. was 'undoubtedly in a depressed mental state. Sits in a listless depressed dejected mood, answers questions in a very depressed manner... has no delusions... the case is one of mental depression and tendency to melancholia.'[61] James died four years later in the hospital.

Tommy P., a 43-year-old Māori man, was one of the first patients at Auckland mental hospital to be diagnosed with mental depression.[62] Tommy said that 'his inside is all on fire down to his legs. His heart is burning and he is frightened all the time he will hurt someone. He wants to be secured as to prevent him hurting his wife or children.'

Asylum staff saw that Tommy was 'labouring under a great sense of fear and is very apprehensive about himself and other people. He said he is compelled to copy animals.' Significantly, Tommy's medical diagnosis was recorded as depression in 1913, but earlier observations described him as suffering from dementia, and being in a maniacal state. This shows not only the crossover between terms for mental illness, but also how diagnoses for Māori in particular were often imprecise or superficial.

Historian John Weaver found that witnesses at suicide inquests in Aotearoa during the twentieth century mentioned depression and sometimes linked this with stress. With 'public recognition of depression as an illness, the word "depression" had multiple applications. Sometimes it merely summarised a short-term emotional state, and in these instances it is hard to separate reactive depression, from sadness.'[63] Reactive depression was considered to be a response to life events or the environment, rather than being biological in origin.

Dr I. M. Allen provided an insightful account in *The New Zealand Journal of Medicine* in 1933 about the clinical features of depression. After graduating from the Otago Medical School, Allen spent five years in Europe and was admitted to the Royal College of Physicians in London, where he made observations about depression that remain relevant within many cultures in Aotearoa.

> [I]n most cases it is worse early in the morning and the patient feels that his night has done him no good. In others it may be worse in the afternoon, and in many, late in the evening when the patient feels that he is only to go to sleep to wake early to face another day of misery. During the day it may improve considerably, especially when he is in company or occupied, only to reappear in its full force when he is alone even for a short time. The depression varies considerably in intensity.
>
> In some it is merely absence of the *joie de vivre*, low-spiritedness, or a feeling of misery or unhappiness. By some it is described as a long attack of the 'blues' or a feeling that life is not worth living. For many it is associated with a feeling of isolation; of being shut off from the world round about; of being unable to come into contact with people they meet; and, often with good cause, of being misunderstood by those and their own household to whom they look for understanding and help.
>
> The patient feels that he may go mad. He may try to relate his symptoms to some definite cause such as the loss of a relative, financial anxiety, domestic trouble or overwork, but has little faith in this explanation and still feels that they are beyond all understanding.
>
> Fear haunts the patient day and night, but most often when he is alone. It varies from what he calls nervousness, anxiety or loss of confidence to an indefinite dread or a fear related to a definite

> object . . . Often there is a fear of the future, which seems to hold nothing in store and makes life not worth living. There is a fear that normal health will never return. Sometimes the fear is related to the patient's occupation — that he will spoil his work or fall out of work. More often it is related to his actions, such as a fear of going to the door, of going out, of crossing the street or of traffic. Most commonly it is expressed as a fear of the patient himself and that he may do wrong, which in more severe cases becomes a fear that he may do himself harm . . .
>
> Often the patient wants to weep as he feels that if only he does so he will feel better. Often he cannot do so and then complains that he can have no feeling of any kind. Sometimes he weeps for no adequate reason, and when it is over feels that his final state is worse than the first.
>
> He has no energy either of mind or body. He cannot fix his mind on anything . . . He becomes irritable with anything he tries to do, and most often with those who unwisely urge him to pull himself together and tell him that if he does so he will be quite well.[64]

Depression, like melancholia, underwent changing reiterations of diagnostic symptoms and medical and lay classification into sub-types. One of the earliest expressions was constitutional depression. In 1871 *The Nelson Evening Mail* reprinted an article from London's *Saturday Review*,[65] which claimed that the children of upper-class alcoholic mothers would probably suffer from constitutional depression. In his dictionary published in 1901, the American philosopher and psychologist James Mark Baldwin classified constitutional depression as:

> a pessimistic temperament that is inclined to see the dark side of everything and is led to gloominess and despondency upon slight provocation. Such moods or periods often present a temporary character in the form of more or less periodic exacerbations, which . . . rather readily pass off with an improvement in the circumstances of the patient. Such attacks are occasionally accompanied by marked feelings of anxiety.[66]

Constitutional depression appeared as a cause, and from the 1940s was a diagnosis at Ashburn Hall in Dunedin. Other descriptors of depression recorded in Ashburn's case books were 'depression with hysterical features' and 'anxious depression'. A 1968 Kingseat Hospital survey listed multiple types of depression: neurotic depressive reaction, depressive, puerperal, epileptic (with depression), manic depressive psychosis, hypomania, involutional melancholia, endogenous, agitated, anxious and reactive depression.[67]

Two separate tragedies in December 1928 were attributed to acute mental depression. Twenty-one-year-old Stanley, who was in charge of the family farm in Tīrau, Waikato, when his father was ill, had become worried about it being overrun with rabbits. He shot himself in a paddock after shooting and killing his brother in his bedroom.[68] The coroner determined that Stanley had been in a state of acute mental depression. His family suggested that his mental condition may have been affected by inhaling carbon bisulphide fumes, used for poisoning rabbits, when he had not taken the proper precautions. Dr S. L. Hazlett had found Stanley to be 'perfectly normal'. He had previously suffered from two nervous breakdowns — the first when he was 15.

Acute mental depression was also the cause given when 18-year-old Harold Wood jumped off a wireless mast on Mount Victoria in Wellington in 1928.[69] He had been ill, possibly with meningitis, but some time after resuming work as a clerk he returned to the family home feeling unwell. He rested that day, but then insisted on going for a run, during which he climbed the mast. Was this an impulsive or a predetermined act? It seems that both his physical and his mental state drove his decision to jump.

By the mid-twentieth century, the earlier demarcation between psychotic (usually associated with delusions) and neurotic depression (seen as a reaction to external circumstances) had been replaced when psychiatrists drew a distinction between endogenous and exogenous or reactive depression.[70] The former might be considered to have a genetic, biological or physiological basis, even from development of the child's personality during their formative years, while the latter was seen to be caused by events outside the individual; for example, unemployment or rejection or the death of a loved one. External stress could be social, economic, political or environmental.

During the 1960s a general practitioner testified that his patient's suicide was explicable because her history of endogenous depression surfaced before menstruation and during and after pregnancy. She had given birth to four children, who were aged between 18 months and 4 years when she ended her life. The doctor described her mental condition with the ambiguous term 'hysterical depression', possibly insinuating that her mental state was an exaggerated emotional response.[71]

In practice, it proved difficult to separate endogenous and exogenous depression. In 1958 a doctor said that the cause of a colleague's suicide was 'while the balance of his mind was disturbed [by] an acute attack of endogenous mental depression . . . a mental illness which arises from within a person rather than being the result of external circumstances'.[72] His wife confirmed that her husband had 'periods of great depression' and 'periods of almost over confidence, these moods changing without warning', but she also attributed the depression to worry over financial matters, and recent worry over his inability to treat his patients correctly. Internationally, the distinction between endogenous and neurotic reactive (exogenous) depression was questioned, but these terms continued to be used in Aotearoa by doctors and laypeople.[73]

As we have seen, the many diagnoses and classifications of melancholia and depression in Aotearoa were often influenced by research and diagnostic standards from overseas, but what were the causes of New Zealanders' depression? Were they specific to Aotearoa? And did they change as melancholia was replaced by depression as a diagnosis? Causes, like diagnoses, were subjective, often crossed between different clinical categories, and included heredity, the body, worry and stress, masturbation, and women's biology and minds. Loneliness, isolation, grief and poverty were other causes; these are explored in the following chapters. Cultural and spiritual causation are considered in chapters 2 and 6.

Whether certain people and their behaviours induced the 'blues' or whether melancholia was a universal condition was a question posed in

1876 when the Otago newspaper the *Bruce Herald* reprinted an article from the British *Liberal Review*:

> There are certain sorts of people who are supposed to be peculiarly subject to what are popularly called the 'blues.' Persons who drink too much and those who are unable to comply with the demands of their creditors are among these. Yet it is a mistake to assume that only individuals who play fast and loose with their constitutions, and are not in a position to liquidate their liabilities, are in the habit of taking gloomy views of life and things generally — men who live in the lay of luxury, and exist in a quiet and regular fashion, being often the first to fall victims to hypochondriacal attacks. Perhaps, indeed, it is the almost universal tendency to melancholy which leads to many of the excesses which are alleged to produce mental depression.[74]

Despite suggestions that melancholia and depression may have affected all sorts of people, hereditary (or heredity) was a common cause given during the nineteenth and twentieth centuries in Aotearoa. In 1869 *The New Zealand Herald* reported 'a partner in a large firm, committed suicide, owing to the depression of mind caused by a supposition, alleged to be unfounded, that his business affairs were in an unsatisfactory condition . . . evidences of what is called a suicidal tendency in a family. The deceased's father hanged himself about four years ago, and his grandmother drowned herself.'[75] In 1898 17-year-old Alice poisoned herself by swallowing 130 matchheads. Her fits of melancholia were considered to run in the family; her father had committed suicide a few weeks earlier.[76]

Until the 1940s, notes at Ashburn Hall included family trees so that insane ancestors could be traced. Even in the late 1940s, depression with links to heredity was still being recorded at Ashburn. Elsewhere heredity might be given as a cause of melancholia even when there was very little evidence for doing so, or when the patient spoke very little English, such as when a young gumdigger from Dalmatia was committed to the Auckland asylum in 1911 and was almost incoherent when talking to an interpreter. It was established that worry over a debt of £20 was another cause of his condition.[77]

Somatic, or physical, causes of melancholia and depression have been most often associated with non-Western cultures. Somatisation of mental distress was when patients presented to a doctor with a physical malady that might also be due to emotional and mental factors. Chapter 2 indicates how somatic illnesses, such as bodily pain, might induce some Māori to seek Western medical help for depression while at the same time they continued to be cared for within Māori health systems, which considered physical, mental and spiritual aspects in a holistic way. Chapter 6 discusses somatic expressions of melancholia and depression within other ethnicities in Aotearoa.

But, as several cases in this book indicate, Pākehā could also cloud their mental distress within physical illness and seek relief through bodily treatments. In an inaugural address to the Wellington Philosophical Society — part of the New Zealand Institute — on 29 June 1898, the scholar, writer and social and political reformer Edward Tregear referred to the connection made by the Scottish physician Alexander Haig between increased amounts of uric acid and disease, 'associated with many phenomena, all morbid, both of body and mind, and notably with headaches, melancholia, depression of spirits, epilepsy, and, in general, with a lowered tone of consciousness'.[78] Tregear asked the audience to consider the reverse: how mental disease might induce physical disease.

> People, too, die from homesickness — that intense desire and longing for their native country and friends . . . in this the mental illness soon reacts fatally on the physical forces. We know also that gloom or despair may induce jaundice; that good news will make the heart beat vigorously, that cheerfulness will calm and regulate its beat; that fear and anxiety may paralyse digestion.

Even the advent of the electric light was considered a cause of melancholia. In 1916, at a meeting in Dunedin, electrical expert F. R. Sheppard claimed that the brilliancy of the tungsten lamp 'must have a serious effect on the eye which is perhaps the most sensitive organ in the human body, and is undoubtedly responsible for a large percentage of headaches which in many cases lead to melancholia, neurasthenia and other nervous disorders'.[79]

Many physical causes of depression were attributed to influenza. When a 46-year-old Tīmaru coal merchant committed suicide in 1923, the coroner ruled he was in a state of great mental depression caused by the lingering effects of the influenza epidemic as well as business worries.[80] Dr Vivian from Taumarunui testified at an inquest in 1928 that 'an influenza patient usually suffers more or less from mental depression and the best remedy for such a condition is absolute rest'.[81] Similar advice was given during the twenty-first-century Covid pandemic, when the links between viral infections, low mood, fatigue and depression were widely recorded.

The link between anxiety and depression now receives much publicity, but worry or anxiety and their manifestation as depression, and suggested links with depression, have been evident in Aotearoa since the nineteenth century. In 1872 the body of John Diddams was found by a 13-year-old in the Mechanics' Institute's library in Auckland.[82] Diddams was a frequent client, and the librarian had noticed that he was melancholy, appearing 'under some heavy mental depression'. Isaac Worthington Harrop, the treasurer of Auckland's City Corporation (the forerunner to the city council) testified at the inquest that Diddams had been neglecting his duties as a rate-collector and valuator and was facing dismissal.

When William M., a farmer from Southland, was admitted to Dunedin's Seacliff Asylum in 1900 'in an earlier stage of melancholia' than was usual for admittance to an asylum, the cause was financial worry.[83] His doctor said that for several weeks William had been very despondent about his work and had threatened to commit suicide, but that all his affairs were in fact in good order. His worry was a complete change from his usual 'tone of mind'.

Alcohol abuse and addiction were correlated with cases of depression and suicide, either as a cause, a symptom or as a means of coping. Alcoholism, too, was often considered hereditary. In a sample of 16 patients admitted to Seaview with melancholia during the years 1869–1876, in five cases (31 per cent) alcoholism was listed as a cause, including a woman who died from dementia. In contrast, alcoholism was listed as the cause of 10 per cent of 28 patients with melancholia at Seacliff in 1915.

A 61-year-old unmarried farm labourer, and a 'heavy drinker for many years', spent five months in Seacliff.[84] He was from Hokonui, near Gore, once renowned for its illegal liquor stills hidden among the hills. He told doctors that he would rather commit suicide than go back to Hokonui.

He was very depressed, 'tired of the world as things are going against him and he has no money', his notes said. George P., a former accountant, also spent time in Seacliff over 1915–1916 because of melancholia, attributed to heredity and alcoholism. He and his wife then lived apart and George found it difficult to find employment. In 1917 he took his own life.[85]

Masturbation had frequently been identified by European doctors in the past as a cause of melancholia and depressed mood, especially for males. It was considered that this 'unnatural practice' could cause 'enfeeblement, weakness, listlessness, passivity, and idiocy'.[86]

From the age of 14 Frank M. had worked as a sharebrokers' clerk at Reefton.[87] When he was admitted six years later to Seaview Asylum in 1887, he was described as an 'unhealthy looking youth whose facial appearance and furtive manner suggest the existence of a history of self abuse . . . addicted to masturbation'. His religious delusions may have caused him to feel guilt, and to attempt suicide by drowning, but he was also worried about his debts. Frank was sedated and wore glove restraints to stop masturbating. He was considered incurable, and within four years was diagnosed with chronic mania. Frank lived until 1934, dying in the asylum aged 67 of secondary dementia, a term then used to refer to the symptoms of gradual mental and physical decline.

William S., who had begun to 'self-abuse' at the age 15, was admitted up to four times to Auckland's asylum and to Sunnyside in Christchurch suffering from melancholia and depression. Two years after he stopped the 'practice', 27-year-old William was admitted for four months at Ashburn Hall as a voluntary patient.[88] He revealed to a doctor that 'the sexual cause is wrong with me'. William's case notes also show that he had been subject to attacks of depression since he was a schoolboy and he considered that he was not 'brilliant at anything'.

In the first half of the twentieth century in Aotearoa masturbation continued to be considered wrong, and a possible cause of mental illness, by some religious and medical circles. In 1928, at the family's cowshed in the Waikato, Chester swallowed a lethal dose of cow douche tablets that contained chloride of mercury.[89] He told the police, who were called to the farm after he was found, that he 'was very depressed and thought that he was going blind following self abuse'. Chester died the following day. At the inquest his father told the coroner that he had 'accused [Chester] of it at various times and tried to check him. I suspected it when he was about 14 years. I did not think it advisable to speak to him about such a thing. I did give advice about his sexual organs.'

Masturbation is recorded as a cause in only a few instances of women's melancholia.[90] In 1911, 25-year-old Clara M. was admitted to the Auckland asylum with acute melancholia: 'She has constantly bad thoughts in her mind connected with her sexual organs. She says she has had constant sexual desire but that she would not allow such a thing because she knows that it is wrong . . . she says she cannot settle to work, and must not be left alone,'[91] her case notes record. She was described as a 'nymphomaniac who was depressed and delusional'. Clara tried to tear her vagina and bite her lips, and was put in a straitjacket and her lips padded.

Although masturbation or alcohol abuse do not much feature in the causes of women's admissions to asylums for melancholia and depression treatment, their bodies and hormones certainly do. Women's melancholia and depression have long been linked to their menstrual patterns. Medical and family observers equated women's depression with their bleeding (in early asylum records called 'catamenia'), rather than mood fluctuations before the onset of their menstrual flow. In 1912 a 29-year-old asylum patient was said to become 'quite deranged when she has her periods'.[92]

The terms for melancholia and depression associated with pregnancy and childbirth fluctuated from 'puerperal insanity' and 'antenatal depression' to 'postnatal depression', and were cited as causes of depression along with miscarriage and lactation. During the late nineteenth and early twentieth centuries 'puerperal' or 'puerperium' was often given as a cause, although the duration of the puerperal period was vague. This period conventionally referred to six weeks after childbirth, but puerperal insanity/mania/melancholia/depression could extend from early pregnancy until long after the postpartum period.[93]

From 1916 to 1919, 35-year-old Christina D. was treated at Sunnyside for melancholia (puerperal) caused by the puerperium.[94] She had been a patient at Seacliff during 1911–1914. Christina was an unmarried mother of two children but assumed a married name. Four days after her third baby's birth she left it on her own doorstep, saying that she would nurse it 'for the mother'. She denied the baby was hers, and threatened to kill the child and herself. Unmarried mothers suffered severe stigma in the past, and this could be especially so within some religions and cultures. Women also faced financial and emotional stress as unmarried mothers, but so, too, could married mothers, especially if their partners were unsupportive or unable to help because of work commitments.

Yet the history of melancholia and depression connected to childbirth reveals that although women may have been depressed or suicidal after childbirth many, as we will see in chapter 5, lived long lives.[95]

The cessation of menstruation, or menopause, was often cited as a cause of melancholia and depression. This link was tenuous, and other pressures clearly were significant, even if not prominent in the medical records. Often melancholia and depression were noticed by family members or doctors several years before menopause. The climacteric was listed as the cause of 42-year-old Janet C.'s admission to Sunnyside in 1889, although she had experienced four melancholia 'attacks' since the age of 21.[96] Sarah Y.'s notes for her resistive melancholia and general depression in 1913 suggest the cause was possibly due to the 'change of life', even though they noted that she had been melancholy for around 15 years.[97] She had given birth to 10 children, and by the age of 47 was very emaciated. Sarah died in Auckland Mental Hospital four years later. At Ashburn Hall in 1905, Phoebe B. aged 52, had melancholia (climacteric) recorded as both a cause and a diagnosis,[98] but her depression was also linked to the death of a daughter several years prior.

An Otago medical school student dissertation written in 1972 outlined the widely held gendered stereotypes, both in Aotearoa and globally, about depressed middle-aged women.[99] It was assumed that 'Middle aged women find themselves with little to occupy them beyond cooking and housecleaning.' Depression was described as:

> unnecessarily disabling, especially to ageing women whose physical attractiveness and position in the family, determines her general status. The types of depression affecting women of this age used to be explained by changes in the hormonal environment, but now have been divided into reactive,

endogenous, and agitated depression. All types manifest themselves with changes in the vegetative functions i.e. changes in sleep patterns, appetite, weight and libido and diurnal variation . . . Chronic frustration in work or family life, unexpressed grief associated with bereavement and constitutional factors all play a part. It shows first as sadness, dejection, feeling of hopelessness, self reproach and a general loss of self esteem.

Mental functioning is affected often with extreme boredom and lassitude, decreased concentration and memory, with an inability to make decisions. It is physically manifest, often by fatigue, headaches, dry mouth and anorexia, diarrhoea, constipation, menstrual irregularities . . . muscle weakness, dizziness and many cardiovascular changes. The patient often does not realise she is depressed, she just feels very ill. The less literate patients phrase their misery in symbolic physical complaints, leading to tests and operations . . . During the forties and fifties a person's sources of social prestige and economic security may be threatened or actually disappear . . . at this stage of her life a woman easily grows fat, her voice may become deeper, she may become increasingly hirsute, at the same time that her hair grows thinner . . . They get a depressive illness in which hypochondriasis, hostility, demanding behaviour, dependence, anxiety, and manipulation of their environment become manifest when they find that they cannot get the ideal life situation.

Involutional melancholia is an old term applied to an illness occurring at middle age when the patient becomes painfully aware that youth has gone and that their remaining lifetime has become limited. The pain is increased and enervated by the cessation of the menstrual cycle, possibly due to hormonal changes at the hypothalamic level, which is experienced by many women as a diminution in her femininity and self esteem and this makes her increasingly prone to depression. Menopause itself causes no psychological illness or abnormal emotional state,

> but the folk belief persists that the change of life is bound to be unpleasant and may even drive a woman insane.

This chapter opened with the language of depression used in reference to the Great Depression of the early 1930s. By then 'depression' was also a common diagnosis within clinical settings, although, as much of this chapter and book traces, this was often as a descriptor of a symptom of the more frequent term 'melancholia'. During the twentieth century, melancholia fell out of use as a diagnosis, and in Aotearoa, as globally, depression was ascendant. By the late twentieth century, depression was precisely defined according to a range of symptoms.

New Zealand's mental illness classifications followed the International Classification of Diseases, Injuries and Causes of Death (ICD) adopted by the World Health Organization in 1948. The American Psychiatric Association's DSM codes for mental illnesses (*Diagnostic and Statistical Manual of Mental Disorders*) appeared in classifications of depression at Seacliff by 1957 — early, given that the DSM was only introduced in 1952.[100] Both ICD and DSM codes were revised several times over the following decades.

In 1994 the American Psychiatric Association released DSM-IV (the fourth edition of the *Diagnostic and Statistical Manual of Mental Disorders*). In 1996 these criteria were applied in Aotearoa when some of the earliest guidelines for identifying a major depressive disorder were published there.[101] Ten years later, *Te Rau Hinengaro: The New Zealand Mental Health Survey* reiterated the criteria of DSM-IV.[102]

A major depressive disorder entailed an individual: (1) experiencing at least one of the two following symptoms during a two-week period — a depressed mood most of the day nearly every day, and a marked loss of interest in all or most usual activities; and (2) having at least four symptoms every day or most days — a change from previous functioning, significant weight loss or gain, insomnia or oversleeping, psychomotor agitation or retardation, fatigue or loss of energy, feelings of worthlessness or excessive/inappropriate guilt, diminished ability to think or concentrate, or indecisiveness, recurrent thoughts of death or suicidal thoughts/actions.

The DSM standards for identifying symptoms of depression have been heavily criticised, not least because of the lack of attention to cultural nuance and local circumstance. Even so, while the medical discourse of melancholia and depression was transferred from Europe and North America to Aotearoa, the application of that usage was also shaped by local medical institutions and personnel, as well as by laypeople and the media.

In 2001, the psychiatrist and academic Sir Mason Harold Durie (Rangitāne, Ngāti Ḳauwhata, Ngāti Raukawa) offered another schema — one that provides a more holistic summary of depression derived from kaupapa Māori, but which is also applicable to other cultures.

Mason Durie's meanings of depression[103]

Broad conceptualisation ***Depression as a . . .***	**Features**
Response to traumatic events	Unhappiness, grief, remorse
Reaction to physical illness	Sadness, mood change, introspection, in the presence of a definable physical illness
Mental disorder	Psychological and mood abnormalities (guilt, self-accusation; despondency) Clusters of specific signs and symptoms, recognised natural history
Physical disorder	Altered energy levels Weight change Appetite and bowel dysfunction
Reaction to societal adversity and oppression	Unemployment, poverty, powerlessness
Spiritual response	Cultural alienation, loss of capacity for self-respect and respect of others

While boxes that define depression appear clinical, the confidence of clarity they provide are useful tools for practitioners, even if the longer history of melancholia and depression shows that discourses change, and that typologies have to be reformulated. Behind these boxes live those with their own or others' experience of depression. These people, as well as, for example, medical and legal experts, academics, clerics, philosophers and artists, have long asked whether depression is madness, a moral failing, a mental disorder, a biological condition or simply the black cloud that closes in as we face life's challenges. The following chapters uncover the human narratives in New Zealand's past that speak to melancholia and depression.

2.

Rāwakiwaki

Waata (Walter) Pihikete Kūkūtai, a prominent Ngāti Tīpā rangatira in Waikato, was highly regarded by the British as a Māori magistrate and government advisor and became a major in the New Zealand militia. In 1854 Kūkūtai, a convert to Anglicanism, moved his hapū to Te Kōhanga, where he would oversee the building of a church and donate land to the Crown so that the Church of England could build a school.

Between 1865 and 1866 Kūkūtai wrote several letters to Bishop George Selwyn, the first Anglican bishop of New Zealand, requesting support for the project. In a letter dated 4 October 1866, he told Selwyn that he was full of despair because his wife, Mihi Kūkūtai, was ill and close to death. On 3 December 1866 he confessed in a further letter to the bishop that such was his grief that he had sinned by consuming a lethal poisonous medicine.[1]

A contemporary newspaper report stated that the recent deaths of Kūkūtai's wife and nephew had 'deeply affected him and caused him to be in very low spirits'.[2] Kūkūtai died on 8 January 1867, aged around 45. It is unclear whether the poison was the primary cause of his death, as Kūkūtai also suffered from tuberculosis and a severely ulcerated throat.

The same year, several newspapers reported that Wi (Wiremu) Waka, a Rangitāne leader in the Wairarapa, was experiencing 'mental depression'. He had opposed the British and land dispossession, and was a follower of Pai Mārire (goodness and peace), a religion which blended Māori spirituality and Christianity but which many Pākehā of the time regarded as a violent movement.

> Wi Waka looking very ill and the picture of misery. He felt very sick, and begged for spirits and European food, with neither of which we of course could immediately supply him. It was evidently mental depression that affected him. He had received a letter from Mr. Wardell, R.M., directing the unconditional surrender of himself to the Governor, but promising that his life should be spared. His immediate adherents and followers were also to come in and take the oath of allegiance. Wi Waka refused to comply . . . He dares not stir from his hill, fearing capture by the Defence Corps, and is virtually a prisoner in his own castle but he looks so utterly depressed.[3]

Was Kūkūtai's decision to take poison to end his life because of mental depression? Was Wi Waka's depression caused by the profound disruption of colonisation and the sense of despair, caused by knowing he would have to surrender to the British who had taken Māori land and would try to suppress Maōri identity?

Any history of depression and melancholia in Aotearoa must consider mental health within the context of Maōri or tangata whenua. Today, Māori have very high rates of depression, but research suggests that few suffered from melancholia or depression before the twentieth century, reflecting the small number of mentally distressed Māori who came to the attention of the colonial medical establishment, the racial framing of mental illness, the complexities of cross-cultural diagnosis, and the paucity of detail within asylum and coronial records about the mental state of Māori and any others who were not European.

Mason Durie has written extensively about how physical, mental and spiritual health are entwined within Māori and Māori mental health.[4] Ideally the balance is between wairua (spiritual wellbeing), hinengaro (intellectual wellbeing), ngākau (emotional wellbeing) and tinana (physical wellbeing).[5] Anthropologist Sir Hirini (Sidney) Moko Mead (Ngāti Awa, Ngāti Tūwharetoa, Ngāi Tūhoe, Tūhourangi) regarded health and wellbeing in relation to 'hauora' as the 'spirit of life, health, vigour', or 'healthy, fresh, well'.[6]

According to Mason Durie, before contact with Western medicine and even long after, Māori distinguished between physical accidents (mate taua) and mate atua (illnesses with no obvious physical causes). Depression and madness, or wairangi and pōrangi, were usually explained as:

> an infringement of the laws of *tapu* or of the sensitivities of powerful others whose retaliation could produce derangement even without a physical confrontation. Although there was a spiritual basis to the condition it was also closely linked with accepted social values and often suggested a departure from community norms either by the patient or the wider family. Individual and family distinctions were not sharp, the health of one being regarded as a symptom of the other.[7]

Durie also placed Māori health within modern circumstances:

> [P]sychological well-being is related to personal encounters, developmental experiences, societal values and equity, stress, genetics, culture, standards of living, physical health, and political influence. The foundations for mental health are to be found as much outside the mind and the body as within. They lie with families, communities, jobs, decent homes, schools that value children, reliable transport, policies for health, equity and fairness, access to goods and services, safety and security, and experiences carried over from earlier times.[8]

Māori had several terms equivalent to mental depression that varied between iwi, over time and according to context — pōkē, pōuritanga, tiwhatiwha, whakapōuri, poururu, mate pāpōuri and rāwakiwaki. In 2007 Hāpai Te Hauora consultants Leonie Pihama and Paul Reynolds described āhua pōuri, another Māori concept for depression, as:

> dark, unclear, not sure where you're going, your thoughts aren't all together, you're trying to find, you're closed in, with nowhere to go, depending on how dark it is. You're not feeling good about anything actually about yourself, about where you are in life.[9]

Hākerekere, a compound word made up of hā (breath), and kerekere (dark), is often used as a translation for depression. An expression to capture the psychosomatic nature of depression is 'te haumaruru o te ngoikore' (debilitation and weakness).[10] Although Durie wrote about the need to consider mental health for Māori within a holistic framework, he also cautioned against making a diagnosis of depression based on emotional symptoms and observable mood changes. 'Māori patients who have a depressive disorder are not necessarily overwhelmed by symptoms of sadness, hopelessness, or unhappiness. Those emotions may not be significantly distinguishable from the range of feelings experienced as part of normal living. Nor does guilt or self-accusation dominate the picture', he wrote in his 2001 book, *Mauri Ora.*[11] A depressive disorder could manifest through somatic symptoms, such as appetite or weight loss, bodily pains, reduced libido, loss of energy and a feeling of coldness. Manawa-pōuri, a term for sadness, literally translates as 'sad heart'.

In a holistic view in which spiritual, physical and mental health are entwined, spirits were prominent in early accounts of mental health, depression and melancholia, as well as in the overall health among Māori. The causes of mental illness often were located within the spiritual world, especially with transgressions of tapu (social mores and laws).[12]

Durie has explained how mate atua (illness with no obvious cause) could be caused by mākutu, through spiritual powers or a spell that had been cast by a tohunga:

> A person or family who had committed an offence could become distraught in either physical or mental terms, by a tohunga, often from a distance. The victim might have transgressed while visiting another area or might have given serious offense within the family or tribal context. In any event makutu produced a serious state of disability which without intervention from another tohunga, could lead to death.[13]

In 1882 Dr Edward Shortland, a scholar (possibly New Zealand's first anthropologist), administrator and medical doctor, provided a detailed example of the ritual and karakia that might be offered by a tohunga to cure pōrangi caused through mākutu in his book *Maori Religion and*

Mythology. An authority from Te Arawa told Shortland that the last part of this karakia was a curse directed against some tohunga who had supposedly imposed the disease. This information was published many years later:

> When anyone becomes *porangi* or insane, as not unfrequently happens, he is taken to a *tohunga*, who first makes an examination as to the cause of the disease. He and the sick man then go to the waterside, and the *tohunga*, stripping off his own clothes, takes in his hand an obsidian flint. First, he cuts a lock of hair from the left side of the sick man's head, and afterwards a lock of hair from the top of his head. The obsidian flint is then placed on the ground, and upon it the lock of hair which had been cut from the left side of the head. The lock of hair cut from the top of the head is held aloft in the left hand of the *tohunga*, while in his right hand he holds a common stone, which is also raised aloft . . . the *tohunga* breathes on the flint, and smashes it with the stone held in his right hand. After this he selects a shoot of the plant *toetoe*, and pulls it up, and then fastens to it both the locks of hair. Then diving in the river, he lets go the *toetoe* and locks of hair, and when they float on the surface of the water, he commences his great *karakia*;
>
> This is the *Tiri* of Tu-i-rawea,
> This is the *Tiri* of Uenuku.
>
> Where lies your fault?
> Was eating a *kutu* your fault?
> Was sitting on *tapu* ground your fault?
> Unravel the tangle,
> Unravel, untie.
> Take away the fault from the head
> Of the *Atua* who afflicts this man.
> Take away the disease,
> And the *mana* of the curser.
> Turn your *mana* against your *tohunga*,
> And your *whaiwhaia*.
> Give me the curse

To make as cooked food.
Your *Atua* desecrated,
Your *tapu*, your curse,
Your sacred-place-dwelling *Atua*,
Your house-dwelling *Atua*,
Give me to cook for food.
Your *tapu* is desecrated by me.
The rays of the sun,
The brave of the world,
The *mana*, give me.
Let your *Atua*, and your *tapu*
Be food for me to eat.
Let the head of the curser
Be baked in the oven,
Served up for food for me
Dead, and gone to Night.[14]

But in many whānau, mākutu was not, and still is not, openly spoken about. The practice was never advertised, and often only male specialists could practise.[15]

In 1962 Laurie Kalman Gluckman, later to become a prominent psychiatrist who practised mostly in Auckland, wrote an important dissertation on mākutu and psychiatry.[16] Several of the Māori patients Gluckman treated were depressed; others were suffering from different psychiatric and physical conditions. Many considered that they were under mākutu, and they were afraid to discuss this with a Pākehā. Most of the Māori patients Gluckman met were given the then gold-standard psychiatric treatment of electroconvulsive therapy (ECT), as outlined in chapter 7.

Gluckman, who worked within Western psychiatry, used terms in his dissertation and publications such as 'witchcraft', 'superstition' and 'cultural indoctrination'. Some patients agreed to talk with him about their belief that their actions had led to mākutu. Keira, for example, who was admitted to hospital during the 1950s with acute depression and a physical illness,[17] was assessed as having reactive depression due to an unhappy marriage. Gluckman decided on a course of electroconvulsive treatments to alleviate her depression.

After the first electroshock, Keira started eating, talked with other patients and read her prayer book. But after the next day's electroshock, she reacted with acute apprehension, hyperventilated, trembled, sweated and sobbed. She refused further treatment and demanded to leave the hospital, stating that otherwise she would die. Keira told Gluckman that she did not have mākutu when she was initially admitted to the hospital, but that it had emerged after she had made negative comments about a tohunga. She considered that her faith and modern medicine could not protect her, and she insisted she was not pōrangi or insane. She was discharged from hospital but readmitted after a domestic dispute.

Another Māori woman, whom Gluckman described as 'grossly depressed', attributed her mākutu to having done something wrong or evil; possibly from eating an apple, potato or kūmara that had the power to make her ill.[18] Gluckman reported that she appeared somewhat better after ECT, and after talking about her difficult marriage and about being a mother to three children by the age of 22. She appeared to recover within seven days of her admission.

Some depressed patients believed that others' actions had put them under mākutu. One patient, aged 36, had been seeing images of his grandmother or great-aunt during the night ever since he was nine years old. His father had broken a tapu, leading to mākutu.[19] Eliza considered that her de facto husband's new partner had put a mākutu on her.[20] She was admitted to hospital with depression and because she refused to eat. Eliza had become aware of mākutu when young. Gluckman stated: 'Atua could affect her physically and emotionally either as spirits directly or by the spirits being incarnated in animal forms (Tohu or Tokana), indirectly.' Eliza began to heal during a brief stay in hospital.

Mākutu has remained implicated in causes of depression for some Māori since Gluckman's research. During the 1980s, a Māori man who had held a responsible position but committed suicide put his overwhelming depression down to a curse (mate Māori).[21] In some whānau there may be levels of 'wrongdoing', such as long-term adultery or the theft of taonga tapu, which may have caused depression. As Maata Wharehoka (Ngāti Tahinga, Ngāti Koata, Ngāti Apakura, Ngāti Toa, Ngāti Kuia) explained to me: 'Mate Māori might be used to avoid the truth or to prevent the spread of malicious conversation in the whānau or community.'[22]

This phenomenon was well known to Dr Golan Maaka (Te Kōrana) (Ngāti Kahungunu, Ngāi Tahu), who graduated from the University of Otago Medical School in 1937. He found that mākutu was active in his practice with Māori, especially in Matahi and Waimana in the Bay of Plenty, and Te Urewera. His biographer Bradford Haami recounted: 'Golan would come across old people who knew they had been placed under makutu and were just sitting in the forest waiting to die. Golan recognised immediately the effects of makutu — advised them to return to the old tohunga(s) he knew in the area . . . He tried to teach or tell the old people that it was actually "the fear of makutu", that killed them, not the makutu itself.'

Many of Golan's patients were sent to sanatoriums like Tokanui (the psychiatric hospital near Te Awamutu), where they would remain for the rest of their lives. Golan tried to prevent people who were pōrangi being admitted to psychiatric hospitals, because he knew that they were likely to be treated in a Pākehā way, whereas they could be cared for within the Maōri way by tohunga. 'Golan also believed in the importance of dreams and the natural signs of nature which the old people read, studied and drew conclusions from as to the fate of a person or people. He recognised the need for karakia and the right of the tohunga to perform the old kawa (ceremony) and tikanga for the people,' Haami wrote.[23]

Whakamā or feeling ashamed can also mask depression for some Maōri. This is associated with a sense of helplessness, being unable to control the situation or 'feeling like someone is trampling on our mana (prestige) or the mana of our whānau'.[24] Psychiatric survivor Iwa Stewart was only 14 years old when admitted to Kingseat Hospital at Karaka, south of Auckland, with a diagnosis of a depressive illness. Stewart explained in a 1998 issue of *Mental Health Quarterly* how whakamā and depression are linked:

> The inner feelings of whakamaa are displayed by shyness, uncertainty, inadequacy, embarrassment, fear, hurt and shame. These feelings left unchecked can become chronic. The outer signs of whakamaa are seen in the physical appearance of a person and encompass hunched shoulders, eyes darting to and fro, downcast eyes, at a loss for words, physically avoiding people and crossing arms. We all experience the inner feelings and outward signs of whakamaa to different degrees . . .

> Although whakamaa is not considered a mental illness, a person suffering from it is deemed to be weak and vulnerable. The symptoms associated with most depressive disorders are similar to those of whakamaa, such as anxiety, sudden mood-swings, feelings of worthlessness and loss of meaning in life. Hopeless despair like this may lead to suicidal thoughts and attempts. There does seem to be a link between chronic whakamaa and depression.[25]

Stewart questioned the initial assessment of depression: 'the symptoms I displayed as a child, young adult and even to some extent today, were the result not of a depressive illness but of chronic whakamaa'.

The word 'depression' was not often used by Europeans about Māori in a medical sense, but instead to describe negative attitudes held by the 'Natives'. William Searancke, a district commissioner in the Land Purchase Department in Wellington who lived in the Wairarapa, wrote to the native secretary in 1860 that 'The Natives are all now perfectly quiet, and their late self-confidence has been succeeded by a sulky depression.'[26] European discourse about Māori and depression was also entangled with the assumption that Māori were a 'dying race'.

In 1924 the British anthropologist George Pitt-Rivers pointed out that Māori would reveal depression and despondency 'to a sympathetic observer', but he added that Europeans tended to attribute this to 'the Maori's incurable laziness'.[27] It should be noted that 'laziness' could be a form of exerting agency through submission or non-compliance with controlling colonists.[28] But an examination of the historical and social pressures caused by colonisation in Aotearoa offers more complex and less ethnocentric understandings of despondency among Māori.

Colonisation by Europeans induced poor health, including mental depression, for most Indigenous people throughout the world.[29] Colonisation could be through 'informal' encounters, whether violent, negotiated, religious or transactive (through trade). Formal imperialism and the annexing of colonies by colonial powers followed European exploration and settlement, and was tied in with the expansion of global capitalism, with the conversion of Indigenous people to Christianity being a major catalyst. This does not, however, deny Indigenous agency, through co-option or resistance to colonial encounters and rapacious European dominance. Anthropologists Frederick Cooper and Ann Laura Stoler summed up anthropologist Talal Asad's insight into colonisation:

> monumental destruction at every level, precisely because it attempted to reorganize not only the polity, but social relations, economic structures, and values. It was not just the violence of pillage, but the violence of self conscious and self righteous transformation of social life. And its destructiveness was not just a question of conquest but of law: an attempt to redefine norms as well as practices.[30]

Colonialism was pervasive, imposed not only through brute violence but also through the word of God, colonial pacification and commercial development. It penetrated into the most intimate spaces to pervade the lives, minds, bodies and spaces of Indigenous peoples.[31]

Māori may have first arrived in Aotearoa during the thirteenth century, sailing from East Polynesia. The Dutch explorer Abel Janszoon Tasman was probably the first European to reach Aotearoa, in 1642, but Europeans did not actually set foot on Aotearoa until 1769, when Englishman Captain James Cook and his crew came ashore. During the late eighteenth and first half of the nineteenth centuries, Māori encountered others they termed 'Pākehā', including sealers, whalers, missionaries, traders and settlers from Great Britain, Ireland and the United States. Some lascars and sepoys came from Asia. Thus Aotearoa shifted from being a land of Indigenous Māori to a colony of the British Empire in which Pākehā dominated.

Unlike many colonies, New Zealand has a founding document, Te Tiriti o Waitangi (the Treaty of Waitangi), which was signed in 1840 as a partnership between the British Crown and a number of, but not all, Māori chiefs.[32] New Zealand became a colony of Britain, with Māori as British subjects. There are many contested understandings of Te Tiriti, many created by the differences between the English and Maōri versions. Although ostensibly intended to protect Māori, the treaty was soon breached by the Crown as European settlers demanded more land. Māori also lost considerable land during the New Zealand Wars, which were fought between iwi and the British Army — and then a volunteer militia — and their Māori allies in various districts of the North Island from 1845 to 1872. Massive Māori land confiscations (raupatu) followed the wars, enabled through the workings of the Native Land Court.[33]

By the end of the nineteenth century very little land came under Māori title. In addition to the devastation wrought by land dispossession, there was a drastic decline in the Māori population, due especially to introduced diseases, lifestyle changes and psychological despondency. The Māori population estimated by James Cook to be 100,000 in 1769 had fallen to between 70,000 and 90,000 by 1840, and by 1896 numbered around 42,000.[34]

In 1934, the psychologist Ivan Sutherland testified to the Native Affairs Commission that there was no other future for Māori than a life based on the land: 'When the Maori wars were concluded in 1872, the state of the Maori people was for the most part deplorable in the extreme. Their best land had been confiscated from a number of the tribes, and these tribes felt a strong sense of defeat, injury and injustice. A period of profound depression in the mental outlook of the Maori followed.'[35] Despair and culture were entwined: land for Māori was not simply a resource or commodity, but had cultural and spiritual meaning.[36]

Archival evidence of the relationship between mental depression and land dispossession for Māori is patchy, but it was recorded in a few case notes of the Auckland mental asylum. For example, in 1897 Hirini T. indicated that his melancholia may have been caused because 'his people are worrying him by selling all his land for drink'.[37] A preoccupation with land featured in Ariani P.'s delusional melancholia in 1914.[38] She may not have personally possessed land, but she insisted on travelling to Auckland from Morrinsville to sell her large block of land. She had also tried to kill her sons, but denied this after admission to Auckland Mental Hospital in 1914. Ariani remained a long-term patient in Auckland, and in 1935, aged 58, she was transferred to Tokanui Hospital.

Māori also suffered melancholia or depression as a result of the prolonged fighting of the New Zealand Wars. The wars had a profound effect on 35-year-old Tamihau from Waikato, for example. When first admitted to a hospital he refused to talk or eat. He was diagnosed with melancholia and confined to the Auckland asylum from 1869 until his death in 1878. When Reverend McDonald was visiting the asylum in 1869, he succeeded in conversing with Tamihau, who 'Spoke in bitter terms about the war and the natives engaged therein'; '[h]is motto was "Peace" and he took it very much to heart that there should be any fighting'.[39]

Colonisation radically changed the practice of Māori healing. In 1907 the Tohunga Suppression Act outlawed traditional healers.[40] A combination of reasons for this included settler prejudices, the perceived risk of charlatans taking advantage of vulnerable people, and particularly the ineffectiveness of many forms of traditional Māori medicine against introduced infectious European diseases, such as tuberculosis. Many leading Māori reformers, including Māori parliamentarians, supported the Act.[41] Nevertheless, some tohunga continued to practise away from colonial eyes, where traditions were passed on.

Healing was never just the preserve of tohunga, but was sustained on marae communities, where kaumātua and kuia treasured ancient health knowledge. Karakia could also be offered to cure insanity.[42] Rongoā (Indigenous medicinal plants) treated many illnesses, but there is no written record of a treatment for depression.[43] Symptoms of depression, such as bowel complaints and general weakness, could be alleviated with pirita (supplejack) and kawakawa (pepper tree), which were usually drunk as infusions.[44] In the 1960s Laurie Gluckman described a ritual at Ahipara in Northland to treat mākutu for a Ngāpuhi patient whom he had diagnosed with clinical depression.[45] An eel was caught and cut in half, with the tail portion applied to the patient's head and the head portion sometimes cooked and eaten, or sometimes buried. The total remnants had to be buried. Other elderly Māori described similar rituals to Gluckman.

The most common treatment for mental disorders and depression among Māori was care by whānau. There were limits to tolerance of aberrant behaviour by those with mental disorders, however, especially when tapu was violated or there was unacceptable violence within whānau. As colonial law became imposed, so were rules about when insanity absolved a crime. If colonial subjects were considered not guilty on these grounds, then appropriate institutional confinement within an asylum was usually advocated.

The story of Watene reflects the complicated transition between traditional ways of dealing with violence and mental illness and the fledging colonial mental health infrastructure.

Watene — called 'Old Cranky' by whānau at Wakapuaka (near Nelson) — suffered from melancholia. His episodic and strange behaviour was tolerated even when he tried to assault a woman and later tried to drown himself. Watene was eventually arrested in 1858 after murdering his wife, Kahiwa, and then attempting suicide.[46] The coroner assessed his insanity as 'melancholy madness', but suggested that Watene may have also suffered from monomania, considered during the nineteenth century as a psychological obsession in a sound mind, when a sane person might commit a bizarre act.[47] Monomania was sometimes called 'partial insanity'.

The warder of Nelson Gaol, William Rodgerson, observed that Watene 'was melancholy, very silent, and very much reserved. He was now in better health both bodily and mental. There was at first a good deal of wandering of the eye: his features were vacant and melancholy: had frequently spoken to him: prisoner had generally a very vacant smile.' Nelson doctor Theodore Bernhard Thebing agreed: 'These symptoms are very characteristic of melancholia, one form of insanity; this form of insanity, more than another, frequently results in violent acts of frenzy: those acts are mostly sudden as a flash of lightning: this form of madness is often caused by jealousy.' Thebing suggested: 'Confinement in a prison might account for the sullenness shewn by the prisoner.'

The jury found Watene not guilty on the grounds of insanity, but rangatira Emanu reminded the jury that in earlier times Watene's murder of his wife (who was Emanu's sister) would have had dire repercussions.[48] 'Had we been still living under Maori customs, the prisoner would have forfeited his life . . . probably most of the tribe to which prisoner belongs, would have been slain,' he told the court. Emanu considered that many of Kahiwa's whānau 'may still adhere to their Maori customs' and not understand English law.

He hoped that Watene would be sent far away so that Māori would not be 'grieved or angered by the sight of one whom we must still regard as the slayer of his wife, and that wife a chief's sister'. Watene was sentenced to two years' imprisonment with hard labour. At the time there was no mental asylum in Nelson, and the few asylums elsewhere were administered by provincial governments.

My sampling of melancholic Māori patients committed to the Auckland asylum found that violence and disturbances within their community could precipitate admissions. In 1900, for example, William C. threatened to kill his parents and whānau, but he became quiet and solitary within the asylum.[49] Kii Kii, a 25-year-old labourer and gumdigger from Ōhinemuri (Coromandel), died after five months there.[50] Although people had been afraid of his violence, it was only after he suddenly attacked a companion in church that he was admitted to an asylum.

Tio P. was first admitted to the Auckland mental asylum in 1907 and discharged, but after his wife's death he became violent, leading to another admission in 1915.[51] He frightened people on the marae and threatened to 'kill for other natives' as soon as he returned from the mental hospital. Tio was observed as melancholic, depressed, taciturn and morose, and probably also had aural and visual hallucinations.

Another Auckland asylum patient, Morrinsville woman Ariani, was violent towards her sons, and burned her whare, confirming her husband's conviction that she was 'as mad as possible'. She also wandered away from home at night. Violent and mentally disturbed wanderers were considered unacceptable among Māori. In 1911 whānau and neighbours feared Hepita M.'s wandering when he became maniacal and violent.[52] He was brought from Kohukohu to Rāwene, in the Hokianga, and then admitted to the Auckland Mental Hospital with mania. A doctor stated that he was obviously mentally depressed. Hepita had two further admissions, in 1914 and 1916, and was diagnosed with melancholia.[53]

Wandering seems harmless, but was sometimes indicative of mental distress.[54] Excessive mobility was not necessarily odd among Māori, but might be considered so within dangerous places, without resources and, importantly, without whānau. Mākutu or fear could lead to wandering, as when 49-year-old Frank Travers (Te Wharau Whareiti) believed he was being pursued by a taipō (ghost). During the winter of 1912 he tried to cross the hills from Paparamu to Kihikihi, in the Waikato — a walk of at least 13 hours — to see his mother. He had no food or shelter and was almost naked.

After Frank was found at Maungatautari, near Te Awamutu, he was sent to Hamilton hospital, weakened from his nights in the bush.[55] This was not the first time he had wandered from his wife and whānau into the bush, without food and clothes. His restlessness continued in the Auckland Mental Hospital, where nurses reported that he disturbed patients, shouting, roaming at night, and crawling on the floor because he believed that the devil was in his skin. At other times Frank, who was diagnosed with melancholia, was 'very dull and depressed'. He was discharged from the hospital in 1919.

A few widowed Māori women who wandered were committed to mental hospitals with melancholia. One woman was 'always trying to run wild over the country and without food'. In 1900, aged 70, she was committed to the Auckland asylum after searching for her husband, who had been dead for six years.[56] Her friends tried to keep watch over her, partly because some whānau members had been 'pōrangi'.

Herina K., a widow from Manutūkē, Gisborne, wandered from her home for some years before her committal in 1913 to Auckland's asylum with delusional melancholia.[57] She believed that there was poison in the houses of nearby strangers, and that, because she owned the mission on the marae, she could enter other people's homes. According to her son, Herina thought that she and her ancestors owned these houses. 'She digs in the ground, saying that she has a house there and she wishes to get it.'

After Herina entered farmer John Clark's house at night and lit dangerous fires, he filed papers to have her committed to an asylum. He knew that she had been looked after by whānau at Manutūkē, but, because her children could not pay for her care in a hospital, Clark did. A few weeks after admission, Herina told an attendant that she was 'no more porangi' and felt 'kapai'. She died in the asylum from phthisis (tuberculosis) in 1918.

Until the Second World War most Māori lived on rural marae, which enabled strong ties to whānau and culture and provided crucial psychological care and support. Residential and cultural patterns for Māori shifted during and after the war, and became accelerated with the rural-to-urban migration from the 1960s.[58] In the 1980s, lawyer, activist and scholar Moana Jackson (Ngāti Kahungunu, Ngāti Porou) highlighted how cultural isolation, alienation from land and from traditional family structures had an impact on the mental health of Māori offenders.[59] Loneliness and isolation are at the root of much depression, and for Māori this often meant disconnection from whānau, hapū, iwi and community.[60] Those ties have been through profound change, and the lack of wider support for Māori from society in general has also adversely impacted Māori wellbeing.[61]

International Indigenous literature refers to 'cultural depression', which is sometimes described as 'trying to live in two worlds and fitting into neither'.[62] Recent scholars have referred to intergenerational depression as another effect of the historical psychological trauma of colonisation for Indigenous peoples.[63] Some researchers argue that the experiences of cultural trauma caused by colonisation exacerbate health-related disease among Indigenous populations, via epigenetics,[64] which claims that history, society and environment can impact on the way in which people's genes work and their bodies respond. Depression as 'cultural grief' and 'collective post-traumatic stress disorder' is explained by the Māori leader, health advocate and researcher Keri Lawson-Te Aho (Ngāti Kahungunu ki te Wairoa, Ngāti Pāhauwera, Rongomaiwahine, Ngāi Tahu, Ngāi Tūhoe, Ngāti Porou, Rongowhakaata, Ngāti Tūwharetoa) as:

> a form of cultural depression, variously called sub-clinical depression, acculturative stress, cultural grief and collective post-traumatic stress . . . This psycho-pathology (mental illness) is thought to be characterised by self-destructive behaviour (such as drug and alcohol abuse) and negative ideation (thinking) (such as low self-esteem, feelings of worthlessness, feelings of inadequacy, feelings of hopelessness, and depression) . . . There is a point beyond which individual behaviour becomes a deficient explanation for widespread indigenous mental illness. Indigenous mental illness is thought to be related to the outcomes of trying to live in two worlds and fitting into neither, coupled with histories of cultural genocide over which indigenous peoples have been not able to exercise sufficient control. This carries an idea of intergenerational, collective cultural suffering.[65]

Pōuritanga (darkness) or depression could be passed down to subsequent generations if left unaddressed.[66]

Before the twentieth century, many 'experts' considered mental illness as a 'white man's burden'. Early British psychiatrist Daniel Tuke considered in 1878 that Indigenous people did not suffer mental illness or depression.[67] American physician Edward Jarvis suggested in 1852 that insanity was 'part of the price which we pay for civilization'.[68] Suicide was once considered an index of civilisation.[69] The medical doctor and anthropologist Peter Henry Buck (Te Rangi Hīroa) drew upon his Māori (Ngāti Mutunga) and Pākehā heritage when he articulated mental disturbance within both Māori beliefs and a Western racial evolutionary framework in his MD thesis submitted in 1910 at Otago Medical School.

> The nervous system of the savage, along certain directions, is more unstable than that of the more civilised races. To a certain extent it is more liable to respond to stimulation of an emotional or exciting nature . . . The lack of judgement of the higher centres, combined with defect of inhibition or of control by the higher over the lower centres which exists in childhood, is true to a large extent of the less educated brain. The result is that some powerful emotional stimulus such as that of fear of witchcraft or the transgression of tapu, owing to defective inhibition or control of the higher centres, is communicated to the lower centres. The vital processes are depressed; shock and fatal melancholia are produced.[70]

Some Pākehā were hesitant to apply Western definitions of madness to Māori, as evidenced in Watene's trial, during which jurors were asked to decide 'whether or not he suffered from melancholy madness when he murdered his wife'. The defence counsel reminded the jury 'to decide, upon one of the most painful cases ever yet brought before the notice of a jury in this province . . . the prisoner was a member of another race, and there was a great difficulty in getting at facts'.[71]

The facts of mental disturbance across cultures were imbued with racial stereotypes and the perceived shortcomings of non-Western cultures. In 1912, for example, Travers was described in his notes at Auckland Mental Hospital as 'An aboriginal native with the usual dark skin, dark eyes, and dark hair.'[72] 'His knowledge of English does not appear to be expansive enough for an accurate investigation of his mental condition but possibly this is due to a large extent to his mental condition. Very dull, depressed and confused, hardly speaks at all.' He also spoke incoherently in te reo Māori. In 1900, Kii Kii's medical notes at the Auckland asylum depicted him with a 'wild ferocious look, gesticulates as if performing Haka, seizes food like a wild beast'. He talked Māori to himself in the asylum. A fellow patient, Pare T., from Tuakau, was said to be 'garbling in Maori and English; the English at any rate being disconnected and foolish'.[73] It is not clear whether these assessments about melancholic patients were made by speakers of te reo Māori.

Withdrawal is common among many depressed patients of all cultures. Was this reaction among Māori also cultural withdrawal — possibly whakamā — or from the institutional regime?[74] Or were some Māori patients withdrawn because they considered their sickness was due to mākutu or because they had violated tapu, either within iwi, hapū or whānau or to themselves?

'Whakamomori' is a widely recognised term for suicide among Māori. Whakamomori has also been associated with depression, 'the desperate state when something horrific has happened to us, like losing someone we're really close to. It might even make us feel as if we are cold to touch. People say whakamomori is like being somewhere between life and death.'[75]

Mason Durie suggests that there was no traditional cultural understanding or general sanctioning of suicide among Māori apart from self-strangulation linked to bereavement. Widows occasionally strangled themselves to join a dead husband, but this was not usual if they were caring for dependent children.[76] Other factors, including suffering from depression, were cited in coronial inquests into probable suicides by Māori. In 1917, for example, a Māori widow committed suicide 'by hanging herself with a piece of flax' at a 'native settlement' in Waiuku. She had become depressed after her husband's recent death.[77]

In 1942 Maki Pihiri of Pātuharakeke at Takahiwai near Whangārei hanged himself from a pūriri — a sacred tree associated with the mourning and burial of the dead. *The Evening Post* reported that the 72-year-old had followed 'an ancient custom'.[78] At the inquest his wife, Hera, and their son Henry emphasised that Pihiri was depressed. He had suffered from ill health during the last year, and his depression was compounded by another son's death in the war.[79]

In the past, suicide among Māori was possibly culturally sanctioned, but early colonial Eurocentric perspectives suggested that for Māori suicide was a cultural or impulsive response to avoid shame, confrontation, punishment or as an act of revenge. This oversimplified suicide as well as the way in which depression could lead to extreme consequences for Māori.

In a comparison of suicides between the 1930s and 1980s, historians John Weaver and Doug Munro have suggested that Māori suicides were probably undercounted, and that the majority of those who took their lives were mostly young rural males.[80] Among the samples I perused of Māori suicide until the 1980s, coroners often ruled the cause 'great mental depression' or a 'severe state of mental depression'.[81]

Other factors could be alcohol abuse, ill health, grief, family and marital conflict — no different from Pākehā. In 1942 *The Gisborne Herald* reported the tragic death of a 30-year-old woman on a farm in the Bay of Plenty under the sensational headline 'Human torch. Maori woman's fate. Set light to clothing'. When her husband had returned from a visit to Te Teko, he found that she had locked herself in her room. He broke the window, but she had already soaked her clothing with kerosene and set herself alight. Her husband pulled her from the blaze, but was unable to save her life.

The inquest revealed that she had left a suicide note describing severe marital tensions and feelings that she was not being treated properly. Police stated that she had been 'labouring under severe mental strain'. The night before her death she was upset because her husband had stayed up late at a dance. The coroner 'returned a verdict of suicide while in a severe state of mental depression'.[82]

During the 1930s the tragic suicide of Louis Potaka and the attempted suicide of George Rameka revealed in very different ways how depression could be entwined with racism.

On 2 October 1936, Dr Louis Hauiti Potaka and his friend David Mason (Rawiri Meihana) were driving over Tākaka Hill, near Nelson, when Potaka asked Mason to stop the car because he wanted to burn some papers.[83] After they both got out of the car, Potaka got back in and drove away, leaving his companion behind. Following on foot in the direction the car had gone, Mason was informed by a man that he had seen Dr Potaka drive past on the road to Canaan. Mason and two others went up this road and saw Potaka emerge from the bush. Potaka was taken to Nelson Hospital, where he died of self-inflicted morphine poisoning.

Potaka was aged 35. His parents were Esther Potaka (née Caselberg) and Arapeta Tapui Potaka (Ngāti Hauiti). Potaka had been a stellar student at Wanganui Collegiate, and in 1930 had graduated from Otago Medical School as the fifth Māori medical graduate in the nation. He practised in Murchison, Nelson and Tākaka, and famously was the doctor on Admiral Richard Byrd's Antarctic expedition of 1934–1935. He had been appointed after answering a newspaper advertisement for an urgent replacement for the expedition's original doctor, who had withdrawn because of health problems. Potaka was posthumously awarded a United States congressional medal for his service. Potaka Inlet on Thurston Island in Antarctica was later named in his memory.

Why did this talented and popular general practitioner end his life? The coroner put it down to being in a state of deep depression. Potaka's biographer Bruce Young claims that Potaka may have first considered suicide after contracting ultraviolet keratitis (snow blindness) in Antarctica. His eyesight was severely impaired, but he avoided examination by an ophthalmologist when he returned to Aotearoa in 1935. In a final note Potaka said that he had not slept properly since January 1935 (when he was still in Antarctica), and that death would be a relief. He was also anxious about his finances and professional future, which journalist Gerard Hindmarsh, in a story written about Potaka for *The Nelson Mail* in 2020, claimed was due to 'institutional racism . . . that finally brought him down'.

In April 1930 Potaka had taken up a contract to practise as a general practitioner in Murchison, but the county council refused to renew his three-year appointment. Hindmarsh considered this was because of resentment that a Māori held a high position.

Five years later, when Potaka returned from the Antarctic, he became Dr Edward Bydder's locum and the Native Medical Officer at his private hospital in Tākaka. Potaka's appointment was terminated once Bydder learned of conflict between Potaka and the matron, Lynda Hyland. When Potaka, popular with patients, started a practice nearby, Bydder reported him to the Nelson Division of the British Medical Association, which decided that such behaviour by a locum was unethical and that Potaka should close his practice or face deregistration. He refused, and instead committed suicide.

The Tākaka community showed its support and love for Potaka at the large funeral held before his burial at Rototai Cemetery. His mother received hundreds of condolence letters, including one from Byrd. Louis Hauiti Potaka was, Hindmarsh says, 'a great, inspired man who gave his life to serving others, loved and accepted by the common people, but who faced incredible adversity from the powers that were simply because he was Maori'.

The 1931 trial in Auckland of relief worker George Rameka (Pahara Rameka Kere) for murdering his lover Gwendoline Johnson, whose husband was working abroad on a ship, attracted widespread attention throughout Aotearoa. Readers of the newspaper reports of the trial were titillated by lurid details of a fatal fall-out between a Māori man and an English immigrant.

Dr Robin Martin Beattie, a former medical superintendent at Auckland Mental Hospital, testified that Rameka was mentally unstable but he 'found Maoris as a rule emotional and intensely sensitive'.[84] Beattie added that Rameka was suicidal and suffered from 'abnormal depression'. It is not clear why this depression was abnormal, and Rameka's defence of hereditary insanity was hardly abnormal for that time. Nor were the psychological effects of war trauma.

Through an interpreter Rameka stated that he had gone to war at the age of 15, and for over two years had dug trenches and maintained wire entanglements in 'no-man's land'.[85] After being gassed at Messines he was hospitalised in New Zealand with war wounds. He claimed that since the war all of his 16 brothers and sisters, with the exception of one sister, had disappeared. 'Sometimes I suffer from depression and it seems to darken my outlook,' he said. Rameka's defence lawyer described his client as 'solitary'.[86]

The day before Rameka, who was separated from his wife, killed Johnson, the pair had been at the horse races, where she had asked him for money. He told her he was 'broke'. The next day, 'in a fit of depression',

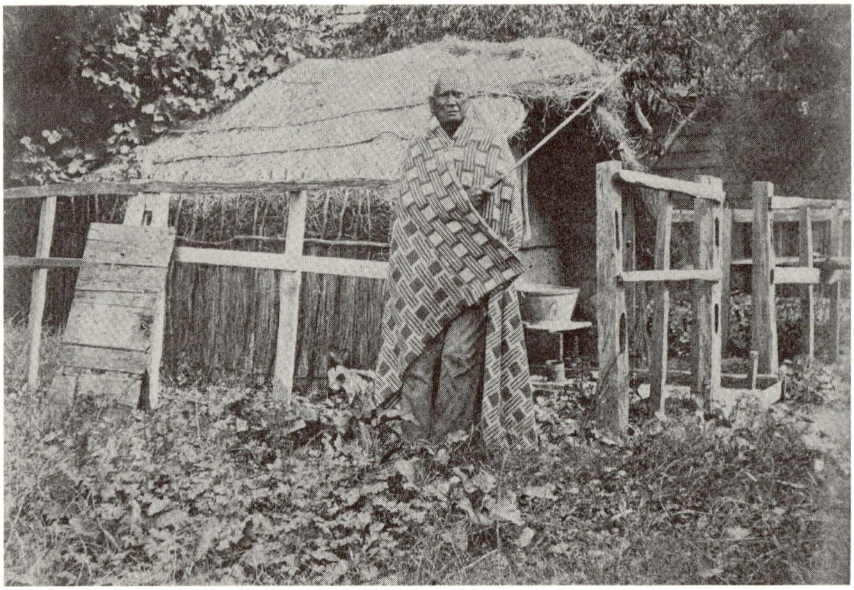

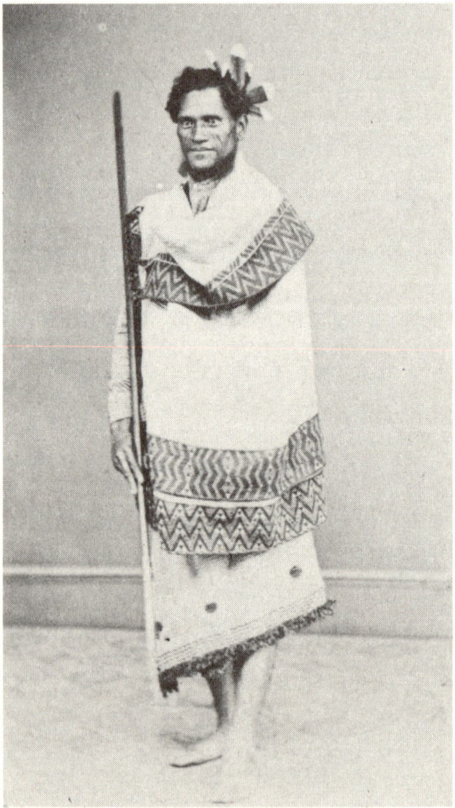

Above: In traditional Māori culture tohunga could both treat and induce mental ailments. *Right:* Waata Pihikete Kūkūtai, a prominent Ngāti Tīpā rangatira, suffered profound grief after his wife's death, and consumed a lethal poisonous medicine.

Opposite, clockwise from top: Dr Louis Hauiti Potaka (right, with Ivan Rankin and Frank Bruning at Canaan Downs, Tākaka Hill, c. 1935) had severe sight problems and was subjected to racist treatment; psychiatrist Laurie Gluckman wrote a dissertation on mākutu and psychiatry in 1962; depression and being subjected to a racial slur were presented as mitigating factors at George Rameka's murder trial in 1931.

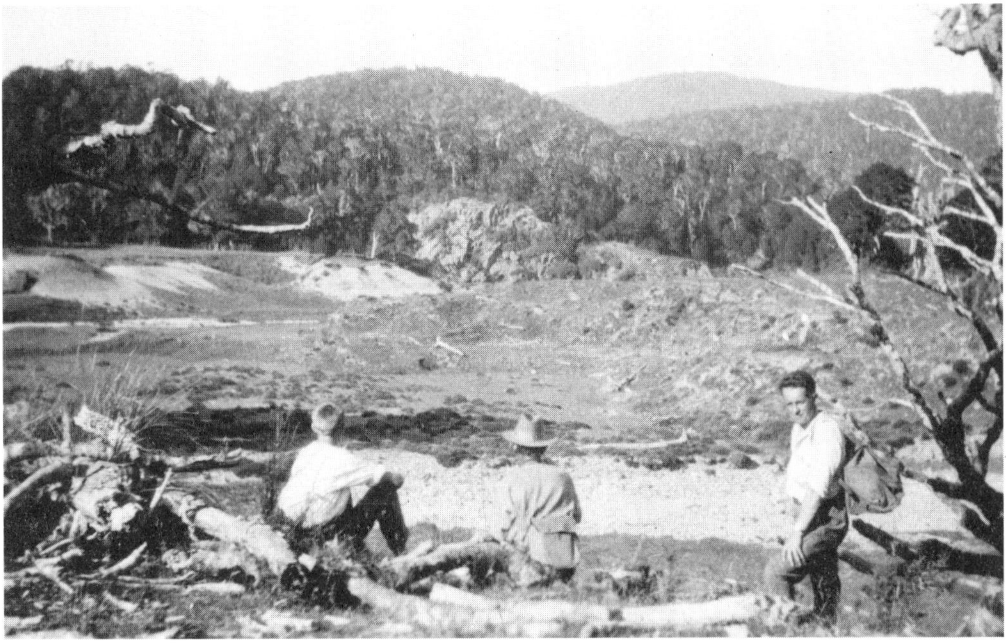

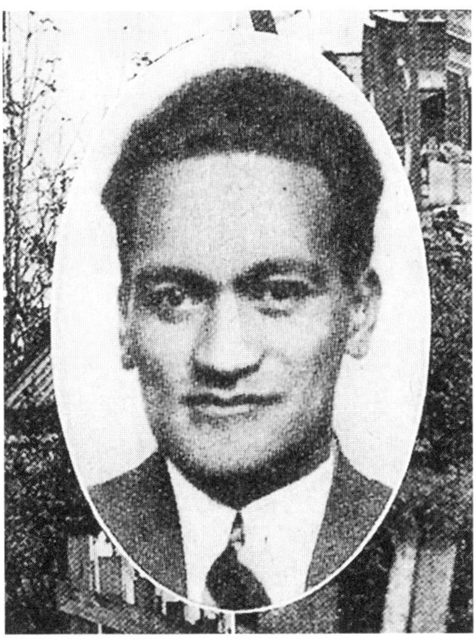

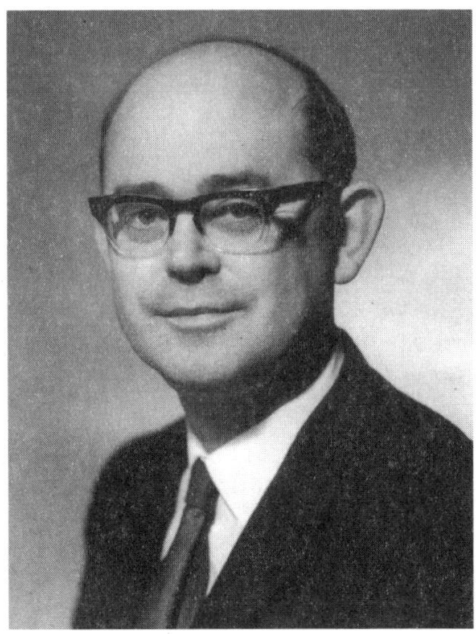

Rameka bought a bottle of the poisonous disinfectant Lysol, contemplating suicide. That evening Johnson told Rameka she 'did not want him anymore' because he 'had showed her up at the trots'. Rameka, 'full of jealousy and temper', threatened suicide.[87]

The next morning he went to Johnson's room and drank the Lysol. His throat and stomach were burning. He had a knife in case the poison did not kill him. As Rameka told the court in English, when he opened the door 'She looked at me and said: "What do you want here, you black nigger?"'

Beattie considered that Rameka stabbed Johnson after he 'was called a name that all Maoris resent, and he got into an irresponsible maniacal condition'. However, Dr H. M. Buchanan, Auckland Mental Hospital's superintendent, considered that Rameka had committed a conscious act. The jury found him guilty, but on the grounds of mercy he was sentenced to life imprisonment.

Until the late twentieth century, the rate of Māori admissions to psychiatric institutions and for mental health treatment was lower than that of Pākehā,[88] but, as early as 1858, Staff-Surgeon R. K. Prendergast of the 65th Regiment observed that Māori 'were very backward in making known cases that occurred among themselves'. He was not sure whether this was because of 'their putting them aside' or from the infrequent occurrence of insanity among Māori.[89]

Around a century later, mental distress among Māori was still underreported. This was put down to a reluctance to access hospitals, but also because 'psychoneurosis' tended to be treated within communities.[90] Many Māori remained sceptical or unaware of psychiatric institutions and what they felt were the strange methods used to treat the insane. As has been noted, mental illness was not a separate component within Māori ontology, or ways of being, and an individual's malaise was considered in relationship to others. Melancholia and depression were entwined with spirituality. As Mason Durie has noted, 'explanations that fail to take account of cultural norms will inevitably make little sense to the Maori view of health — and ill health — as a product of spirit, mind, body and the social environment'.[91]

An important caveat in measuring the prevalence of mental illness and depression is how official statistics classified Māori. It was only in 1995 that the census changed ethnic classification from a biological ('blood') quantification of 50 per cent to self-identification,[92] and until the 1960s official recognition as Māori was narrowly determined.[93] Mental health statistics for Māori have therefore been 'lost' for those of Māori descent and other ethnicities, even if they identified or were recognised as Māori according to iwi protocol. Historians Lorelle Barry and Catharine Coleborne found that Māori admission rates to asylums in 1880 were very low compared to non-Māori: 4 per cent of patients at Auckland Mental Hospital, and 1 per cent of the total asylum population in Aotearoa.[94] There were only a few Māori patients recorded in the Seacliff asylum.

In 1939 the Wellington psychologist Ernest Beaglehole published an early study of Māori prevalence rates of mental illness, based on his analysis of first-year admissions to mental hospitals between 1925 and 1935.[95] He found a high incidence of manic-depressive insanity among Māori females; much higher than for Europeans, and, except for 1930, considerably higher than for Māori males. In 1952 a student researcher at Otago Medical School, K. M. Mayo, suggested that manic depression was more common among Māori women than Māori men, and that Māori did not show 'schizoid' (psychotic, delusional or unusual patterns of thinking or speaking) traits in their personalities.[96]

Although awareness of rising rates of depression among Māori was growing, by 1994 there was still no empirical data about the prevalence of depression within Māori communities outside hospitals.[97] Hospital data indicated the rates for neuroses and other depressive disorders for Māori females as 36.7 per cent, compared to 28.7 per cent for non-Māori females. Māori male rates were lower than non-Māori (15.8 and 20.7 per cent, respectively), which is possibly indicative of the denial of depression by Māori men.[98] The 1994 data showed that Māori male hospitalisation rates for various psychoses was higher than for non-Māori; police were more likely to intervene with psychotic episodes, while depression was suffered in silence.

A 2007 report by consultants Leonie Pihama and Paul Reynolds and the Mental Health Foundation highlighted Māori men's silence and denial about depression. Participants highlighted aspects of Maōri masculinity in relation to depression.

> There is a sense that men don't talk about depression, don't show emotion or discuss what's wrong with them. The interviewee had mentioned that he 'was brought up in an era where man was you know, the rugby playing, beer swigging' type. He was unable to talk to others about his problems. One of the reasons why some men do not open up relates to the feeling of not wanting to burden whānau members with their problems. Other reasons relate to the 'get hard' mentality amongst some men.
>
> Historically we've never wanted to talk about it. They'll punch you in the bloody head. Give you a hiding, tell you to fuck off, you know, that sort of thing. That's how we were, and I know a whole lot of, some of my uncles were like that. Some of my own whānau, they'd rather sort it out, 'Toughen up.'[99]

Although these responses apply to many 'Kiwi blokes', they also partly speak to a violent Māori masculinity emanating from cultural disconnection when living in an urban setting, as depicted in Alan Duff's 1990 novel *Once Were Warriors*,[100] and in the 1994 movie of the same name. While generalisations and stereotypes about this portrayal of Māori masculinity are questionable, the 2007 report did stress that the repression of men's depression could be both an unspoken trigger for, and a consequence of, violence.

═══

By the twenty-first century there was clearer documentation of the high rates of depression among Māori treated in general practice.[101] In 2005 the University of Otago's Mental Health and General Practice Investigation research group found an alarmingly higher rate of major depression among Māori clients who attended general practices (46.4 per cent compared to 15.4 per cent in non-Māori).[102] The rate for female Māori patients was 55.2 per cent, and the greatest disparity was between Māori and non-Māori women. Another study in 2010 found lower rates of diagnosis and treatment of depression by general practitioners among Māori compared to non-Māori patients.[103] The doctors reported greater stigma around depression among Māori patients, and that Māori patients were less likely to talk about being depressed compared to non-Māori patients.

Mason Durie's earlier observation that Māori had a different mental illness profile compared with non-Māori — such as tending to present at a later and more severe stage for treatment — was reiterated in later research.[104] Whakamā or shame may have been a factor in avoiding treatment, but economic pressures and poverty played a significant role, too. Medical fees could constitute a considerable proportion of family income — and depression was often lower on the priorities of a family's more immediate health needs.

For those in employment, taking time off work to see a doctor or counsellor might reduce wages. Government health statistics from 2013 to 2014 suggest that the diagnoses of anxiety or depressive disorder among adult Māori males were around the same rate as for women, with this being twice as likely as among non-Māori males. Māori were about 1.5 times as likely as non-Māori adults to report a high or very high probability of having an anxiety or depressive disorder.[105]

Questions remain as to whether the increased rates of depression among Māori men is due to there being more depression, a greater willingness to seek treatment and talk about their mental health, or because general practitioners were more sensitive to the cultural nuances of depression. Meanwhile social, economic and political contexts remain powerful issues in addressing the increased and high rates of depression among Māori. This follows from the earlier discussion about the impact of colonisation and the need to locally historicise mental health. There are now initiatives to introduce Māori cultural beliefs and perspectives into mental health treatment and care.[106] To conclude with Mason Durie's wisdom:

> Mauri Ora practice assumes that identity, self-knowledge and idiosyncratic behavioural patterns are a reflection of a complex interaction between the individual and the wider environment. Gaining access to those key institutions — be they whānau, marae or ancestral land — and experiencing relationships in a positive manner generates opportunities for improved mental health and a greater capacity for problem solving.

3.

≡

The lonely land

> Insanity is much more common in this country than it is at home, chiefly on account of the limited range of sympathy which the isolation of individuals and families in the country gives rise to, and also on account of the oppressive loneliness which many newcomers experience even in our crowded towns.[1]

In September 1877 Constable Porter found Julia and Thomas Rowan and their five young children living in a small tent at the top of Maclaggan Street in Dunedin's town belt. It would have been very cold, especially at night, more so for children with inadequate clothing and crying from hunger.[2] The year before, Julia had been living with her children in a small tent in the bush at Pūrākaunui, 25 kilometres north of Dunedin's city centre.

In 1872 in County Mayo, Ireland, Julia had bid farewell to her parents and four siblings and boarded an immigrant ship, the *Euterpex*, bound for Wellington.[3] After they arrived, the family travelled south and settled at Green Island, near Dunedin. Thomas found a job as a labourer at the Dunedin railway workshops. Julia and Thomas 'bore very good characters' and their future as workers in the colony seemed promising.[4] This prospect changed after Thomas was seriously injured at work, was laid off and was then unable to find employment. He set out for Wellington, looking for work there, leaving Julia and the children in makeshift conditions at Pūrākaunui. Thomas sent money to Julia, but she 'gradually fell into melancholia'. When she was admitted as depressed to the Dunedin Lunatic Asylum in 1876, she was physically emaciated and had been breastfeeding the baby, John, for the past 14 months. She remained at the asylum for seven weeks.[5]

Julia's admission records report that she had attempted to kill her children, but as a Roman Catholic, she said, she was only making the sign of the cross on them. Her physical health rapidly improved after admission to the asylum, probably because she was eating regular meals and had been relieved of the exhausting task of caring for young children in a demanding environment. In 1876 Julia and her children were under the care of Mr Quin, master of the Benevolent Institution at Caversham, Dunedin, but a year later, when Thomas had returned and they were charged with having no means of support, she refused to return.

On 14 September 1877 the couple appeared at the Dunedin police court, where they told the presiding justices of the peace Charles Reeves and Edward McGlashan that they were determined to remain in the tent in the Dunedin town belt 'until they died'.[6] Thomas was adamant that he would not live in the Benevolent Institution. He told Reeves, 'You can punish me if you like. Put me into gaol, and I'll work any way you like. You can put me to death, your Worships, and I'd be quite willing to do it.'

Julia refused to be separated from her husband, and would not allow her family to be placed under Quin's care: 'But that I was a good Christian, I should have been dead long ago. My body and bones are worn away to nothing. My husband has good health now, and if he had food he could work . . . I will do anything you like. I am doing the Lord's work, and would not like to go against the Lord,' she told the court.

Julia and Thomas were committed to the local lunatic asylum and the children were sent to the Industrial School at Caversham. Thomas was diagnosed with melancholia with delusions, and described as depressed and refusing food in his admission notes. He died in 1886 at the Seacliff asylum of exhaustion from epilepsy.

Julia was readmitted to the Dunedin Lunatic Asylum in 1877, and then transferred to Seacliff.[7] On 21 June 1898 the Industrial School's manager wrote to Seacliff's superintendent, Truby King, asking if Julia could live with her daughters, who by now were between 27 and 33 years old. Julia was reunited with her children and died in 1905. This disturbing narrative is but one of the many stories of the forgotten immigrants to Aotearoa who became depressed, medically diagnosed as melancholic or sent to mental asylums.

Julia's family was among the nineteenth-century waves of migrants to New Zealand, predominately from England, Scotland, Wales and Ireland, with much smaller numbers from continental Europe, North America and elsewhere.[8] The 1860s gold rushes also enticed 2000 Chinese, and even more Europeans. Between 1871 and 1875 289,026 immigrants arrived in Aotearoa, but during this period around 40 per cent left, as discussed later in this chapter, often because of disappointment. Immigrants came here seeking a better life than the one they had left — Thomas and Julia, for example, had hoped to leave rural poverty behind them — and some early settlers had visions of becoming grand landowners. But, for most, their new lives would be as farm labourers, artisans or working in the bush.

A minority of very early immigrants were motivated by missionary zeal — the first being three artisan missionary couples from the Church Missionary Society (Church of England) who arrived with Reverend Samuel Marsden in the Bay of Islands in 1814. Trading opportunities also attracted early immigrants. After the signing of the Treaty of Waitangi in 1840, and the creation of a Crown colony, the trickle of arrivals became a steady flow. Immigrants numbered around 2000 in 1839, but by 1852 there were 28,000, the increase in part driven by the New Zealand Company, which during the 1840s recruited settlers, mainly from England and Scotland, to its settlements in Wellington, Nelson, Whanganui, Taranaki, Canterbury and Otago.

After the collapse of the company in the 1850s, the provincial governments stepped up the drive for British and Irish immigrants during the 1850s and 1860s by offering free or assisted passages. Single women, such as Mary B. from County Kerry, Ireland, were recruited as domestic servants or potential settlers' wives. Mary arrived in 1892, much later than those who came as part of the early schemes recruiting single female immigrants. She was initially very cheerful aboard ship, but after a few weeks became sullen, 'dull and wretched'. After arriving in New Zealand she lived with her uncle at Maheno in Otago. He said that Mary had been 'depressed since landing here . . . due to absence from her family in Ireland'. Twenty-year-old Mary threatened suicide and was committed to Seacliff asylum suffering from melancholia on 31 May 1893.[9]

Small immigration schemes operated in Hawke's Bay, Southland, Nelson, Taranaki and Wellington, with much bigger ones in Otago and Canterbury. Some settlers in Auckland and Waikato, including those fighting in the New Zealand Wars, were offered land grants or confiscated land. The 1870s and early 1880s brought an unprecedented number — around 289,000 — of new immigrants to Aotearoa. Assisted by the sometimes exaggerated hype of agents in Britain and Ireland, the New Zealand government offered assisted passages as part of Treasurer Julius Vogel's vision to attract workers to develop the country. A few settled on land confiscated from Māori, but most worked building roads and other infrastructure, or in the factories and commercial enterprises of the new towns.

Even Edward Gibbon Wakefield — the founder of the New Zealand Company and thus the architect of assisted emigration to Aotearoa from Britain — suffered 'bouts of depression that would take weeks to lift'.[10] He finally settled in New Zealand in 1853, and began what would be an ambitious but tumultuous political career. His depression firmly descended after rheumatic fever forced him to resign from the House of Representatives and the Wellington Provincial Council in 1855. He had previously experienced depression, but from 1855 until his death in 1862 he became reclusive, staying mostly in his Wellington home and seeing very few people. In 1990 the historian Miles Fairburn wrote: 'Day after day he sat brooding on his remoteness from his London friends and the squalor of frontier Wellington, his creation and now his prison.'[11]

Wakefield's depression, like that of so many migrants, was tinged with nostalgia — a longing for a past that was linked to culture and place. Nostalgia also infused the mind of the prominent New Zealand Liberal politician and writer William Pember Reeves when he was New Zealand's agent-general in London.[12] His nostalgia came initially from longing more for England than 'my own New Zealand',[13] but later his gaze reverted to his birthplace, Aotearoa. He recalled having been born in a lonely land with a childhood 'among vast empty spaces' in rural Canterbury.[14]

Reeves admitted to passing 'fits of depression';[15] during a stay in England beween 1874 and 1876, when he was to study at Oxford University, he suffered ill health and what his biographer Keith Sinclair suggests was some sort of 'nervous breakdown',[16] a euphemism usually reserved for the genteel who were suffering mental distress, depression or melancholia.

Reeves abandoned his studies and returned to New Zealand to live on a Canterbury farm — 'a life of secure, unbroken monotony, the perfection of unvaried dullness'[17] — and wrote about that lonely land with affectionate nostalgia in *The Long White Cloud Ao Tea Roa*, which was published in London in 1898.

To be an immigrant was to suffer a form of shock: they had been lured to Aotearoa with the promise of a utopia, an arcadia, but for most the reality was rather different. But at least immigrants from Britain and Ireland all spoke the same language and shared a roughly similar heritage. As will be discussed in chapter 6, immigrants from non-European and more specifically non-English-speaking countries had to battle cultural isolation, too. Several of the challenges outlined in this chapter are common to all immigrants, regardless of culture, time and place, and they include the rigours of travel to Aotearoa, isolation and loneliness, lack of networks of family and friends, difficulty finding and keeping work, and the general 'strangeness' of a new environment.

When she researched the impact of the three-month voyage of immigrants to New Zealand and its impact on their mental health, Angela McCarthy, author of *Migration, Ethnicity and Madness: New Zealand, 1860–1910*, found that little was known.[18]

Most migrants had to be considered fit enough to be accepted as assisted passengers, but some suffered from mental illness before embarkation. In 1873 the Imbecile Passengers Act enabled New Zealand provinces to exclude 'mad' immigrants who had not been detected as such before or on disembarkation, but even the colony's agent-general in London, Julius Vogel, found it was not easy to have bureaucratic control over 'latent insanity' in migrants.[19] Mental depression is often not visible, nor does it constantly affect mood or behaviour, so it was not always easy to identify those who might periodically suffer from bouts of depression.

It was also inevitable that the voyage was traumatic for some. They would have witnessed or experienced sickness, childbirth, death and violence. Passengers also endured challenging maritime environments, ranging from freezing and wild storms to the stifling humidity of tropical calms.

Despondency could set in during the endless weeks at sea, when there was plenty of time for the reality of having severed ties with kin, community, and familiar places and activities to hit home. Monotony and the close confines of shipboard life, especially in the dark and stuffy steerage, might alone induce depression.

Some immigrants eagerly anticipated a new start, but others were anxious about the future: they either had little knowledge of New Zealand or had heard alarming reports about the environment and life there. On migrant ships, as in many situations, anxiety and depression were usually confined within an individual's thoughts. Such feelings were possibly shared with a loved one, expressed through a song or a poem, or diverted into daily routines and caring for others. But they could also manifest in alcohol consumption and, occasionally, in violence.

Shipboard depression is largely absent from the records, except when it erupted as melancholy that disturbed others. Angela McCarthy's research located a rare instance of 'shipboard insanity': in 1875 John Hassard, the surgeon superintendent on the *Merope*, recorded Jane T.'s swings from noisy and restless behaviour to melancholia and being depressed during the three-month voyage to New Zealand. On arrival at Lyttelton, she was committed to Sunnyside asylum in Christchurch, where she died in 1888.[20]

A Miss Chapman had also been in a state of 'deep melancholy' during the voyage on the *Wave Queen* from England to Auckland in 1874, and had attempted suicide. On her arrival in Auckland in February, she was examined by Thomas Philson, the port health officer, who found her 'calm and rational'. The historian Jennifer Kain noted in her 2019 book *Insanity and Immigration Control in New Zealand and Australia, 1860–1930* that this first attempt by authorities to invoke the Imbecile Passengers Act failed, and Miss Chapman was able to disembark.[21]

The British historian Janet Oppenheim has noted that doctors sometimes advocated sea voyages to their patients as a way to relieve melancholia and restore mental health.[22] In 1884, Edgar Bastings, hotelier and writer for the stage — he was the proprietor of Dunedin's Robin Hood and Oriental hotels and the Lake Hotel in Waihola — travelled across the Tasman to Melbourne on the *Ringarooma* in 1884 to restore his health and relieve his melancholia.[23]

But ships could also present opportunities for suicide.[24] A witness saw Bastings 'walk aft and seat himself on the taffrail. Then, perhaps in keeping with his theatrical inclinations, he waved his hat frantically in the air, let out a cheer and jumped into the sea.' Bastings was buried in his father's plot in Carlton cemetery in Melbourne. His family remained in Otago, and his wife took over the Lake Hotel.

In 1865, 22-year-old Alfred D. jumped from the *Ida Zeigler* during its voyage from England to Auckland.[25] He was rescued but 'became greatly depressed in spirits', and soon after arrival tried to slit his throat. Alfred was a patient in the Auckland Mental Asylum from 1867 to 1872, before joining his family in Melbourne.

John King, the inspector of asylums, recommended to the colonial secretary that, where possible, sufficiently recovered patients should return to their native countries if they had near relatives or friends there.[26] King also suggested that the homeward voyage (under a guardian's care) could be restorative. An unknown number of early immigrants to Aotearoa who were depressed did return to their original countries or relocated elsewhere — usually where they had kin. A 33-year-old Scottish widow, admitted to the Dunedin Lunatic Asylum for five months from 1864 to 1865, for example, was discharged into her brother's care in Victoria, Australia.[27] Henry P., aged 22, a metalworker who emigrated from England to Dunedin, was a patient in the Dunedin asylum between 1867 and 1868, after which, similarly, he departed with his brother for Victoria.[28]

Other patients with melancholia were repatriated to their birthplaces, whether in Scotland, England, Ireland or China. It is not clear whether Adam F. was ordered to, or chose to, return to Caithness in Scotland after a year in the Dunedin Lunatic Asylum in 1877.[29] He had immigrated to Otago 20 years earlier, aged 19, and had worked on the goldfields, saving enough to buy 88 acres and run a horse and cattle farm at Flag Swamp, Waikouaiti. He had been 'a hard drinker', but in 1876 became a Good Templar and teetotal. This did not stop his depression, however, and he was found wandering in the countryside after he had cut his own throat. Despite this episode, he returned to Caithness and married. He died after falling down a well in 1902 while suffering from what was documented as an attack of paralysis. It is not clear if this term referred to a stroke or the complications of a mental disorder.

'Man alone', a rugged individual living in a harsh, remote environment, is a trope of New Zealand literature.[30] But man alone was often a lonely condition. Historians Angela McCarthy and Catharine Coleborne have documented how isolation and estrangement from home in an unfamiliar country could lead to mental breakdown for immigrants in the Australian and New Zealand colonies.[31] Whether in the fledgling cities and towns, on farms in the back blocks, or in camps in the bush, Aotearoa could be a lonely land. The predominately masculine composition of early Pākehā colonial society intensified this estrangement.

In 1867, for example, European males outnumbered females 3:2. The ratio remained unbalanced until 1906.[32] Historians have noted that single immigrant men were more likely to be committed to mental asylums.[33] Wellington surgeon, politician and prominent Catholic Dr Morgan Grace even suggested to New Zealand's Joint Committee on Lunatic Asylums in 1871 that when men in the 'lonely land' became depressed, it could lead to masturbation, and then to insanity.

> An ignorant man goes into the country, and from comparing himself with himself, and contemplating in solitude the grand sights of nature, he becomes depressed; his hard fare and constant exposure, and the newness of everything around adds to his depression; he becomes careless of food, and occasionally goes without, then gets dyspepsia; he grows weak and miserable, a terrible craving for excitement seizes upon him, and if he cannot get to a public-house and company, he commonly practices masturbation. The seminal discharge for a time does him good, but very soon he is quite exhausted; then comes the loss of the balance of reason, and insanity is at hand. The whole of his self respect is not yet quite gone; he has the grace to wish to conceal his degradation, and often succeeds in doing so for years; but when, from some quasi involuntary eccentricity, he is discovered and informed upon: that man becomes violent on the spot, and immuring him in a dismal lunatic asylum makes him almost incurable.[34]

The early colonial society of Aotearoa may have been predominately masculine, but, as McCarthy and others have shown, many single men had families, workplaces and community networks, and were not necessarily socially isolated from one another or from women.[35] A consideration of how the colonial environment may have induced melancholia and depression also needs to take into account locality, material circumstances, employment, and political and other issues.

In 1872 Richmond Beetham, the warden, or officer-in-charge, of Lake Wakatipu's goldfields visited remote Martin's Bay on the South Island's West Coast and later submitted a report to Sir George Bowen, governor of New Zealand:

> At the date of my visit there were four families resident at Jamestown, or near it, besides other parties working singly or without families; including those settlers who were at Big Bay, occupied in gold mining, there would be about forty souls in the settlement . . . despite its great natural advantages, the settlement appeared to be in a languishing condition. The inhabitants, while they one and all spoke in the highest terms of the spot which they had cleared as their home, appeared to be in a despondent state . . . the settlement had not made the progress which might have been fairly expected from it. I attribute this—1st. To the utter isolation of the settlement, resulting from its uncertain and unfrequent communication with, other portions of the Province. 2nd. By reason of the unsatisfactory working of the Land Regulations, . . . 3rd. To the absence of any settled industry, by the means of which labour and capital would be introduced into the settlement.
>
> The absolute isolation of the settlement has, I think, had a great deal to do with its slow progress. Not only have the settlers been unable to obtain regular supplies, but they have actually been reduced to the very brink of starvation. This uncertain and irregular communication has exercised, in my opinion, a very depressing influence upon the settlers; they look upon themselves as deserted and uncared for, and, as a natural consequence, they lose that push and energy without which

> progression is impossible . . . The settlers also complain that the steamers do not bring for sale numerous necessaries which they require . . . The settlers say, and with truth, that they cannot do a fair day's work on such food as this. An enfeebled condition of body results inevitably in a depression of mind, and it is not in this state that men should exist who have to fight and overcome the primeval forest of New Zealand.[36]

By the mid-nineteenth century, the struggle to tame the bush appeared ceaseless. Native forest could regenerate on land that had been cleared, mostly by burning, only years earlier, and introduced weeds such as gorse and thistles grew abundantly and became a pest in a way they had not been in their original British ecosystems.[37] Introduced animals, such as rabbits, stoats and possums, also proliferated, and had to be controlled. The labour to do this might come from farm workers, forestry gangs or lone bushmen. Solitary, tough work in harsh environments could be a choice, or be taken up as a result of unemployment or family circumstances. Unsurprisingly, long, hard days in the bush could induce gloomy thoughts and mental depression. Or were some men with melancholy souls drawn to the bush?

It was common in the nineteenth century for newspapers to note when local people were sent to mental asylums. In 1886, the *Bruce Herald* reported that James Ritchie, a rabbiter on a station in Mossburn, Southland, had fallen 'victim to melancholia . . . brought on by the isolated life he led'. Ritchie had emigrated from Suffolk, England, in 1872. His case notes at Seacliff Lunatic Asylum revealed other factors besides isolation leading to his melancholia. He was in feeble health upon admission, was a widower, and two months before entering the asylum he had fallen and injured his head, resulting in numbness in his limbs, giddiness, mental confusion and a loss of memory.[38]

William W., a bushman, was admitted to the same asylum with melancholia when living in 'a lonely part of the country' in Southland.[39] Like James, William was a widower — his wife had died before he immigrated to Otago from Scotland in 1875, with his two children and his sister. He saw the children weekly at their home near Invercargill, but otherwise he lived and worked alone. His poor diet of mostly tea and bread probably contributed to his declining mental health and emaciated physical state. At some stage William was 'shocked' to learn that his sister had an illegitimate child, news that may have tipped him into a melancholia severe enough for him to be committed to the Dunedin Lunatic Asylum, his 'mind depressed, expression despairing', as his notes stated. He was recommitted at least four times, sometimes in a manic state, and diagnosed with melancholia.

Injuries and the hard physical nature of most work could exacerbate or even cause depression, especially when there was no other financial support. Until the Workers' Compensation Act, which covered death or injuries at work, was passed in 1900 and the Social Security Act was introduced in 1938, most people who were unable to work had to rely on family or charitable bodies. An Irish immigrant, John S., who lived in Makarewa, near Invercargill, was 18 when he began to experience 'attacks of melancholia'.[40] In 1898, aged 24, his skull was fractured, and an eye and an arm were paralysed in an accident. Two months before John was admitted to Seacliff in 1900 with melancholia, he suffered another injury to his head. Yet the cause of John's 'madness' was attributed to masturbation. While in the asylum he had wanted to destroy himself because he was tired of life. After he cut his throat, he was restrained with 'locked gloves'.[41] John was discharged later that year, but was readmitted in 1907, and again in 1911.

One example of a lonely but significant life in the bush is that of Richard Treacy Henry, one of New Zealand's outstanding bushmen and an important early conservationist. Like some workers in remote places, Henry was prone to depression. His story is a mix of his experiences living and working in isolated parts of Aotearoa and his despair at the decimation of indigenous birds.

Henry was born in County Kildare, Ireland, in 1845. His family immigrated to Australia in 1851, but his mother and infant brother died during the voyage. Another brother died in 1867. In 1874 Henry sailed to New Zealand and, among many jobs, worked as a rabbiter in Southland. It appears his love for a woman was unrequited, and by 1883 he was working as a guide and explorer based at Lake Te Anau. Henry became increasingly involved in conservation and worked with the Otago Acclimatisation Society. After his anticipated appointment as a curator of a sanctuary for flightless birds

— the first in the world — on Resolution Island in Dusky Sound in 1891 was delayed because of factions within the conservation movement, his depression intensified and he moved to Auckland.

Henry became more depressed as his concerns for endangered indigenous birds, notably the kākāpō, fell on deaf ears. His biographers Susanne Hill and John Hill depict him as feeling 'unwanted and forlornly alone'.[42] In 1893 Henry attempted to shoot himself, failed, and admitted himself to Auckland Hospital to have the bullet wound treated. He wrote to his friend Edward Melland, a Te Anau runholder and member of the Otago Institute: 'I have often been dissatisfied with myself and that is the principal reason that I have got tired and gave up the business.'[43]

In 1894 Henry was finally appointed as caretaker and curator of Resolution Island, to where he transferred over 700 endangered native birds from the mainland, especially kākāpō, takahē, tīeke and kiwi. He also wrote several articles for newspapers and scientific publications, and the book *The Habits of the Flightless Birds of New Zealand*, which was published in 1903.

A significant threat to these flightless birds were the mustelids — stoats, ferrets and weasels — that had been introduced to the country to control rabbits. A key rationale underpinning these offshore bird sanctuaries was to separate and protect the vulnerable birds from these ruthless and voracious predators. Henry's depression returned when he found himself unable to prevent stoats, ferrets and weasels from swimming from the mainland to the island, attacking the birds and eating their eggs. He moved north to work as curator of the bird sanctuary established by the government on Kāpiti Island from 1908 until 1911, before retiring to Katikati in 1912, and then moving to Helensville in 1922. He died aged 84 at Auckland Mental Hospital on 13 November 1929.

Although Henry's long life was marked by depression, no doubt exacerbated by living alone in extremely isolated places, he found beauty and meaning in the environment and through working to protect native birds (a 'modern St. Francis'),[44] and communicating this mission to the public. His contribution was remarkable. He had introduced and operated 'the first programme of systematic bird transfers anywhere in the world. Nothing like it was attempted for another 70 years.'[45] When the last kākāpō in the South Island was captured in Fiordland in 1975, it was named Richard

Henry in his honour. The bird was transferred to Maud Island, where, like its namesake, it lived a long life, dying in 2010 aged about 80 years.

Not all bush workers led solitary lives, but other circumstances could push them into melancholia. John F. was born in Durham, England, in 1840, and immigrated with his parents and siblings to Australia, where he worked on the Scarsdale gold-diggings near Ballarat. He married another English immigrant, Kate. After his father died in 1869, John and his family sailed to New Zealand and settled in Kumara on the West Coast, where he worked as a woodcutter. Kate died in 1879, soon after her fifth baby was stillborn, and John was left to raise five children, including the child of his eldest daughter, on his own. He was deeply 'troubled' by these family and financial responsibilities.

An Anglican by faith, he turned to reading the Bible and *The Pilgrim's Progress*, and became concerned about his own 'wickedness', believing that he had 'ruined his children', and became suicidal. In June 1888 his admission notes record that he was committed to Seaview Asylum in Hokitika 'dull and depressed'. Although he could be tearful or would break down sobbing when friends visited him, he was allowed to work outside the asylum and played draughts and billiards with the other patients. John was discharged to his brother's care, but he died two years later.[46]

In 1871 Dr Morgan Grace told the Joint Committee on Lunatic Asylums that 'the migratory population from our goldfields, excited, by the varying chances of their fortune, and exhausted by hardship and exposure, swell the numbers of our lunatics out of all proportion to the population'.[47] Fourteen miners were among the 54 males admitted to the Dunedin Lunatic Asylum during 1871,[48] although not all were diagnosed with melancholia.

Edward Peters (born in India of European and Indian heritage) discovered gold at Tuapeka in Otago around 1857, but it was Gabriel Read who registered a viable mining claim in 1861 that led to the Otago gold rush. Mining communities soon rose to around 14,000 at Tuapeka, and by 1864 there were 22,000 miners in Otago. From 1865 the rush for gold extended to the West Coast, and the following year to Thames and Waihi on the Coromandel Peninsula in the North Island. Initially in Otago and the West Coast, alluvial mining in riverbeds was done by individuals, but by the 1870s companies had established more mechanised operations. Gold mining was tough work in harsh, isolated environments — whether the hot, dry summers and freezing winters of Central Otago, or the wet, cold bush and windswept beaches of the West Coast. Nevertheless, this labour was crucial to Dunedin's prosperity, and to the establishment of other lively towns and ports, such as Queenstown and Hokitika.

It is impossible to gauge the prevalence of depression among mining communities, as many would have simply lived with their despondency or possibly diverted their woes with alcohol. Both men and women featured among the early diagnoses for melancholia in the asylums at Dunedin and Seaview, which catered to the large mining communities in Otago and the West Coast, respectively. (These patients included Chinese miners, discussed in chapter 6.) In the North Island during the late nineteenth century, mining, along with forestry and gumdigging, was significant at Thames and Waihi. Those working there were not immune to mental distress either. One sufferer of melancholia, who was sent by steamer in 1870 to the Auckland asylum, tried to jump overboard. He died three years later in the asylum from apoplexy (a cerebral haemorrhage or stroke).[49]

Eleanor Catton's Booker Prize-winning novel *The Luminaries*,[50] which is set during the era of the Otago and West Coast gold rushes, revolves in part around the story of the fictional Anna Wetherell, an Irish immigrant who worked as a prostitute in Hokitika and who, while suffering from depression and opium addiction, was incarcerated in the Seaview gaol awaiting trial for various crimes. On 23 July 1868, in real life, 29-year-old Irish woman Bridget McMahon was the first patient diagnosed with melancholia to be admitted to the lunatic ward at South Spit Hospital in Hokitika. She had been living in the West Coast gold mining town of Ross, and the cause of her insanity was given as prostitution.[51]

A sample of Seaview's records from 1869 to 1876 reveals 15 patients who had been diagnosed with melancholia. Four of the nine men were miners, the others were a carpenter, saddler, shoemaker, brewer and engineer. The carpenter was Joseph Evans Whidby [Whidbey], a 'man of colour', who had emigrated from Victoria, Australia. He spent four months in the asylum in 1871 with a diagnosis of melancholia, before being discharged, as his notes record, to 'coloured friends in Hokitika'.[52] After this he visited the town's library, where he hid letters that he had written to his wife in Melbourne.

Did this mean he was depressed, eccentric or, as the police said, 'a lunatic'? Regardless, Whidby was arrested and charged with vagrancy because he could not pay for his accommodation at a boarding house. He was sentenced to three months' imprisonment and then 'chased out of town'. In 1880 he was imprisoned in Christchurch for six months with hard labour, as he had been 'sleeping out' and had been in gaol on previous occasions.[53]

The case records of miners admitted to the Dunedin and Seacliff asylums with melancholia show that they were not always lacking mates or family. In 1863 Michael J., an Irish immigrant, and five other miners each obtained around 60 pounds of gold from the Shotover River. The men embarked on a 'spree' at Bracken's Hotel in Queenstown, but returned to the river 'determined to brave out the [winter] season and not leave the spot until they had made their pile'.[54] Two years later Michael was admitted to the Dunedin Lunatic Asylum for almost four months with a diagnosis of melancholia.[55]

Men living alone in remote areas, especially if regarded as eccentric, were sometimes called 'hatters' (from the saying 'as mad as a hatter').[56] In 1876 a vivid description was given of a hatter who roamed the Central Otago town of Lawrence and its surrounding hills.

> Lawrence boasts of a veritable wild man of the woods in the person of a 'hatter' named Armstrong. This man, who was in the habit of visiting the township clothed in bags fastened together with flax, much resembling the cut of a modern Robinson Crusoe, has without doubt become a prey to melancholia. Recently he was seen on the ranges near Bungtown by William Brown, a digger there, and on his trying to get within speaking distance, Armstrong fled like a wild deer, making pursuit hopeless. He is said to be covered with hair. A gentleman who has been in the habit of supplying the solitary diggers in this inhospitable region with rations, says that Armstrong has not purchased food for four months.[57]

When a 29-year-old miner from St Bathans in Central Otago was committed to Seacliff in 1900, his melancholia was attributed to leading a solitary life, despite his having family nearby. Five weeks earlier he had stopped working, kept to his hotel, and, although he left his room for meals, he spoke to no one. He had lost interest in caring for his two horses. He was transferred to Sunnyside Lunatic Asylum in Christchurch in 1907.[58]

Not all immigrants within gold mining communities were miners. Police Inspector William Nixon Morton and Dr John Rutherford Ryley, both professionals in the goldfields, were admitted to the Auckland lunatic asylum with melancholia and depression during the 1870s. They later spent a period away from New Zealand in Fiji; Morton took up cotton farming and Ryley continued to practise as a doctor, even being appointed as Fiji's chief officer of health, as well as a brief stint as a member of Fiji's parliament in 1871.

That same year, Morton was admitted from Fiji to the Auckland lunatic asylum because of his mental depression.[59] Only a decade earlier he had been a shining star in Geelong, to where he had emigrated from Ireland around 1854. He was described as 'a remarkably handsome young man', and as a cadet in the Victorian Mounted Police was 'one of the smartest and cleverest of colonial detectives'.[60] Victorian Police Commissioner Captain Standish from Australia later admitted to St John Branigan, the Otago police commissioner, that Morton had been 'always eccentric and betrayed a morbid disposition'.[61]

In December 1863 Morton was appointed police inspector of Wakatipu and worked alongside Branigan to police the Otago goldfields. He was briefly redeployed to Marlborough, and while there he married Mary Charlotte Pickering, who was from a Pākehā settler family. Morton's star began to fall when he was charged with assaulting James Grant, editor of the *Otago Witness*'s *Saturday Review*, in Dunedin in December 1864.[62]

In 1867 Morton was retired because of his health. Like many, he was attracted to the South Pacific by the prospect of making his fortune from the global shortage of cotton during the American Civil War, and he sailed with his family to Fiji in 1868. Cotton had been recently introduced as a cash crop to Fiji, but the cotton boom was short-lived and by early 1872 around 600 plantations in Fiji had folded, partly because so many prospective planters, like Morton, had no experience of tropical agriculture. Morton's case notes

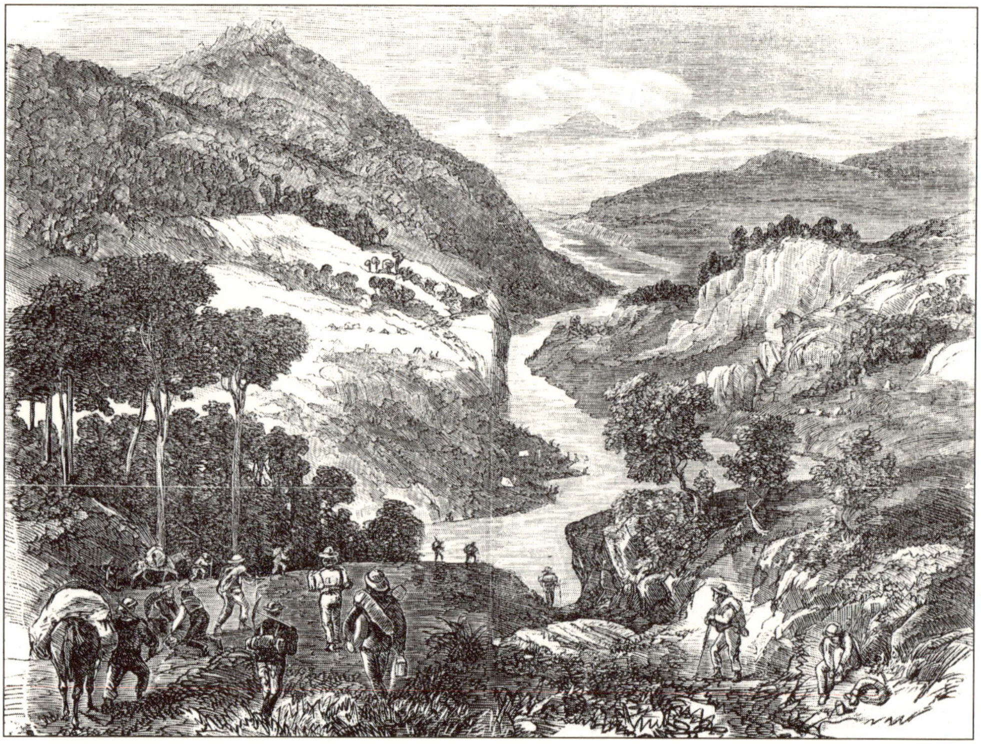

The Dunstan goldfield,
Otago, 1862.

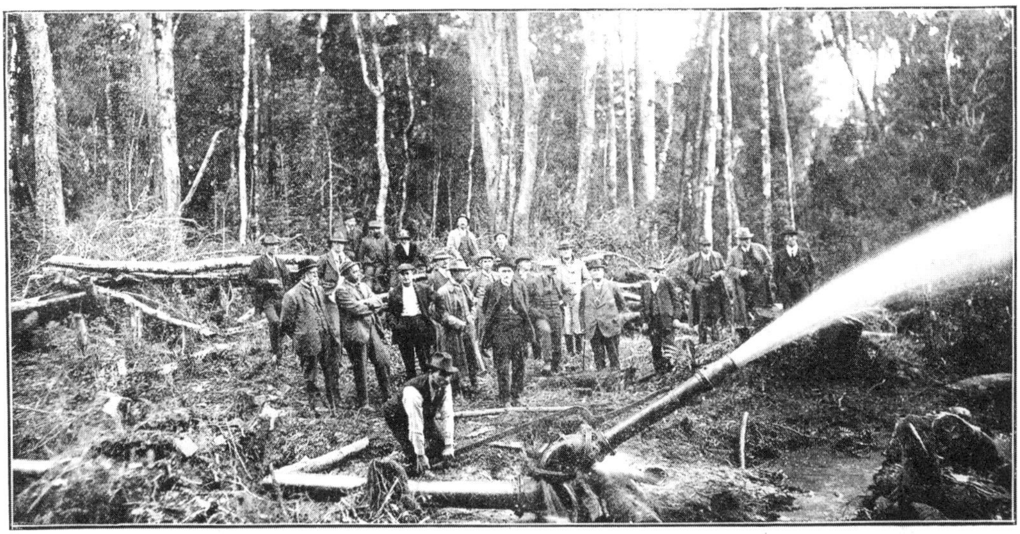

A gold mining field is opened near Lake Kaniere, on the West Coast, in May 1919.

from the Auckland asylum described him as a 'professed melancholic' until July 1872, when he changed to a 'very marked degree', becoming excited, noisy and refusing to eat or drink. He died there soon after, a death the inquest attributed to dementia, although he was aged only 39.

Branigan, who had been transferred from the Seacliff mental asylum, was also a patient in the Auckland asylum. *The Nelson Evening Mail* observed on 23 July 1872: 'Passing strange that these two — who were the founders of a police system of which every province in New Zealand is reaping the benefit to this hour — should, a few years afterwards, come face to face with each other, both confined as lunatics in the Auckland Asylum.'[63]

Ryley, another Irish immigrant, was also briefly committed to the Auckland asylum in 1870 with melancholia. A surgeon, he had cared for miners in Otago, Hokitika and Thames, and is renowned for introducing antiseptic surgery to New Zealand.[64] Ryley published several medical papers, including his observations about typhoid fever on the West Coast. When he was discharged from the asylum, his case notes recorded that 'longer incarceration would be likely to convert a case of slight mental irritability into confirmed lunacy'. It is unclear what was meant by 'slight mental irritability'.

Ryley's first wife had died in Scotland, and he had left his son in her parents' care while he worked as a ship's surgeon. In 1863 he married 17-year-old Charlotte in Invercargill, but he physically and mentally abused her, especially after his second son's birth in Hokitika, when he was the surgeon superintendent at the local hospital, gaol and asylum. Charlotte filed for divorce, but after Ryley was discharged from the Auckland asylum he left for Fiji, taking their child.[65] He lived in a relationship with a woman in Levuka, Fiji, until 1873, when he returned to practise in Australia. In 1879 he was a civilian surgeon in the Zulu War in South Africa. In Sydney, in February 1884, Ryley swallowed a mixture of morphia with prussic acid and was transferred to Sydney Hospital, where he died the next day, aged 46.[66]

This chapter has looked at life and mental distress in a lonely land — whether lonely through place, work, lack of (or from) social and family networks. So far the focus has been on isolated locations, the camps and the bush, but what of life within the colonial towns? *The Luminaries'* fictional Anna Wetherell found these spaces could be both welcoming and dangerous, especially for lonely, vulnerable and transient women. Other immigrants brought more skills, or capital, and family support to the towns, but even this was no guarantee of avoiding either physical disease or mental anguish.

Anne and John Mollison emigrated from Montrose in Scotland, arriving in 1851 in Dunedin, where during the following decade they established a successful boot- and shoemaking business, a general store and the 'Diggers' Mart', which catered to the burgeoning gold mining population.[67] Anne gave birth to a daughter, Elizabeth, in 1851, and three years later to a son. Another son was born in 1857, but died two days after birth. Then both John and Elizabeth died in 1862 from gastric (probably typhoid) fever. It is perhaps not surprising that Anne fell into a melancholic state; she was one of the first patients admitted to the Dunedin Lunatic Asylum, located near Stuart Street, on 21 November 1863.[68]

She spent around two weeks there before being discharged as cured. Most of the early patients in the asylum diagnosed with melancholia were there for only a brief period, presumably because the treatments and the medical expertise available were very limited (see chapter 7). So unless patients were a danger to themselves or to others they would be released, especially women who had young children to care for. Anne had a nine-year-old son, and, it seems, was financially secure and had the emotional support of many friends. She lived for another 24 years, and died in 1887, aged 71.

Hugh Coolahan, an Irish immigrant, arrived at the other end of the country, in Auckland, in 1841. In 1847 he established a bakery on Shortland Street, becoming very well known through his investments in mining, finance and railway construction. He served on the Auckland Provincial Council and was extremely active in Auckland's Catholic Church.[69] Like Anne Mollison, he spent only a brief period in an asylum: one month in the Auckland asylum in 1871, aged 69, where he was admitted as 'much depressed', perhaps because of financial problems. He was given comfortable accommodation, away from the other patients, possibly because of his status but also because he was physically very ill. After his discharge, he wrote a letter thanking the doctors for the 'happy times which I enjoyed (from the cares of the world)'. He said that he was 'still labouring under the malady in my head', but not getting worse.

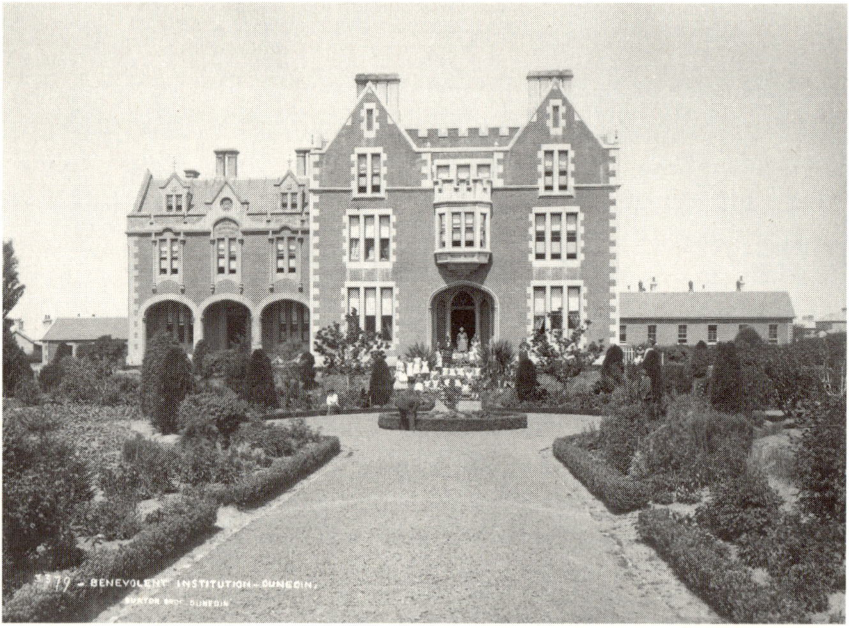

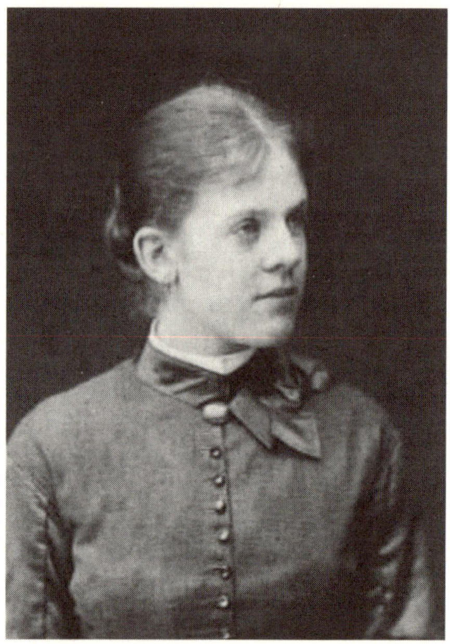

Clockwise from top left:
Julia Rowan and her children were sent to the Dunedin Benevolent Institution after her first admission to the Dunedin Lunatic Asylum in 1876; colonial promoter Edward Gibbon Wakefield was sometimes prone to depression; Richard Henry, conservationist and caretaker of Resolution Island, suffered from depression; Jane Jeffries, who migrated to New Zealand after marrying soldier John Dick in 1919, was a patient at Seacliff, Orokonui and Cherry Farm from 1923 to 1975; profoundly disappointed after immigrating to Aotearoa in 1903, Ingeborg Stuckenberg committed suicide in 1904.

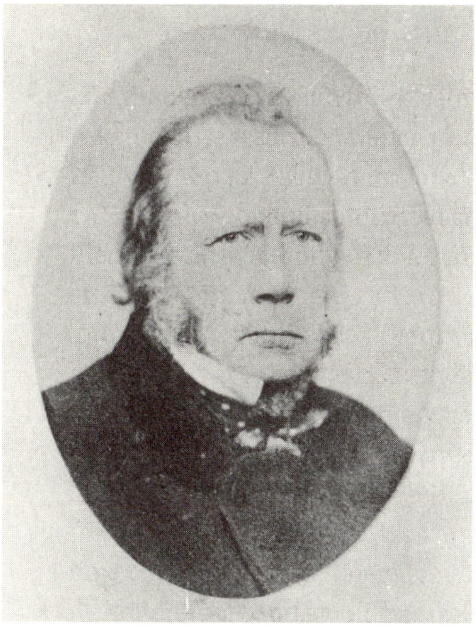

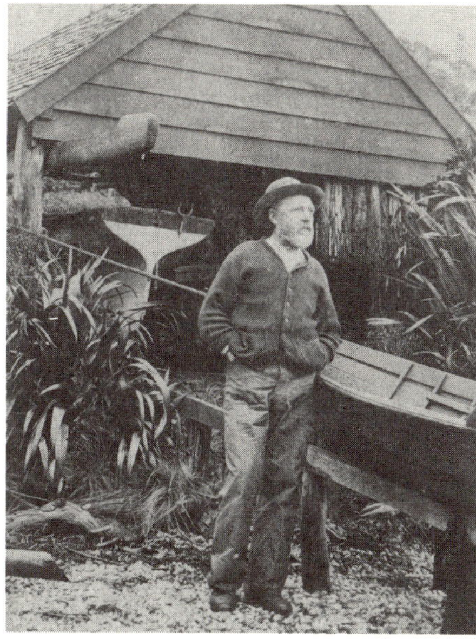

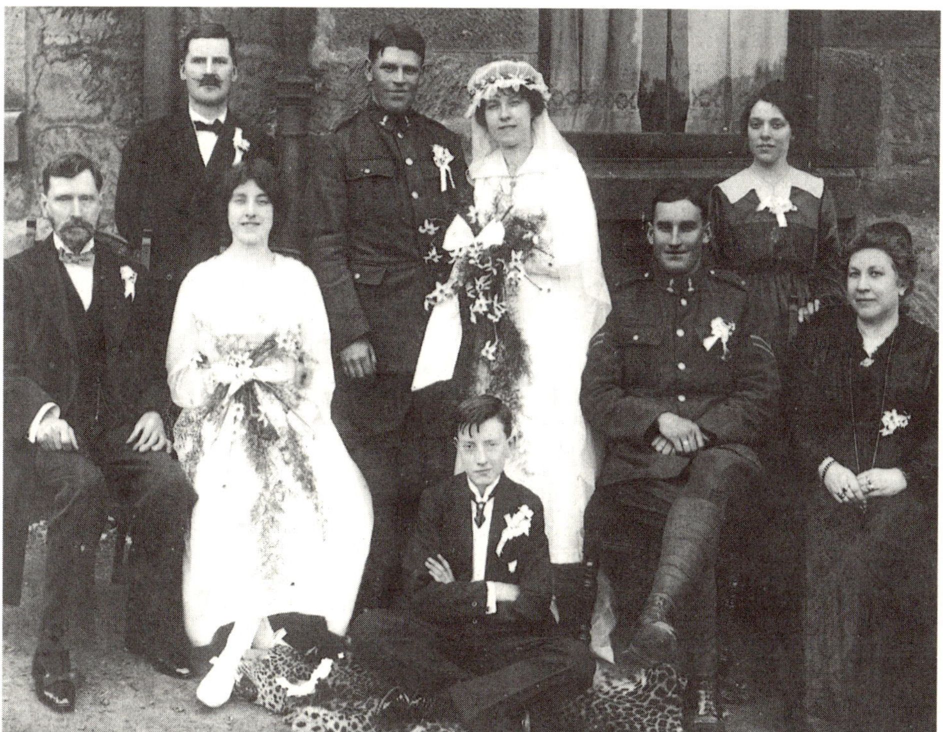

Other colonists, despite their early promise and respectability in urban New Zealand, died in mental asylums after being admitted with melancholia. Charles C., from London, who married in 1885 at the synagogue in Hokitika, was one such case. He was a respected stationer in Reefton, but fell into bankruptcy before attempting to drown himself, 'very depressed in spirits'. He was admitted to Seaview Asylum in 1905, and again in 1908: 'a typical case of melancholia'. He became very emaciated, and his death in 1914 was from marasmus (undernourishment).[70]

Richard Feltus was one of the more unusual cases of melancholia in colonial Auckland.[71] He was admitted several times to the Auckland mental asylum, where he eventually died in 1914, aged 69. On 7 December 1883, *The New Zealand Herald* reported concerns over his safety: 'being out of health, and somewhat depressed in spirits', he had sailed from Auckland to the Wade River (Weiti), just north of the city.[72] He was found in the bush and admitted to the asylum.

Richard's father, George Feltus, had been recruited from Ireland to join the Royal New Zealand Fencibles, retired soldiers from Britain and Ireland who enlisted as a military reserve to protect early settlers in southern Auckland,[73] but he had died from typhoid during the voyage out in December 1846 and been buried at sea. However, Richard's origin story, as recounted in 1883 by Pollex (a writer for *The New Zealand Herald*) was that the child 'was also thrown overboard with his father three days before arrival in New Zealand, but the child somehow landed in Auckland. The facts concerning a child being thrown overboard and Richard's arrival in New Zealand are certainly mysterious.'[74]

Feltus worked as a clerk in the military stores in 1863–64, during the New Zealand Wars, and then subsequently worked for Ridings and Dowden, from whom in 1866 he pleaded guilty to embezzling money.[75] At his trial, witnesses testified to his good character and potential. The judge treated the case with leniency and sentenced him to six months' imprisonment in Auckland with hard labour. On his release Feltus began to lead a vagrant life, sometimes sleeping in the Auckland Domain, wandering the streets and not eating. Meanwhile, almost annually, he petitioned Parliament for compensation for the house and land his father had been promised as a Fencible, and for compensation for the death of his brother, who had died aged 20 from a fever at Drury.[76]

Melancholia and depression often descended when the expectations and hype of migration were not realised. Morgan Grace reported in 1871 that many immigrants 'form the most extravagant anticipations of their new home, and are proportionably depressed by the result of actual experience'.[77] The same year, in a letter to the editor of *The Daily Southern Cross*, a military settler wrote that in Kihikihi in the Waikato 'I have not for the last five year known so much mental depression as exists at the present here amongst our independent farmers, on account of native matters.'[78] But, as we saw in chapter 2, the mental effect on Māori, whose lands were appropriated and lives were uprooted by the same settlers who spoke of depression, would have been far more profound and enduring.

The Danish writer Ingeborg Stuckenberg, who arrived in Auckland in 1903, wrote to her sister Agnes Schwarz about being unable to find work, and at the lack of the rich social, intellectual and creative life she had enjoyed in Denmark.[79] 'The traveller stands alone and looks with hate-filled eyes at the much-praised beauty; no money, no work, not even his daily bread. Like a terrible sarcasm in all this misery the land surrounds him — wonderful, sunlit, with its blue mountains and glistening fjords, and on all sides, the sea.' Ingeborg explained to Agnes that suicides in this 'Promised Land' were because of sorrow and disappointment, not madness. Did this explain why Ingeborg fatally shot herself in 1904?

Nostalgia and depression were also cited as reasons for the suicides of other immigrants. When Louis Derecskei, a Hungarian circus employee, hanged himself in Dunedin in 1911, the coroner surmised that he had been in a 'state of acute depression and suffering from extreme nostalgia, as so many foreigners did in strange lands'.[80]

Sarah had emigrated from England and settled in Lower Hutt in 1925, when she was in her sixties, and had spent the next year unhappy and depressed. Her husband, her son and her daughter-in-law, with whom she lived, were concerned but she was not treated for her depression. After a brief period of seeming more cheerful, she hanged herself in 1926. At the inquest her husband said that she 'did not like the life out here; having left her friends and a married daughter in England'.[81]

In Taihape, a domestic servant jumped from a bridge into the Hautapu

River in 1928. Her employer stated at the inquest that: 'For some time she has been complaining she could not sleep, and at times she appeared to be much depressed. I think she suffered from loneliness, and wanted to get back home to Belfast.'[82] Also in 1929 in Aparima in Southland, a farm labourer ingested the lethal poison strychnine. His peers recalled at the inquest that he 'did not like New Zealand and would like to get back home to Ireland'; 'he would have been better if he had stayed at home'.[83]

These sad stories notwithstanding, very few immigrants to New Zealand committed suicide. Feelings of depression and doubts about emigrating were most likely left unspoken or were expressed within the confines of family and confidantes. Only a small minority were ever committed to mental hospitals. One of these was Ellen R., who, after her admission to the Dunedin Lunatic Asylum in 1868, seldom spoke, except to tell staff that she should have never come to New Zealand from Ireland.[84]

A photograph posted on Ancestry.com shows Pansy M., a smiling young woman who had immigrated to Auckland from Canada with her family in 1909, when she was 17.[85] In 1913 she attempted to commit suicide by swallowing matchheads and trying to drink Lysol. Pansy was admitted to the Auckland Mental Hospital in a poor physical state and suffering from melancholia. She had warned her mother that 'Auckland will drive her mad'. Her case notes recorded that she 'did not like the place and people and said that their narrow mindedness and lack of sociability would "drive her off her head"'. During almost eight months in the asylum Pansy's physical and mental state improved, and she was able to sing at the asylum's New Year concert. After being discharged in 1914, Pansy settled in Auckland, where she married in 1921 and later had two children. She died in 1946.

The knowledge we have of melancholia and depression in colonial New Zealand suggests that women were more likely to be diagnosed with these conditions than men.[86] Catharine Coleborne found that, in a sample of every third year between 1873 and 1910 at Auckland mental asylum, of the 113 diagnosed with melancholia, 47 were women and 66 were men. These samples should be placed against 4037 cases (including readmissions) during this period, of whom just over a third were women,[87] suggesting that women were proportionately more likely than men to have melancholia.

The significance is in the world 'proportionately' — the numerically higher numbers of men with melancholia in these asylums simply reflect the greater number of men with all diagnoses who were committed. These ratios began to even out by 1900. Although the sample from Sunnyside may have been an exception, the majority of patients with melancholia were women.

Samples of asylum patients diagnosed with melancholia by sex

Asylum	Date	Male	Female	Total
Seaview	1869–76	9	7	16
Auckland	1853–71	29	13	42
Dunedin	1863–77	29	10	39
Sunnyside	1900	2	8	10
Auckland	1900	15	12	27
Seacliff	1900	12	11	23

Source: Samples from asylum registers and case books. Some years are missing for the Auckland sample, and a case book is missing for Seacliff.

These numbers are an indication only; not all patients were given diagnoses, while patients with another diagnosis might also be described as melancholic and depressed, and diagnoses could change with re-admissions, or according to the medical superintendent's bias.

Although there are limits to how much asylum records can be extrapolated to reflect the extent of depression within the general population, these records are one of the few written sources we have. Along with letters, diaries and creative material, they provide some insight into depression among women in colonial New Zealand.

As with men, accounts written by women represent only a small number of immigrants. Among the educated and literate, missionary Hannah King — who was part of Samuel Marsden's first mission station at Hohi in Pēwhairangi Bay of Islands from 1814 until 1832 — and Charlotte Kemp — who was at Marsden's second station in Kerikeri from 1819 until 1848 — were both prone to 'nervous disorders'. These conditions were probably anxiety and depression, exacerbated by the demanding lives they led as mothers of large families, cooking and caring for extended households that included the children of iwi leaders, teaching in the mission schools and attending to the sick. Conflicts among the missionaries, and the snobbery of those in more senior positions, may have also induced despair.

Then there could be the terror of sudden violence, so often directed at women, that loomed for Pākehā and Māori during those colonial times. When Hannah's husband, John King, was absent from Hohi in November 1822, a large taua (war party) threatened to kill and eat Hannah and her children, and ransack and burn the house. John wrote in his journals that this had a great effect on Hannah's mind.[88] Historian and archaeologist Angela Middleton suggests, in her book detailing the missions and Māori at Pēwhairangi, that Charlotte Kemp needed the constant attention of her husband, James Kemp, after their eighth child, Samuel, died in 1834, aged only seven months. 'Within a few months, she recovered sufficiently to carry on with the girls' school, although intermittent bouts of mental breakdown recurred throughout the rest of her life.'[89]

The extent to which women were depressed by life in a new land could be revealed in the letters they wrote to close family members. The act of writing surely helped to release frustration and despair, but, as Sarah Stephens — who arrived in Motueka in January 1842 to join her husband, Samuel, a surveyor with the New Zealand Company who had arrived four months earlier — reminded her mother in September 1843, some of her letters were written 'when my mind was somewhat depressed . . . Many months pass before the letters arrive so you should hope that circumstances have changed as to make me feel and see all things more bright around us'.[90]

The life experiences of Julia and Jane, which open and close this chapter, highlight the depression and melancholia that both immigrant women and those born in the new colony experienced. Loneliness in a lonely land, the expectations and demands of care, domestic and paid work, and the stresses and gender-based violence, economic insecurity and the absence of other women's support in strongly masculine environments — all took their toll.

Even those living in a 'comfortable home' and surrounded by beautiful scenery could be caught up with depression, as Taranaki nurse Margaret Bilton recalled in the New Zealand nursing journal, *Kai Tiaki*, in 1913, when she described caring for a depressed patient.

> My first trip over Mt. Messenger — where a coach road is cut out of the mountain side with the loveliest bush on either side of it — was on a pouring wet day in September, when it took four coach horses all their time to plough through the mud, axle deep in many places. On arrival at my destination up the Moki road, I found my patient (a neurotic woman) suffering from influenza and despondency, verging on melancholia. She could not believe that I saw any beauty in the bush — all she could think of was the mud and the rain, and her one idea was to get away from it.[91]

Bilton's patient was depressed but not hospitalised. Case books from New Zealand's asylums record many women with melancholia associated with living in lonely places — although other stressors are also implicated.

Among a group of female patients from South Spit who were admitted to Seaview Asylum in Hokitika on 31 July 1872 was Ellen M., who, her case notes recorded, had 'lived a solitary life at the Greenstone'.[92] Maybe so, but she had lived with her brother, and it was his sudden death to which her neighbours attributed her insanity. When police found her, a bag containing about 100 sovereigns was tied around her waist. Much of this considerable sum went to paying for her care in the asylum, where 'the chances of her leaving are slight indeed, hers is truly a case of profound melancholia. She never speaks unless spoken to and then answers in a half vexed manner.'[93]

Loneliness was also compounded by the misfortune, abuse, trauma and stress that many immigrant women experienced either before migration, during travel or after their arrival in the colonies. Although doctors did not usually attribute women's insanity to material hardship or money in the same way that they ascribed this stress to men,[94] asylum records reveal that women who were deserted by their partners or who were widowed suffered economic hardship that could induce melancholia.

In 1867, for example, Elizabeth J. was found wandering Auckland's streets with no money and 'depressed in spirits', after disembarking from Sydney.[95] She had migrated to Sydney with her husband, but he had soon after deserted her and their children. Elizabeth was unable to find work and had reluctantly left the children in a charitable institution in Sydney to seek employment in Auckland. Her mental and physical state improved after spending almost four months in the Auckland Provincial Lunatic Asylum. Having 'recovered' from melancholia and considered a 'model patient' who had assisted the matron, Elizabeth returned to Sydney with a grant of £2 from the government and £2 from Bishop Selwyn of the Anglican Church.

Bridget E., who had emigrated from Ireland in 1884 aged 18, spent nearly two months in Seacliff Asylum in 1900, suffering from melancholia caused by 'domestic anxiety'. She had filed a gold-prospecting claim for Cardrona — a tough, remote location —and had given birth to three children within four years.[96] She was admitted after apparently threatening one of her children with a knife. Her husband told a doctor in Dunedin that his wife was a 'whore and that she lived a life of drunkenness and sin', but he also stated that she was fond of reading novels, and could be shy, retiring and affectionate. A sign of Bridget's 'abnormality' was that she roamed the hills, 'to the alarm of her neighbours'. A lone 'wandering woman' was considered abnormal in colonial Aotearoa, as it was in many colonies and cultures.

Rachel B. was married to a man working in another tough, remote location — in her case a gumdigger in Northland.[97] Her neighbours reported her nocturnal wandering, and that she was living alone in a gumdigger's hut. Her hospital case notes stated that this was because she was afraid that her husband would murder her. Rachel was sent to Auckland Mental Hospital in October 1913 diagnosed with acute melancholia, and soon improved. She was quiet and reserved, but took interest in the other patients' welfare and assisted in feeding them. However, a year later she was still melancholic and having delusions. She died in the mental hospital in 1922.

Some women bore the brunt not only of economic hardship but also the shame of giving birth to a child out of wedlock. In 1867, 24-year-old Irish immigrant Elizabeth O. was working as a domestic servant in Auckland when she became pregnant to a male servant in the household.[98] He refused to support the child or marry her. After a court appearance, he was prosecuted and ordered to pay maintenance.[99] Not long after, the baby died and Elizabeth was committed to the Auckland asylum in 1868 with melancholia. Her case notes record that she 'became greatly depressed in spirit saying she was lost and that people were trying to keep her out of heaven'. She remained in the asylum until her death 33 years later, in 1901.

Jessie G., a migrant from Scotland, was admitted to the Dunedin Lunatic Asylum in 1874, after her husband died, leaving her with a two-year-old daughter.[100] A year later, Jessie was discharged and got a job as a washerwoman. She became pregnant in 1876, but the father rejected her and the baby, despite her attempts to seek legal restitution. Jessie became seriously depressed and at times manic. She was again admitted to the Dunedin asylum in 1877, after being charged with lunacy and neglecting her two children. The youngest was only four months old, and her five-year-old daughter had been found wandering the streets.[101]

They were sent to the industrial school for seven years and ordered to be brought up in the Roman Catholic faith, despite Jessie being a Presbyterian. A factor may have been that she had melancholia and mania with religious delusions. It is not clear whether Jessie ever saw her children again; during the 1890s she was transferred to the Porirua asylum, north of Wellington.

Helene M. was married when she was sent from Gisborne to the Auckland asylum in 1912 with 'simple melancholia'.[102] She and her husband had first immigrated to Canada for work, but 'underwent numerous hardships and often had insufficient food', recorded as semi-starvation. Although Helene's husband was a school teacher, he could not find employment in New Zealand and their child remained in poor health. Helene tried to commit suicide and smother the child, but after three months in the asylum, and gaining weight, she was discharged.

Women's reproductive functions were closely linked with diagnoses of melancholia and depression, and a wide range of conditions were labelled as puerperal melancholia, before, during and long after the birth, and including miscarriage and lactation. Menstruation and menopause were also cited as causes of depression. When a woman was sent from Kumara to Seaview Asylum in 1898, her brother said she smashed things during every menstrual period.[103] Another immigrant, from County Donegal, Ireland, was admitted with melancholia to the Auckland mental asylum several times between 1854 and her death from emaciation in 1870 aged 48. Her illness was linked to catamenia (menstruation) — both its absence and presence.[104]

As psychiatric diagnoses puerperal mania and puerperal melancholia linked women's bodies and minds. The puerperal period customarily referred to six weeks after childbirth, but in practice doctors applied this to a much longer period, including extended lactation.

Doctors tended to focus on embodied causes and symptoms, rather than the social and economic issues, and issues that specifically affected women. Catherine F., a 22-year-old immigrant from Ireland, for example, was admitted to the Auckland mental asylum in 1867 after weaning her first child. Hormonal changes and sadness about the loss of the close bond with her child that breastfeeding had given her may have induced her depression. So, too, may have the actions of her unkind husband. Doctors reported that 'She is found often in tears but will not tell the cause of her trouble.'[105] Catherine was diagnosed with melancholia, and 27 years later died in the asylum.

Even when it seemed clear that Auckland asylum patient Sara's melancholia was due to profound grief and 'shock' after the accidental death of her young children, 'puerperal' was listed as a cause. In 1907 Sara had emigrated, aged 19, from Lebanon to Auckland to join her husband. In 1914, two of their young children wandered from their home in Grey Lynn and drowned in a flooded creek. When Sara found the children she screamed for help, but it was too late to save them.[106] According to her husband, during the following months Sara lost interest in her other children, and in housework. She refused to eat and was depressed. Eight months after the tragic death of the children Sara was admitted to the Auckland Mental Hospital.[107]

Loneliness continued to have a severe effect on immigrant mothers well into more modern times. In 1973, a woman who had immigrated to Aotearoa from the United Kingdom in the 1960s, and who had suffered depression for many years, told a researcher that her depression continued in Aotearoa after the birth of another child. She also become depressed around menstruation and had an unhappy marriage. Depression alienated her from both her relatives in the United Kingdom and her co-workers in New Zealand because she did not want to appear depressed.[108]

This chapter concludes with the story of Jane Nimmo Sampson Dick, an immigrant to Otago from Scotland in 1919. Like Julia, Jane was a wife and mother, and also lived in a remote area near Dunedin, but, unlike Julia, Jane was educated and had left a professional career as a nurse before emigrating as a 'war bride' in 1919. Jane was committed to Seacliff Mental Hospital on 8 October 1923,[109] and she spent 52 years there, separated from her children. She died in 1975.

Jane had suffered from postnatal depression after the birth of Jean, her second child with her husband, John Dick, in 1922. The couple were living on a farm at Wickliffe Bay in an isolated corner of the Otago Peninsula, a very different environment from Jane's former life in Scotland. Born in 1888, she grew up in Coatbridge near Glasgow, where her father was an iron roller, and where she would have 'looked right into the face of those huge iron mills which would have been going 24 hours a day with massive furnaces'. Her granddaughter Pinky Agnew made this point when I interviewed her in order to stress the sharp contrast between the industrial environment Jane had grown up in and her life on a farm on the Otago Peninsula.

In 1913, when Jane was 19, she married George Brown Harrison in Scotland, and five months later her first child, Gertrude, was born. Jane may have suffered postnatal depression. The couple divorced in 1913, but an informal arrangement was made that Jane relinquish Gertrude's care to George's mother. After Jane immigrated to New Zealand in 1919, she wrote weekly to Gertrude, but the letters never reached her daughter. Thus Gertrude grew up thinking that her mother had died, unaware that she had a sister and a brother 'on the other side of the world'.

As it did for millions of people, the First World War had sent Jane's life in a new direction. By 1917 she was the sister in charge of surgical wards and a theatre nurse at the County and City Royal Infirmary in Perth, Scotland, where she met invalided New Zealand soldier John Dick when she was among a group of nurses singing Christmas carols to the patients.

The couple married in 1919, and nearly four months later departed

Plymouth on the chartered troopship *Ionic*, destined for Aotearoa. Jane was among the 856 women on board, most of whom were 'war brides'. When the *Ionic* berthed in Wellington, newspapers reported: 'It was with curiously anxious eyes that these women, the majority of whom were very young, gazed over the bulwarks at the city and surrounding hills, dimly wondering perhaps what the future holds for them in the new land.'[110]

Jane's future was as a farmer's wife on the Otago Peninsula, but she was determined to put her skills to use and to establish a lying-in home for pregnant mothers in Portobello. She was a lively and cheerful woman, who had a fine voice and sang in local concerts. In 1920 she gave birth to John ('Jock'), and in 1922 to Janet ('Jean'). But times were tough, and John found it difficult to find extra income to support the family beyond what the small farm could generate. Pinky Agnew recalls:

> He would have to leave her every day to go out to work; she was very unwell, mentally unwell, and she couldn't get out of bed. So, he would tie a rope around Jock's waist so that Jock could get in and out of the window and relieve himself. And he tied the other end onto the bed, and presumably left food out . . . One day, she got up and got dressed, and took the children out for a walk . . . [to the] cliffy house . . . it was very isolated over on the other side of the Otago peninsula, and she was walking across the paddocks, holding Jock's hand and holding baby Jean in her arms.

A neighbour found Jane and the children and persuaded her to return home. She was not to remain at home for long, though — sadly Jane spent the rest of her life at Seacliff, Cherry Farm and Orokonui hospitals, north of Dunedin.

4.

Enduring darkness

> I served three years in the Army; it seemed to take away all my self-confidence, everything I had. Things did not turn out as I had expected when I got back and for the past months I have been in a terrible state of nervous depression which with other things is making life unbearable, for one who was always inclined to be temperamental. I am writing this because I continually have thoughts of suicide and am afraid that in a bad fit of depression I might do this cowardly disgraceful thing, but I hope that the thought of the terrible shock and disgrace that this will bring to my near and dear ones will hold me back, but it seems impossible for me to carry on in my present state.

Twenty-nine-year-old Trevor wrote this note a few days after Christmas Day in 1944, before shooting himself with a rifle in a farm hut in South Canterbury. He was admitted to Timaru Hospital, and died on New Year's Day.[1] After serving one term in the army, he had returned to Canterbury around August 1944 and was working with his brother, planning to start a farm at Waimate and to marry his fiancée. His brother noticed that since Trevor had come back from the war he had suffered 'nervous depression and became very depressed and looked on the black side of everything'.

Before Trevor went overseas he was, his brother said 'a normal type of man' and so he did not take his suicide ideation seriously, but rather just 'thought [he] would get back to normal eventually'. Trevor consulted five doctors after returning to Aotearoa, and although this did not prevent him from ultimately committing suicide, his relentless pursuit of help illustrates the severe, sustained impact that war trauma and army life could have on mental health.

Much has been written about New Zealand soldiers suffering shell shock and neurasthenia during the First World War, but the long-term impact of war on combatants and their families deserves further recognition.[2] Depression was not a common diagnosis for war veterans, but rather was subsumed as a symptom within shell shock, neurasthenia, combat or war neurosis; contemporary terms for this include post-traumatic stress disorder (PTSD) and combat stress reaction.[3]

Many of the symptoms of these differently labelled conditions fit within mental depression. Alongside such factors as physical impairment, unemployment, economic problems and family and personal relationships, it is problematic to ascertain how significant depression was in the reintegration of soldiers into civilian life. The impact of war trauma, leading to depression (and melancholia), featured heavily in the lives of returned service people, and for their families, including 'war brides' such as Jane Dick, whose story is told in the previous chapter.

This chapter covers the First World War (1914–1918) and the Second World War (1939–1945). New Zealand's contribution to these respective wars was significant, not least because so many died. The chapter also speaks to the families, friends and those left behind by war. I focus on these wars because of the paucity or inaccessibility of mental health data for other wars in New Zealand's history. To date, we know very little about how Māori suffered mentally from combat during the global wars of the twentieth century, and about the effects for whānau. If more evidence was available, the scope of this chapter could have been extended to both earlier and later conflicts, where melancholia, depression and suicide also featured.

For example, some Pākehā and a few Māori who fought in the New Zealand Wars (1845–1872) were admitted to asylums. In chapter 2 we encountered Tamihau, a patient at the Auckland asylum at the same time as William Lawton, a discharged soldier in the 14th Regiment, who suffered from melancholia and who spent 19 years in the Auckland Provincial

Lunatic Asylum,[4] from 1870 until he died there in 1889. John K., also diagnosed with melancholia on 25 March 1867, was aged 22 when he was admitted:

> [W]hilst serving at the Taranaki militia [he] became unsound in his mind, deserting into the bush where he was found after an interval of 3 days in a half-famished condition having had no food during that time. He was taken to the hospital where he was treated for some time but owing to his persistent refusal of food and extreme emaciation he was forwarded to Auckland for further treatment. He would not speak or answer any questions, refused his food and lay constantly on the floor stoutly resisting any other attempt to coerce him to swallow fluid nourishment. When left alone he would beat the wall with his feet crying all the time, 'God my God!'. . . Gradually the suicidal tendency wore off and he now eats heartily but is one of the best workmen.[5]

During the First World War over 100,000 New Zealand troops served in Sāmoa, Gallipoli, Sinai-Palestine, Belgium and France. The fatalities and casualties were very high: around 18,000 died in the First World War, and over 41,000 were wounded. About 105,000 New Zealanders served overseas during the Second World War, and around 7000 died on active service. Nearly 16,000 were wounded.[6] The full impact on the mental health of New Zealanders who served in the twentieth century's two global wars remains unclear. This is partly because of the stigma associated with madness; hence those 'mentally disturbed' as a result of military service were rarely medically labelled as lunatics. Instead, a range of changing diagnoses covered those who suffered from war trauma, and who were deeply depressed and suicidal. These terms are vague.

In New Zealand, neurosis and neurasthenia, considered milder forms of mental distress than depression or melancholia, were often applied to soldiers who had suffered from mental disturbances during military combat in the First World War. In 1917 more troops from the New Zealand Expeditionary Force were admitted to hospitals for neurasthenia than with melancholia.[7] Neurasthenia, a term popularised by the American neurologist George Miller Beard around 1869, was considered a more respectable term than shell shock or mental illness, and it included many neuroses. Neurasthenia often referred to those whose mental and physical performances were reduced by 'depression but with an absence of typical anxiety symptoms, obsessions or hysteria'.[8] By the 1930s neurasthenia was almost a meaningless term,[9] although some military medical historians preferred this term to depression.[10]

The British psychologist Charles Samuel Myers coined the term 'shell shock' during the First World War initially to refer to mental illness and various conditions arising from fighting in the trenches.[11] Much later, American attorney and historian Eric Dean Jr. linked the symptoms of shell shock to post-traumatic stress:

> The symptoms associated with 'shell shock' were varied, from vague anxiety, depression, startle reactions, an inability to concentrate one's thoughts, loss of memory, insomnia, nightmares, intense fear, 'trotting heart', and panic attacks to uncontrollable shaking, aphonia [loss of voice], mutism, hysterical blindness, amnesia, partial or total paralysis, and hysterical fits, in which the subject might scream and blindly thrash about in desperation.[12]

Thus, like neurasthenia, depression and shell shock could be interchangeable diagnoses, dependent on the diagnosing doctor and on the individual soldier's psychological experiences and responses.[13] Many families would have watched their returned men exhibit the symptoms explained an article in 1915 in *The Gisborne Times* under the heading 'Shell Fire and Nerves. Noise Causes Madness':

> Speaking of the effect upon soldiers of shell fire, the 'Hospital' says: There is usually depression as a prominent symptom, and with this there may lie hypochondriacal ideas, vague pains and aches, or definite assertions of disease or injury, the presence of which, however, careful examination fails to disclose. There is a feeling of inability to carry on the accustomed work, or adequately to fill the usual duties, and as a result of this there

> may be suggestions on the part of the patient of suicide or even actual attempts at self-destruction. In other cases there is marked confusion; inability to converse coherently; automatism — as in a case reported from the seat of battle of a soldier who sat ceaselessly beating the bottom of a bucket for hours, apparently oblivious of everything that was taking place around him: vague fears and obsessions.[14]

On 9 May 1917, a Sunnyside hospital doctor filed admission papers for two soldiers, Thomas G. and George W., both of whom were suffering from melancholia caused by shell shock.[15] They had each attempted to commit suicide during their voyage on the hospital ship *Maheno* from the European war zone to New Zealand. The notes were similar: 'This is very similar to many others I have examined at the front and Belgium where they have been under heavy shell fire. All tend to become suicidal.'

Both soldiers told the doctor, A. D. Anderson, that they were fed up with fighting. Thomas was very melancholic, morose and had almost lost his memory, 'tired of acting service and I think will go to any extreme to get out of it'. When George was asked by Anderson whether he would like to return to the front, he replied that 'he had had enough and they could play their own game . . . He gave me the impression he would do anything to get out of it.'

Dr Crooke's case notes from Sunnyside describe Thomas and George as melancholic, morose and hysterical. Both former soldiers were later awarded a British war medal and a Victory medal but there their similarities end. Thomas was transferred from Sunnyside to a convalescent home, resumed work as a riveter and married in 1923, dying aged 87. George, too, had a long life, but he never married and died in Otago's Cherry Farm Hospital in 1960, having been institutionalised for 43 years. By then he had been diagnosed with schizophrenia.

Neurasthenia eventually came to be known as 'anxiety neurosis' or 'psychoneurosis'[16] and by the Second World War the term 'war neurosis' was commonly used,[17] although men suffering from this and related conditions such as combat exhaustion or fatigue were classified under the heading of 'Functional Nervous Disorders'.[18] Like earlier terms for the psychological effects of combat, 'war neurosis' was a vague diagnosis, which might, but not always, include depression. A study of New Zealand troops in Italy in 1944 found 'moodiness, loss of interest or "frank depression"' in 53 out of 100 cases. Other major symptoms included sleeplessness, headaches, tremors, diminished concentration, fatigue and anorexia; all symptoms associated with war neurosis.[19]

In 1942, the editor of *The New Zealand Medical Journal* predicted that the impact of combat on the mind would remain long after the war. 'Psychoneuroses have provided an appreciable percentage of the cases invalided, and unless dealt with efficiently and with understanding these will prove a chronic problem after the war.'[20] A paper delivered to the New Zealand Branch of the British Medical Association in Dunedin in 1948 reported that among the approximately 250,000 men who had enlisted in the New Zealand forces, 7308 were discharged with neurosis, of whom 4160 were awarded a war pension, partly because they were unable to work.[21]

The term 'post-traumatic stress disorder (PTSD)' dates from 1980. Psychiatric diagnosis regards the patient as having experienced extraordinary stress outside the range of usual human experience and which would be markedly distressing to almost anyone.[22] PTSD also refers to re-experiencing trauma long after the event, as in dreams, recollections or flashbacks while awake. People with PTSD often suffer depression, among other symptoms and behaviours, including being 'jumpy', irritable or angry. Sufferers may withdraw emotionally, have trouble concentrating and sleeping, or become reliant on alcohol to relieve the pain; these are also common symptoms of depression.[23] Vietnam War veterans in Aotearoa who responded to a postal survey conducted during the 1990s, and were classified as PTSD cases, exhibited high levels of depression and anxiety.[24]

Regardless of the shifting terms for the psychological effects of war trauma, during the twentieth century soldiers with 'invisible wounds' such as depression were disadvantaged in their treatment by the state compared with those who had more obvious physical wounds. An indication of this discrepancy can be found in the statistics of those who received war pensions, which revealed that only a small number of soldiers with psychological disabilities received war pensions as compensation for death, disability or financial disadvantage. For example, in 1925, among the 12,834 men who received war disability pensions, only around 5 per cent were compensated for shell shock and insanity.[25]

In 1993 history student Peter Boston sampled 75 men from the welfare records of 225 ex-servicemen who had received aid from the Red Cross Society or the Returned Soldiers' Association in Dunedin during the 1920s and 1930s. Boston found that 14 per cent had some record of psychological disturbance. This percentage may seem small but, during the same period, 42 per cent of Boston's sample had been classified at varying times by the medical profession as having psychological disabilities — an indication of how on-going mental issues, such as depression, were under-reported in the welfare records.[26]

In 1919 William Field, the member of Parliament for Ōtaki, asked James Allen, the minister of defence, whether he would 'institute some supervision and watchful care of returned soldiers, even after discharge, whose nerves or mental powers are, or may be likely to be, suffering from depression consequent on shell-shock or other terrible war experiences, and thus reduce as far as possible the number of pathetic suicides among soldiers'.[27] Some of this special care was within the nation's existing psychiatric institutions.

The same year, Inspector General of Mental Hospitals Frank Hay outlined how Seacliff Mental Hospital was the main institution to treat soldiers with mental or nervous conditions. As a means of avoiding the stigma attached to mental illness, and because it was considered more therapeutic, three locations (called divisions) were set aside to separate them from other patients or to limit their contact with civilian patients with similar mental conditions.[28] The most liberal space, nearly 6 kilometres away from the main mental hospital, was the holiday house of Seacliff's medical superintendent, Truby King, at Karitane. Treatment here did not require a magistrate's order. Hay called the Karitane house the ANZAC House Hospital, but it was referred to as the Karitane camp in Seacliff's case books. Ex-servicemen suffering from milder cases of war neurosis were treated there.

The house was beside the sea, and provided a calming environment with recreational opportunities. The second division was the Reception Home, known as Clifton House, at Seacliff, where patients, both soldiers and non-soldiers, committed under a magistrate's order were treated. The third division was the library ward at Seacliff. Ex-military patients could be treated here, and it was considered a more secure place for soldiers suffering severe mental or behavioural issues. To oversee the military discipline of the soldier inmates, King was appointed an honorary major by the military, and Maurice Quill, the second head attendant at Seacliff, was given the rank of sergeant specialist New Zealand Army Medical Corp.[29] Hay reported that by 1919 the only other mental institution in New Zealand where soldiers were treated separately from civilian patients, and without a magistrate's committal, was at the Wolfe Bequest Hospital (known as Wolfe Home) at Auckland Mental Hospital.

Soldiers with mental disorders might be shifted between mental institutions, as was the case for Clifford P. After disembarking from a troopship, this 30-year-old former bushman from the Auckland Infantry Battalion was admitted to Seacliff in 1915, diagnosed with melancholia.[30] He said that he had been drugged in Egypt, and he had jumped into the sea on the voyage. At Seacliff he was dull and depressed and in a state of great confusion. In less than two months, because he was 'well conducted', he was able to join the convalescent camp at Karitane, under King's watch.

He still wished to return to the front and denied any possibility of a relapse. He told doctors that at times he could hear his brother, who was still at the front, calling for help, but he also realised that it was impossible to hear him from that distance. In 1916 Clifford was transferred to the Auckland Mental Hospital, from which he was discharged the following year. He served in the Home Service Guard until 1918.

Eighteen-year-old James P., a farm labourer from Southland who enlisted with the Otago Mounted Rifles, also spent a brief period at the Karitane camp while he was a patient at Seacliff, diagnosed with melancholia.[31] He had been invalided home in 1916 following hospitalisation at Abbassia on the outskirts of Cairo, where the Egyptian Army barracks had been converted to a military hospital. James was described as 'dull, slow, depressed and dreamy'. He had also caught typhoid. In Egypt, James had been convinced of being mesmerised, believing that his testicles were wasting away and that he was transforming into a woman. James was described by military and civilian doctors as a 'typical case of adolescent insanity', 'mentally defective and pathetic', and 'confused and somewhat depressed'.

At the Karitane camp he gained 3 stone in three weeks, to get to 12 stone, still not quite his weight of 13 stone when he joined the army. Because of his 'uncouth' behaviour and because he refused to take his medicine or obey those in charge, he was sent back to the stricter regime of Seacliff. He died there in 1920 from tuberculosis, and was buried in the Returned Soldiers' Association (RSA) cemetery in Andersons Bay, Dunedin.

James was in Seacliff at the same time as 25-year-old Southlander William J., who had served in the Otago Battalion 8th Company and was now 'labouring under acute melancholia characterised by extreme depression'.[32] William had worked as a clerk before enlisting on 15 August 1914, only 11 days after Britain declared war on Germany. On 12 April 1915 he embarked for Gallipoli, where he was injured in the Gallipoli campaign and hospitalised in London. In 1916 he rejoined his unit, but he became severely depressed with guilt because he had contracted gonorrhoea.

Like James, William was admitted to the hospital at Abbassia, classified as a melancholic, and invalided to Otago. At Seacliff, William claimed that he had 'committed great wrongs, that he is no good that he might have made good, but he sees now he is no use to anyone, that he has shamed his relatives and friends'. Only four months later, he was discharged and he resumed clerical work. In 1919 he married, and he and his wife went on to have three children. He died of tuberculosis in 1925.

Hay admitted that although Seacliff and Karitane were considered ideal sites of care for mentally unwell returned soldiers, the location did not suit many family and friends, who wanted to visit but lived elsewhere. Requests for loved ones to be treated nearer to family made it futile to separate returned soldiers from civilian patients. The same issue of remoteness from whānau also applied to Queen Mary Hospital at Hanmer Springs, in North Canterbury, when it opened in 1919 to treat war veterans with 'milder' mental disorders.

The treatments introduced at Queen Mary were innovative and progressive, especially considering the state of mental hospitals in Aotearoa at the time. Psychoanalytical methods for the treatment of neurosis were offered by New Zealand and British staff, who had trained at the Maudsley Hospital in South London and similar facilities in Britain.[33]

It has been suggested by history students Russell Clarke and Susan Fennell that the adoption of these methods — which introduced hypnosis and psychoanalysis to the treatment of mental illness during the First World War — was a turning point in the acceptance of modern psychiatry in Aotearoa.[34]

Captain Percy Chisholm, who trained for three months in psychotherapy at various British institutions, was promoted to lieutenant-colonel and appointed as Queen Mary Hospital's first medical superintendent. His colleague Major Sydney Rhind, who served in the army medical corps, found psychotherapy to be valuable in the recovery of 'Private K.',[35] who had served four years in the army. When he returned to New Zealand in 1919 he worked very hard on his new farm. After six months he had developed 'very marked fatiguability, irritability, and mental depression' — all considered symptoms of neurasthenia.

But after three months' hospital treatment, including psychotherapy by Chisholm and Rhind, Private K. was declared 'a perfectly fit and happy man'. Such success undoubtedly contributed to a greater tolerance of psychoanalysis within the wider medical community, although, as discussed in chapter 7, scepticism about this therapy persisted at the highest levels.[36]

Chisholm and Rhind outlined the case of Private N. in a 1920 issue of *The New Zealand Medical Journal* to illustrate psychasthenia, when there are phobias, obsessions or compulsions that the person knows are irrational.

> Patient was admitted here in February, 1920, giving a bad family history. He had four months in France, until buried by a shell at Messines, and was then evacuated, suffering from emotionalism. He was returned to New Zealand as unfit for further service, and he found on his return to work as a teamster that he was unable to control horses and was incapable of trusting himself out at nighttime, when he suffered from illusions. For instance, if he went out for a walk after dusk, he imagined that people were following him, because of the rustling of leaves. This filled him with terror, although he realised he was wrong.

> In addition to this he had severe insomnia and marked periods of depression, when he contemplated suicide. General routine treatment was given, and he was convinced that his condition was curable and brought to a more hopeful frame of mind. Following this he was placed in isolation and a psycho-analysis was carried out, when it was determined that he had marked battle repressions, and calling up the memory of the Battle of Messines provoked severe emotionalism.
>
> In the course of a few days he was able to discuss and remember the whole of his experiences and tell them evenly and without distress. It was explained to him that his morbid fear of night was associated with the dawn of Messines Day. Following the rationalism, he was taken out of isolation, and was now much brighter and happier and more sociable, but was still reluctant to go out at nighttime. Plainly, the analysis had not gone deep enough, so, to make a short cut, he was hypnotised, and it was then discovered that the rustling of leaves was directly associated with one particular shell-burst. This incident was easily rectified, and in consequence he left the hospital with a good mental outlook and free from noctiphobia and illusions, and perfectly confident of his ability to perform his work.[37]

Private N. was discharged from Queen Mary Hospital, and received a small war disability pension. Other soldier-patients may have benefitted from these new therapies, but routine was considered equally important in treating soldiers at Hanmer. A patient should:

> follow the regular routine of hospital life, to regularise his life, to make him live by the clock. His day is kept filled by outdoor sport and graduated gymnastic work. A man is taught to swim and to play golf, and these exercises stimulate him from his apathy and restore his self-confidence. All men must spend part of their day in doing some kind of work — from leather-work to motor-engineering, practical farming or gardening — and this trains their dormant powers of observation and concentration. All patients are kept up to the mark by firm hospital discipline.[38]

William Field's question about the care of First World War veterans reflected public concern over the treatment of returned soldiers and integrating them back into civilian life. The most ambitious scheme for this was established under the 1915 Discharged Soldiers Settlement Act, whereby the Crown enabled soldiers to be allocated or enter a ballot for low-cost land-allotments and to secure loans to develop farms. The scheme operated throughout the country. But many of these men were inexperienced in farming, and the frustration of breaking in land could compound the mental depression which had often set in as they tried to sustain a livelihood, often with young families, and as they experienced economic and environmental setbacks.[39] In 1929 *The Nelson Evening Mail* reported on the inquest into the death of C. H. Nelson, of Murchison:

> . . . coroner (Mr H. Fraser) returned a verdict that the cause of death was a gunshot wound self-inflicted when in a state of acute mental depression. Case where a man broken in health by war service and not equipped with a great deal of previous experience in dairy farming had attempted to do that which would have taxed to the utmost a man with wide experience and blessed with good health and a sound constitution. The disastrous flood of 1926 when the Buller river changed its course and washed away a considerable area of his farm added materially to his worries. Foredoomed to failure from the outset, he kept on, valiantly striving to overcome insuperable difficulties, until, broken in spirit as well as in health, he gave up the hopeless battle and brought an honourable career to a tragic end. Such a case in this seemed to prompt the questions to whether close sympathetic investigation into the circumstances of other soldier settlers should not be made to see if they were physically and temperamentally fitted for the 'life they have chosen.' During the difficult period of repatriation, both Government and returned men thought the terms of settlement on the land were satisfactory, but perhaps much good would result now if a general review of every case were made where it is apparent that the man was not succeeding.[40]

Such reports raised the question of whether many repatriated soldiers were simply physically and temperamentally unsuited to a harsh rural life. By 1929, when the Great Depression hit New Zealand, several returned soldiers who had taken up farming were acknowledged as medically unfit for the tasks because of their 'age and the latent effect of war service'.[41]

Living in isolated circumstances probably would not have helped their mental health issues, yet they had few options when no other work was available. The economic precariousness experienced by many exacerbated post-war psychological stress and depression, and could be a factor in suicide.

By the Second World War, the treatment for soldiers with depression and the psychological effects of combat were more embedded within the framework of psychoneurosis (another term for neurotic disorders). Curiously, in 1946 Theodore Gray, director general of mental hospitals, declared that this cause of neurosis was simpler to treat because it was mostly partly reactive in character 'and the outlook better than those arising from peace-time conditions'.[42] Gray's assessment was an oversimplification because the mental trauma of war often remained untreated or was hidden, or might be diverted in other ways, such as through alcohol abuse or domestic violence.[43]

In Christchurch, efforts to treat combat neurosis, especially through psychotherapy, were initiated by Dr Charles Maurice Bevan-Brown and others who formed the Christchurch War Neurosis Group in 1944.[44] A site for treatment was secured when his friends Reverend Frank A. Cook and Dr Enid Cook founded the Cranmer House Clinic in Armagh Street in Christchurch, with Bevan-Brown as the senior physician. When the clinic moved in 1950 to Andover Street, it was renamed the Clinic for Medical Psychology to mark that it was no longer specifically military in focus.[45]

Turning to alcohol was common among those who suffered from depression and war's other psychological effects.[46] At the 1918 conference of the Returned Soldiers' Association (RSA), the medical committee expressed grave concern about the number of shell shock and 'mental cases' who were ruining their chances of complete recovery by overindulging in alcohol.[47] The connection between alcohol abuse, post-war trauma and depression is complex — not least because alcohol can be a means of escaping or temporarily avoiding pain, even if it is a depressant. Returned servicemen often sought camaraderie at the RSA clubrooms, where liquor was often more readily available than in the public bars — which, from December 1917 until October 1967, were required to close at 6 p.m. After the Second World War, RSA clubs were also established in some areas of New Zealand where alcohol was legally prohibited.[48] Depressed former soldiers, like many civilians, might also drown their sorrows at home.

Charles's father noticed that after his son returned to Wellington from the war in 1918 he could be very depressed and had started 'drinking a good deal'.[49] Charles became very upset about the news 'of the death of a mate at the front', and thought he would be better off the earth than on it. After one bout of drinking he became argumentative, struck his father and slashed his own throat with a razor. The coroner ruled that Charles died from shock and haemorrhage following a self-inflicted wound, committed while in a state of severe mental depression caused by war experience.

Likewise, one of Jack's friends noticed that he had started drinking more heavily after he came back from the war, where he had served in the Canterbury Infantry Battalion.[50] According to his friend, a Dr Irwin, and the police, Jack also appeared depressed. Jack lived alone in a tent on 50 acres of land at Spotswood in North Canterbury, and had not been doing well as a farmer and carpenter. In May 1928, after he was arrested for 'helpless drunkenness', he told his friend that he was thinking of hanging himself. During the next month Jack did very little work. Eventually, he fatally hanged himself.

At a 1921 trial in the Waikato Supreme Court of a former gunner, Alfred Joseph Ryan, Dr D. N. W. Murray gave evidence in which he advised that 'No man with shell shock should touch intoxicating liquor in any form.'[51] Ryan had been charged with forging cheques and obtaining money under false pretences. At the time of committing the alleged offences, Ryan had been on a trial discharge from Tokanui Psychiatric Hospital, to where he had been committed in 1919 after being found not guilty of earlier fraud offences on the grounds of insanity. Shell shock, mental depression and alcohol abuse had been advanced by doctors as mitigating factors.[52]

At the trial, Murray testified that he considered Ryan to be a 'genuine victim of shellshock' who 'suffered from depression and morbidity, and this induced him to take drink, under the influence of which he lost his self-control . . . Accused had been injured as a result of shell; explosions on Gallipoli and at Messines. His war neurosis blunted his moral sense, induced him to go to liquor, and then commit acts which he would not otherwise do.'

Ryan was sent back to Tokanui. He appeared again before the court in 1930 with several aliases, but was considered 'young and presentable'. He was charged with issuing bogus cheques and obtaining goods by false pretences, and had masqueraded as a Public Works engineer to defraud a tailor and a grocer. Ryan told the court that he was married and had two children in Australia, and that he was a returned soldier suffering from shell shock.[53] 'Drink had caused his downfall,' he said.[54] This time Ryan was sentenced to six months' imprisonment.

Although the link with shell shock was no longer made, trauma from the Second World War induced what oral historian Alison Parr has termed 'silent casualties'. 'Mark' had been captured in Crete while serving with the 23rd Battalion (New Zealand), and taken as a prisoner of war (POW) to Stalag VIII-A in Görlitz, Germany (now Poland) — a very large and overcrowded camp which housed up to 30,000 POWs.[55]

After Mark was released and returned to New Zealand, he became very depressed, drank heavily, was suicidal and was hospitalised, including for a period at Queen Mary Hospital during the 1960s. How far-reaching and debilitating these after-effects were is evidenced by the fact that 20 years after the war the Dunedin branch of the RSA was providing welfare assistance to Mark and his wife. He died in 1968, aged 52.

Coroners' reports also reveal the long-term effects of war trauma that could lead to alcohol abuse, and eventually suicide. One former POW was prone to moody depression, which was often exacerbated by alcohol. His wife knew that the three-and-a-half years her husband had spent in a prisoner-of-war camp had 'affected his nervous system'. He committed suicide in 1960 in a very remote area of New Zealand.[56]

The camaraderie and resilience of POWs is celebrated in popular culture, but many POWs suffered psychiatric illness, especially upon returning to civilian life.[57] In 1953, a former soldier who had come home from the war with several shrapnel wounds frequently threatened to take his life when he was drinking.[58] His wife and his family did not take these threats

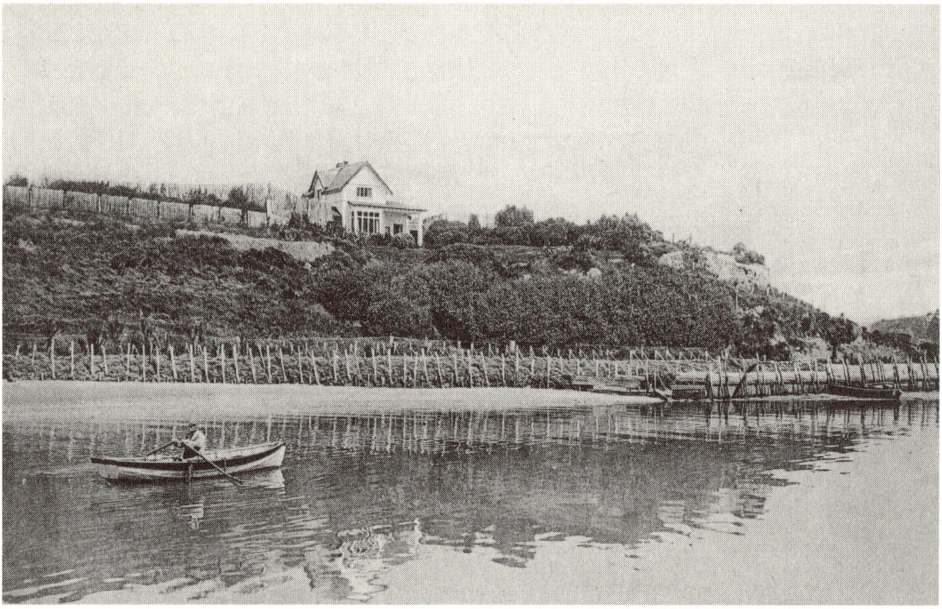

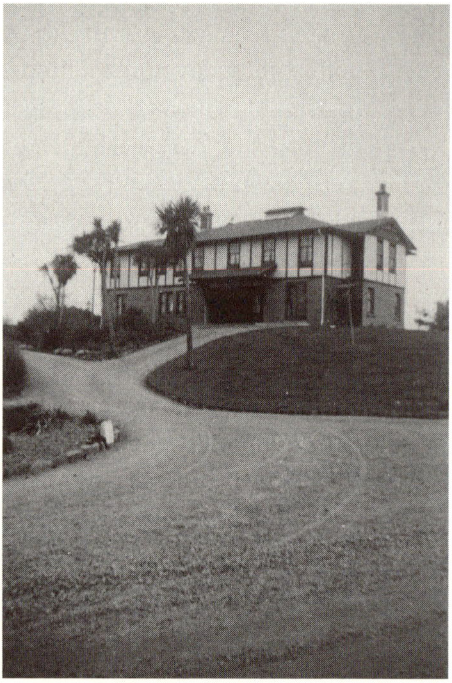

Clockwise from top left: Karitane House, where some of the mentally disturbed soldiers from the First World War were treated; First World War troops at Queen Mary Hospital, Hanmer; soldier resettlement schemes and rehabilitation could lead to depression. This cartoon depicts a returned soldier carrying an axe labelled 'government assistance' being urged over broken fences to the hill of success by a ghostly soldier; a morning at the Henderson RSA clubrooms, 1979–80; Clifton house at Seacliff, to where soldiers were committed under a magistrate's order.

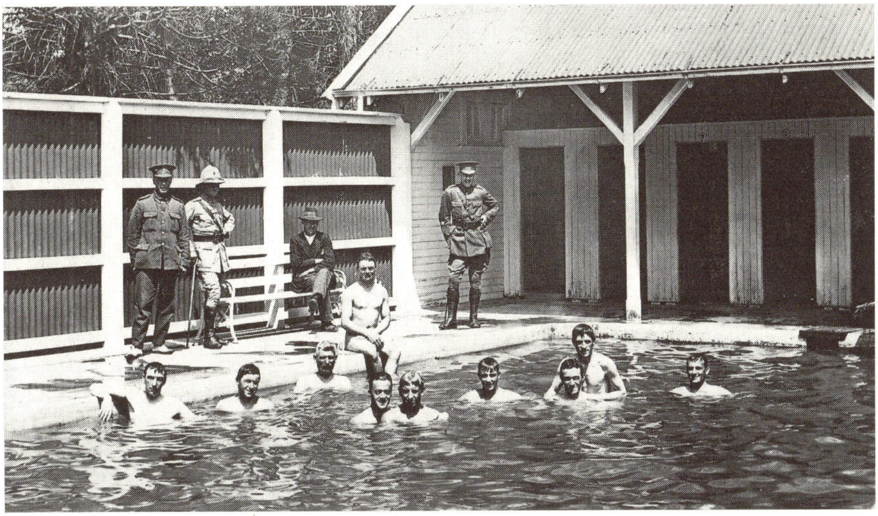

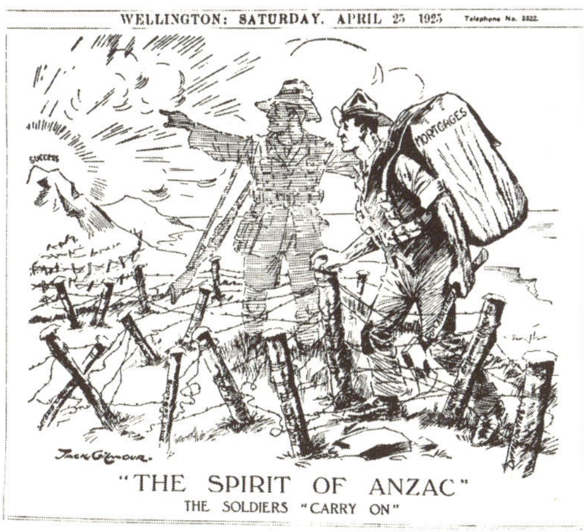
WELLINGTON: SATURDAY. APRIL 25 1925 Telephone No. 3322.
SUCCESS
MORTGAGES
JACK GILMOUR
"THE SPIRIT OF ANZAC"
THE SOLDIERS "CARRY ON"

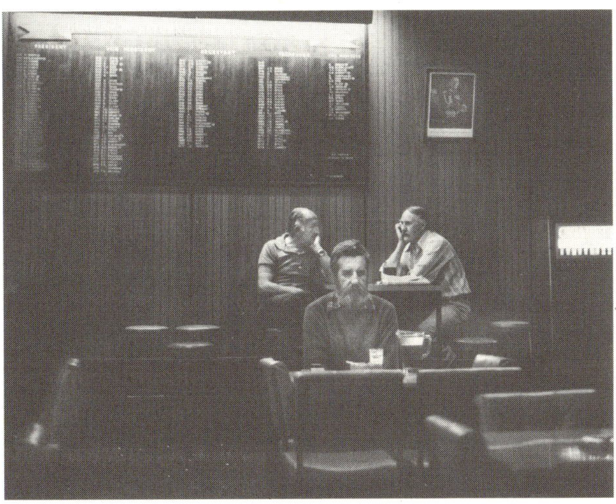

seriously, believing it to be just the drink and depression talking. However, in 1968 he fatally hanged himself.

The fallout from the psychological trauma of war could be ongoing for the partners and families of war veterans. Alcohol abuse was only one among many negative outcomes. Physical and mental impairment often meant that money was tight, especially during the economic downturn of the 1920s and the Great Depression, when unemployment was common and many businesses failed. The financial impact on families was again a serious issue after the Second World War, even during the years when the economy was more buoyant.

Before he served in the Middle East for three years, John had been a small business owner.[59] In 1942 he was shot at El Alamein, and thereafter experienced back and stomach troubles, and bladder weakness. When he returned to Dunedin in 1943, he suffered from 'nerves', and feeling unable to resume his former employment he retrained as a carpenter while also receiving a partial war pension. In 1949 John was briefly admitted to hospital with neurasthenia and depression. The depression became chronic, and by 1968 he was also anorexic and being treated with ECT and antidepressants.

Historian Tiffany Jenks's research into the welfare claims files of the Dunedin RSA reveals how cash-strapped Second World War veterans' families could be.[60] Depression could make it difficult for many men to return to fulfilling work or to retrain,[61] and an inability to concentrate made it hard to hold down a job.

Jenks's and Parr's research also revealed how the care of many returned servicemen fell upon their families, especially their wives, mothers and daughters. But emotional withdrawal or distancing from families was also a long-term effect of war's psychological trauma. Parr interviewed eight Second World War veterans and their wives and families to show how, almost half a century after the war had ended, these 'silent casualties' could still be prone to depression, with symptoms such as nightmares, uncontrollable anger outbursts, emotional withdrawal, war-time thoughts and sleep disturbance.

Tom May, a former tank driver, told Parr that he 'had my own secret little crack-ups where I wasn't bearing up to it and I'd just disappear and I'd have a little weep. You know you generally come right and forget about it — don't be such a silly bugger . . . I didn't want to mix at all. I just couldn't stand it, I couldn't stand people.'[62] After his war service he returned to farm work and married, but although he tried to hide his depression and anxiety, he suffered major breakdowns during the following decades. 'The nightmares, the depressions, the irritability, the emotional withdrawal — have all remained private.'[63] Although Tom was treated by the family doctor and prescribed medication, no link was made to any psychological trauma from the war.

Jack Marshall told Parr how the depression continued for years; he said of one man, 'he weeps easily "for a man"', unlike before the war.[64] There are many stories of Second World War veterans who never discussed their experiences of horrific combat, including having to kill young enemy men, with their children.

Depression could set in even before overseas service, which is possibly indicative of pre-existing conditions. In 1915 a 10th Reinforcements recruit, William H., proudly marched in the bright sunshine to the fanfare of Dunedin's St Kilda band. The soldiers had assembled before a large gathering of well-wishers and then had gone to the Dunedin railway station, where the mayor appealed to the pride of male sacrifice for the empire:

> On the field of battle the New Zealanders had shown themselves to be of indomitable courage, men with hearts of steel who would dare and do anything for the cause of King and Empire . . . Again we had to say good-bye to another band of men who were going out in the pride of their manhood to crush a haughty despot, and show that the men under the Southern Cross were not degenerate, but that the spirit of those who had made the Empire, and who laughed at difficulties and dangers, was still strong and vigorous amongst us.[65]

The mayor's words and the crowd's cheers must have reminded William of his earlier days as a stellar rugby player, a proud representative of the Otago province and his country in the late 1890s. But William had fallen from grace and had been suspended from the national team for drunkenness and bad language. He would never play first-class rugby again, and this probably precipitated his depression. The war gave him the chance to serve his country again, but he did not make it overseas. In 1916 William was transferred from the Featherston Military Camp to Seacliff for a brief period and was then discharged from the army.[66] He was very depressed, had delusions of persecution (attributed to 'alcoholic insanity'), and was diagnosed with melancholia.

William had volunteered for military service, as had Private Thomson in 1941. When he left Burnham Military Camp at 3 a.m. on 6 April to walk to Christchurch wearing only his slippers, he was in a state of 'extreme depression'.[67] He had suffered physical pain after scalding his foot, but his mental state had also deteriorated when he was transferred from a specialised military unit to the infantry.

> That had a bearing on his mental attitude. He was forced to leave his friends and familiar surroundings and was in a distinctly unhappy frame of mind when he took general leave, which itself was a very trying experience, what with the farewells and sadness, for any soldier. The bad scalding of his foot did not improve his outlook. He was caused considerable pain and shock and extreme depression.[68]

The war experience could certainly exacerbate pre-existing conditions, troubles and disappointments.[69] Captain M. H. Aiken, a physician with the New Zealand Medical Corps, found that 68 of the 100 cases of psychiatric casualties he examined among New Zealand troops in Italy had early life histories that were indicative of psychological instability. Sixty-three men had family histories of nervous or psychotic disorders. A startling 93 per cent of Aiken's sample of 68 showed 'evidence of early maladjustment, psychoneurotic family tendencies or faulty environmental factors'.[70]

Aiken outlined case 11, a 21-year-old infantryman who arrived in the Middle East in February 1944, and who from his first experience of action in April was very apprehensive, experiencing tremors, sweating and insomnia. After 10 days he developed cramping abdominal pains and lost his appetite. His dreams were consumed by the battle, and he lost interest and became increasingly withdrawn. On 15 July he broke down. He was admitted to hospital five days later, depressed and with a dull expression. Aiken considered the soldier's background to be pertinent. His mother had suffered a series of nervous breakdowns, and his father had been a chronic alcoholic until heart disease had made him an invalid. Several members of his family had nervous tendencies such as bed-wetting and sleepwalking.

Case 11 came from a 'very unsatisfactory home atmosphere . . . Parents continually at loggerheads. Much strife in the house and restriction of friendships outside the home,' the notes stated.[71] As a child he had wet the bed, sleepwalked, had nightmares and bitten his nails. He was bullied at secondary school, where he found it difficult to socialise. Aiken assessed this patient as having been a very insecure, unaggressive and dependent type. Today we might question whether these personality characteristics were abnormal, and would perhaps be more likely to accept that there were diverse personalities among the young soldiers who fought in traumatic battle conditions.

Perhaps more severe were the pre-existing factors and family circumstances of some of the cases in medical student Edward Hefford's study of 38 returned soldiers who were treated at Dunedin Hospital for war neurosis during the winter of 1942.[72] Case 27 was aged 38 and had served in the medical corps. After nearly a year overseas, he had become very depressed, nervy and uncontrolled, with lassitude and insomnia. A door had fallen on his head during childhood, and in 1938 he had had a 'nervous breakdown' following an unhappy marriage. Case 27 had tried to commit suicide on three occasions prior to his war service but he did not inform the medical board about this when he was accepted for hospital duties overseas.

Another soldier served overseas for nearly a year in the Greece and Crete campaigns without 'breaking down', but after he was admitted to hospital in Egypt with gonorrhoea he became depressed, restless and irresponsible, and showed signs of hysteria and schizophrenia. His father had suffered shell shock during the First World War, and his mother and sister had been patients in a mental hospital.

John Weaver's research on suicide during the twentieth century found that after both the First and Second World Wars returned service personnel had a significantly higher suicide rate than that of their civilian counterparts. While combat 'differentiated them', the researchers could not pin down how many soldiers had committed suicide as a result of depression. During the years sampled, 531 returned soldiers committed suicide; representing one in 15 male suicides (6.9 per cent).[73]

Not all had been diagnosed with depression, but a review of newspapers and coronial records reveals a startling correlation between depression and suicide among returned soldiers. The factors inducing depression and suicide ranged from relationship and family issues to unemployment, work stress and physical or mental problems caused by traumatic events. Many of these (mostly) men had returned to Aotearoa carrying the trauma of shell explosions, being gassed or being buried underneath rubble. Most were young, and lived in an era when the public expression of feelings, let alone any discussion of depression or suicidal ideation, was frowned upon.

Moreover, official figures did not reveal suicides or depression within the military camps. Figures for depression were possibly not kept, while suicides were not made public. Two rare occasions were in 1917 and 1918, when two recruits separately hanged themselves in the bush near Trentham Camp while suffering from mental depression.[74] The verdict 'while in a state of mental depression' was frequently returned at inquests into suicides, and equally applied to returned soldiers. Often the association of depression with shell shock was mentioned, as was ongoing depression that lasted long after the war's end.

News reports were often sensationalist, but many journalists and editors were also sympathetic to the plight of the returned soldier. For example, in 1930 the headline of a report on a suicide in Napier read 'Effects of war. Soldier's sad end. Fought Germans in sleep.'[75] The report of a returned soldier who threw himself under a train in 1925 in Port Chalmers 'while in a state of mental depression' was headlined as a 'sad sequel to shell shock'.[76]

Depression may have stemmed from horrific war combat, the memories of which haunted soldiers for the rest of their lives. Other traumatic crises could trigger a resurfacing of earlier anxiety and depression. Thomas, who was born in Scotland, served in the Highland Light Infantry during the First World War before emigrating to New Zealand in 1919.[77] His right arm had been amputated during the war, and he had been in hospital for two years while also suffering from shell shock. But Thomas's mental anguish and 'nerves' recurred during the Napier earthquake of February 1931, which decimated the cities of Napier and Hastings and killed at least 256 people. He was hospitalised, and in August 1932 he shot and killed himself.

Ben, another First World War combatant, returned to New Zealand suffering from neurasthenia but he had been able to find work. However he was re-traumatised by the Napier earthquake, after which he became dependent on a war pension and his wife for support. He spent six months at Queen Mary Hospital. By 1933 his depression had become so severe that he attempted suicide by taking all the sedative drugs he could find in his home.

Ben entered a mental hospital as a voluntary patient for six weeks, but again attempted suicide by charging his head into a wall. He was treated with shock therapy but discharged himself, against staff advice. Ben's wife, by now 'becoming more desperate', demanded that he be given a leucotomy — an operation in which the nerve fibres in the brain are cut (discussed in chapter 7) — a procedure she had read about in a magazine. Ben underwent the procedure, and awoke from the anaesthetic, in the words of Dr Donald McKenzie, 'chuckling', and returned home.[78]

The mental and physical impacts of war were often delayed or suppressed. Walter departed for overseas service in the First World War, leaving his wife with seven young children to care for. Being gassed in Europe left him suffering 'badly from rheumatism, heart trouble and nerves'.[79] The couple divorced in 1919. Walter worked as a paperhanger and painter, but by 1931, when his new partner could see that 'his war injuries [had] started to catch up with him', she sent him to Sydney on a 'health recruiting trip'. He returned home feeling much better, but within three months he was feeling unwell again and 'was drinking steadily'. Soon after, he had a motor accident and was charged with drunken driving, and in 1938 he committed suicide through carbon monoxide poisoning.

The same year another veteran of the First World War fatally shot himself.[80] During combat he had been buried by an exploding shell. His wife later recalled that at night when he felt depressed, he would often relive his war experiences and say that he could 'hear the shells whizzing. I think his mental condition was caused indirectly through the war . . . His nerves were all to pieces and he would sit with his head in his hands and cry like a child,' she said.

One farmer who suffered injuries and depression from his experience during the Second World War lived with his depression for 40 years before he fatally shot himself. By then his physical health had badly deteriorated.[81]

Charles was an immigrant from England who had lived with his brother. He became depressed when his brother embarked on overseas service. By then Charles was in his fifties and unmarried, and clearly he missed the only relative he had in New Zealand. In December 1942, Charles made the comment to his grocer that 'it was harder for those left behind than for those who had to go away' before fatally consuming the insecticide Blackleaf 40 in his bedroom in Christchurch.[82]

War meant separation, worry and grief — a multiplicity of darkness. Not long after 19-year-old Dulcie G. had married a soldier in 1916, he left to serve overseas.[83] She soon became violent and threatened to drown herself. Three months after her marriage she was admitted to Sunnyside with a diagnosis of sub-acute melancholia. Her husband died in action in Belgium in 1917 — the same year Dulcie was discharged from Sunnyside.

Another woman did kill herself after her husband 'went to the Front'. She suffered from depression due to his departure, 'the change of life' and also 'the strain of running their farm'.[84] In another case, a teenager expressed profound grief and was very despondent after two of his brothers were killed during the First World War. In 1924, at the age of 20, he shot himself with a rifle that had belonged to one of the brothers.[85]

Another farmer on a war pension had suffered shell shock and fever during the First World War. When, in 1944, he learned that his son had died while serving in the air force, he became depressed, and a week after he received a letter informing him that his son's effects had arrived in

Wellington he killed himself. We do not know what impact the double loss of her son and husband would have had on his wife.[86]

John Weaver cites instances of the tragic consequences for those who lost loved ones through war.[87] Thomas said that his wife was 'not in good health and was suffering from a nervous breakdown caused through the death of her son on active service'. She committed suicide in 1946. For others the pain of loss endured much longer than the actual war. Helen had suffered from 'nervous trouble' after learning that her husband had been tortured and murdered by the Japanese during the occupation of the Dutch East Indies (Indonesia). However, it was only six months before Helen took her own life in 1956 that she showed any signs of being depressed.

Guilt and shame about being unable to actively serve in war led some men to depression and even suicide. In 1921, 25-year-old Leslie, who had twice been rejected during the First World War as unfit for service because of his mental depression, shot himself.[88] In 1940 William P. became depressed because he had not volunteered for war service. He was worried that if he were to be selected his brother would be unable to work the family's sheep farms.[89] Instead, William's brother was called up and William then worried about his own capacity to run the farms.

After a suicide attempt, William voluntarily went to Dunedin's Ashburn Hall, and, according to his case notes, soon became 'a favourite with all', as he was cheerful, sociable and a good worker. When he was balloted for military service, the hospital's medical superintendent Dr Alexander Falconer advised the director of national service that William was a voluntary patient who had been overworked and needed a rest. When William left Ashburn, the prognosis was that the depression might persist. He returned to farming and died in 1988, aged 75.

The guilt or sense of failure of not being able to re-enlist and serve their country in the Second World War hit some First World War veterans. Gerald had suffered from shell shock and 'traumatic neurosis' after being buried in an explosion in that war. He was rescued on the verge of asphyxiation.[90] Gerald returned to Aotearoa and married in 1919, cared for two children and worked as a clerk in Greymouth. He was unable to concentrate, and this caused him more worry. When the Second World War broke out, Gerald had been excited about the prospect of rejoining the army, but after finding that he was unable to do this he hanged himself, in 1940, 'while in a state of acute mental depression'. Earlier that year he had also been informed by the authorities of the mental hospital where his wife was a patient that she 'would not recover'.

Another veteran of the First World War who had suffered ill health was also rejected from service in the Second World War. In 1940, and in 'a state of acute mental depression', he shot himself. He had written: 'Having been passed as an unfit Person to defend my country I feel I cannot go on with living on the food that Good soldiers need . . . You have all been wonderful please say good bye to all my Pals and ask them to remember me as they did in the old Days.'[91]

Two years later a grocer's assistant from Tīmaru who was living in Westport also committed suicide a few months after being called up for service. Soon after he entered camp, he was discharged 'as being medically unfit owing to . . . mental lapses'. His 14-year-old-son could see that his father, who had served in the First World War, 'was very depressed . . . He mentioned that he was old and could not get well.'[92]

The First and Second World Wars are pivotal in New Zealand's national history. By looking at wars, and at the challenging ways in which mental depression was manifested, through the lens of mental illness we can see the repercussions for veterans and their families. Some committed suicide, but others were eventually able to speak about, and come to terms with, their war trauma. Nevertheless 'soldiering on' could be a lifetime reality for old soldiers — as it was for many civilians — who suffered depression.

Considering depression in relation to war is complex. Although in many instances there was an obvious correlation with war trauma, sometimes the impact may be also have been connected to pre-existing conditions or earlier life experiences. Certainly, the post-war circumstances — be they personal, economic, physical, or the result of a lonely physical or emotional life — could exacerbate the double darkness of the connection between war and depression.

5.

Living with, and denying, the dark cloud

> One must concentrate on the periods in between — take charge of one's own life in those periods of stability.
>
> — *Meg Campbell*[1]

> This morning I thought I felt a kind of stirring in me — as if my spirit was about to soar, But it came to nothing. I felt like a hurt albatross trying to take off and not succeeding. But I shall soar again I promise you. I am in a kind of intermediate state in that I feel neither happy or unhappy — nor am I numb. Mostly I feel relaxed and secure. However, I'm improving every day.
>
> — *Alistair Te Ariki Campbell*[2]

Many of New Zealand's artists, writers and musicians have given voice to the experience of depression and melancholia through their work. Writers and artists can give us some insight into the ups and downs of depression, and strategies for living with it, and they often reveal a deeper self-awareness of this condition, which can be far more crippling than the profound sadness almost all of us experience.

Later in this chapter we discuss the flipside of awareness — the denial of depression — which is another way of living under the black cloud. While denying depression means that the root of the mental pain is not addressed and may lead to suicide, it equally may be the means through which many people work and create, fall in and out of love, raise children, worry and mourn — and may live into their senior years.

This chapter opens with quotations by Meg Campbell (1937–2007) and her husband, Alistair Te Ariki Campbell (1925–2009), both of whom suffered from depression but in quite different ways.[3] Alistair Campbell, a prominent novelist, poet, editor and playwright, spent a few months in Porirua Hospital as a voluntary patient in 1960. As he recalled in an oral history interview in 2004, he 'didn't go over the edge, wasn't psychotic, got close to it, I was never irrational — had a pain in my solar plexus — churning, churning away. Endless panic in the pit of my stomach. Didn't really "go nutty" at work. I kept it all under control . . . I was ill, I got through it and I found the experience interesting.'[4]

Campbell was born in Rarotonga, Cook Islands, in 1925.[5] His mother, Teu Bosini from Tongareva (Penrhyn atoll), had married his father, John (Jock), a Cook Islands storekeeper and trader who was originally from Dunedin. Alistair's depression may have stemmed from his childhood. In 1932, when he was seven years old, his mother died aged just 27, and a year later his deeply grieving father died from an undiagnosed illness. Alistair and his younger brother, Bill, left Rarotonga to join their older siblings, Margaret and Stuart, who were in the care of their grandmother in Dunedin.

She could not manage, and they were admitted to the Anderson's Bay Orphanage, where Alistair lived for six years, attending the local primary school and then Otago Boys' High School. He was clever, articulate, good at sport and good-looking. Still, he encountered racism. 'I denied my Polynesian heritage and recognised only my European side. I was divided; and this was to land me in a psychiatric hospital. I came right when I recognised what had been troubling me.'[6]

Melancholy is threaded throughout Alistair Campbell's poems, such as 'The Dark Lord of Savaiki' and in this excerpt from 'The Return':

> And again I see the long pouring headland,
> And smoking coast with the sea high on the rocks,
> The gulls flung from the sea, the dark hooded hills
> Swarming with mist, and mist low on the sea.

And on the surf-loud beach the long spent hulks,
The mats and splintered masts, the fires kindled
On the wet sand, and men moving between the fires,
Standing or crouching with backs to the sea.[7]

While he was a patient in the Porirua mental hospital Campbell wrote 'Personal Sonnets', about the deaths of his parents and his brother Stuart, who had died in the Second World War. *Sanctuary of Spirits*, a 1963 poetry collection about the Māori of Pukerua Bay and Kāpiti Island and the Ngāti Toa chief Te Rauparaha, is also very sombre. His novel *The Frigate Bird*, published in 1989, depicts the crazed unravelling of the protagonist, who is travelling to his ancestral home in the Cook Islands,[8] and was based partly on the diary Campbell kept during his first visit to Penrhyn in 1976, when he was mentally unwell. The diary was a 'life-line' to preserve his sanity.[9]

Twenty-year-old Meg Andersen, a drama student, met Alistair Campbell, 10 years her senior and divorced from the writer Fleur Adcock, at a party in Wellington in 1957. Within a year she was pregnant, married and had abandoned her acting career. She was admitted to Porirua Hospital 10 times between November 1958 and 1979; for four of these she was committed, the other six were voluntary admissions. Each of her admissions — from five weeks to two and a half months — were of comparatively short duration compared to many patients and the time she spent with her family between hospitalisations ranged from three weeks to seven and a half years.

During the mid-1960s Porirua Mental Hospital was a large facility with around 1600 patients. Meg Campbell was initially diagnosed with postnatal depression, later puerperal mania, and eventually manic depressive psychosis. She put this 'most unwanted gift — that of a blighted mind' down to heredity, the title she gave to a poem. In 1952 Meg's older sister Jane, aged 17, had been a patient for six months at Porirua, where she was diagnosed with depression.

Although Meg expressed that 'the diagnosis / is cause for anger at those / who brightly say we choose our destinies',[10] she wrote elsewhere that 'This diagnosis led to me being given the right medication, so I had a chance of a near normal life with my family.'[11] Meg credited her eventual recovery to her treatment by a psychologist, and attributed her being able to live with depression (and bipolar disorder) to the support of her 'many level-headed friends' and family. 'My children continued to relate to me as though I was a real person, and their claims, and their sweetness and natural warmth extricated me from the hospital many times. They tended to draw Alistair and myself together again.'[12]

Much later, in the 1990s, Meg wrote about her experiences, and those of others inside and outside Porirua Mental Hospital, with severe depression in an unpublished memoir, 'Arlin'. She wrote this of her friend Lisa, who committed suicide after suffering from profound depression.

> I had never seen anyone — anything — suffer for so long a period.
>
> But Lisa's relationships suffered under the pressure of her illness, as mine did. She sought out those pastimes she had found delightful as I did. She enhanced the lives of our children. She provided fun in her own unique way.
>
> Eventually she couldn't sustain this. Her life was not fun anymore. But she transmitted her vitality to her own lively and capable children. I didn't realise how close she was to death. I only knew that she was very ill, almost frozen in her speech and movements — eyes cast down, head bent. The transformation was quite terrifying. It was easiest not to see — to refrain from realising. I could only urge her to take her drugs, but she was deeply suspicious of drugs. Near the end she said to me, 'I just go to bed all the time. I can't get interested in anything . . .' Her voice was flat. I knew the seriousness of long term depression.[13]

Meg Campbell pinpoints the beginning of her own depression to paranoia after the birth of Aurelian, the Campbells' first child, who was born in 1958, six weeks after their marriage. Following a brief admission to Porirua Hospital, Meg returned to the family home at 245 Tinakori Road to care for her baby and Gregory, the four-year-old child of Alistair and Fleur Adcock. Meg 'was well and the awful depression had gone'. Yet the depression would return:

> Money was short, and I had become increasingly anxious, guilt-ridden and thoroughly depressed. The change in me baffled Alistair. I was a dead weight for him to carry, and he, it soon

> emerged, was also prone to depression. He became tight-lipped, and moody, escaping from me to drink with his friends when he could . . . I knew little about the subjects that interested my husband. I was more timid, and more self-doubting as time went on. I moped about. I was full of regret. None of this made me very attractive.
>
> The atmosphere was terrible. It took so little time for the whole relationship to crumble. I was a great disappointment to Alistair, to myself, and to Fleur who had relied on me to take care of Gregory. And there was Aurelian, yet I could barely find the energy to dress myself and brush my hair. My competence just didn't exist.

After Meg gave birth to Josie in October 1959, she suffered from what was termed 'puerperal mania'. Doctors warned the Campbells that she might suffer from this after each pregnancy. Meg later said, 'Sadly it happened over and over again . . . The family tottered. Time and again the children were split up and sent to stay with friends or were cared for in a foster home.' But in 1969, while in isolation at Porirua Hospital, Meg heard lines of verse in her head; she 'begged a pencil from a nurse, split open the sleeve of my Greys Tobacco packet, and wrote down on the cardboard the first lines' of what became her first published poem.

> **Solitary Confinement**
>
> Like a fisherman I wait
> until the words are caught
> on my line. My bait is silence,
> for between me and the world
> are locked doors, passages
> and more locked doors.
> There is no one else in this wing.
>
> It was peaceful this morning at dawn.
> I was locked up with my thoughts
> catching them on a hook
> as they darted about. My anchor
> settled in bright sand.

In the half light I peered
at the words sprawled on the page.
A bird sang in the hospital garden,
and outside the unbreakable
glass window the flowers grew
without supervision, and the sun
lifted into the sky of its own volition.[14]

Janet Frame, one of New Zealand's most famous international writers, was institutionalised for eight years at psychiatric institutions in Dunedin, Christchurch and Auckland, and vividly depicted mental illness in her books *Owls Do Cry*, *Faces in the Water* and *Scented Gardens for the Blind*, as well as in her three-volume autobiography.[15] When she was 21 Frame was admitted to Seacliff Mental Hospital. She was able to write, and in 1951 she was saved from a frontal lobotomy when her first book, *The Lagoon and Other Stories*, won the prestigious Hubert Church Memorial Award.[16] Frame had been misdiagnosed as schizophrenic but appears instead to have suffered periods of depression and anxiety.

The Aotearoa-born director Jane Campion adapted Frame's autobiography for the movie *An Angel at My Table*, in which Jane's mother, Edith Campion, a prominent actor and writer, played a cameo role as the school teacher, Miss Lindsay. Edith was herself hospitalised for depression at Ashburn Hall in 1980, and at various times at Porirua Hospital.

The academic Alistair Fox has explored how Jane Campion's family dynamics, including her mother's profound depression and loneliness, has influenced much of her work.[17] The writer Frank Sargeson summed up the link between creativity, the ordinariness of existence and depression in Edith's stories from *A Place to Pass Through*: 'the private agonies of the solitary individual made hopelessly lonely and depressed by entanglement in the day-to-day trappings of contemporary urbanised life'.[18] When Edith tried to commit suicide after her divorce from Richard Campion in the 1980s it was not the first time.

Jane Campion's recollection of her mother's 'complete lack of hope' reveals how intimate bonds thread through the ways in which people may be lifted out of the 'dark cloud'. When she was a teenager, Campion offered to help her very depressed mother die. Edith's response — 'I don't want to die, I don't want to die' — demonstrates the ambivalence of depression, suicide ideation and attempts, and how people and their families live through this suffering. In *Brainstorm*, a 1995 Australian television documentary on depression by Lina Safro, Campion recalled: 'I realised that my job was not to sort of see her in darkness, but say, "Oh, it's going to be better, you're going to get better."'[19] Fox suggests that this early insight may have influenced Campion's decision to end the movie *The Piano* with the depressed and suicidal protagonist Ada living instead of drowning.[20]

The writer and journalist Robin Hyde (Iris Guiver Wilkinson) was diagnosed with schizophrenia in 1933. Earlier, after her baby's death in 1927, she had been admitted to Queen Mary Hospital at Hanmer Springs with a diagnosis of postnatal depression. Hyde captured the essence of depression in her letters and publications, as doctoral student Alison Hunt summed up in 1995: 'Tiredness not only in its literal physical sense and in the sense of world-weariness, but also as a symptom of and euphemism for depression.'[21]

In 1933 Hyde, then a journalist working for the New Zealand *Observer* and a single mother, was living in Auckland and supporting her three-year-old son, Derek. These were tough economic times, and she was suffering from 'nerves' and influenza. After a row with her editor, she was walking down Auckland's Queen Street when 'a dark cloud came over her and the next thing she remembers is being hauled into a boat.'[22] Hyde had jumped off an Auckland wharf but was rescued, arrested by the police and then charged with attempted suicide. She was held in Auckland hospital for 18 days before agreeing to voluntary admission to the Auckland Mental Hospital in Avondale, where she stayed from 1933 until 1937. A psychiatrist prescribed 'bed-rest' in a private room in the low-security building known as the Lodge, which was located away from the main building. Hyde wrote that 'it was so very pleasant to lie here . . . The room grew dark and strange, but it was still pleasant.'[23] Her psychiatrist Gilbert Tothill encouraged her to resume writing, especially within an autobiographical genre.[24]

Despite mental and physical pain (an earlier knee injury had left Hyde with permanent mobility difficulties), economic hardship and complicated relationships, Hyde's brief life was one of prolific creative and journalistic output.[25] Alison Hunt's doctoral thesis outlined how the mental hospital provided space and freedom for Hyde to 'devote time to literary writing, which explains her productivity in times of wellness'.[26] Novels such as *The Godwits Fly*, *Wednesday's Children* and the autobiographical *A Home in This World* depict mental suffering and suicide within families, and among those mentally shattered by war.[27]

In 1938 Hyde set off alone for England, probably to gain further writing experience. She travelled across China, then in the midst of a war with Japan. Near the northern border, she was forced to flee the captured city of Hsuchow (Xuzhou) and suffered a serious eye injury.[28] She returned to Hong Kong for more treatment, and then sailed to London, where she continued writing and became active in left-wing groups. But she was virtually penniless and was in and out of hospital, 'suffering from depression, dysentery and anaemia'.[29] In 1939 Hyde committed suicide in London by taking an overdose of the amphetamine Benzedrine.

Creativity and work were often the one constant that kept depressed people going, but, as with Hyde, the pain of mental and physical illness could sometimes prove too much.

During the 1940s the artist Rita Angus also suffered severe depression, and between 1949 and 1950 she became a patient at Sunnyside Hospital, where she was encouraged to keep painting. The art writer Greg O'Brien described her work at this time as 'very calm', but in later years she went on to produce highly original pieces. 'She kept reinventing herself . . . The painting was her lifeline.'[30]

James Courage,[31] the author of five novels set in Aotearoa, considered his family background to be instrumental in his depression and anxiety. Being homosexual in an era when it was condemned as both immoral and criminal created a further strain. He grew up on a farm near Christchurch and in adulthood, under psychoanalysis, he came to view his relationship with his parents as dysfunctional. He was cared for by a nanny and felt that his mother, Zoe, had abandoned him. His father, Frank, 'was a hostile, domineering tyrant' who could not accept that his son had eschewed

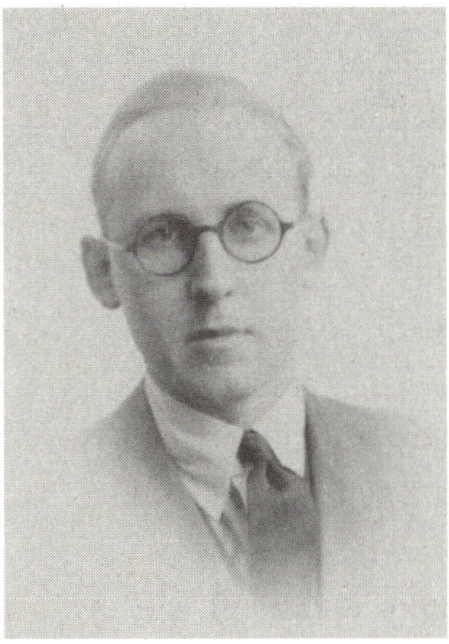
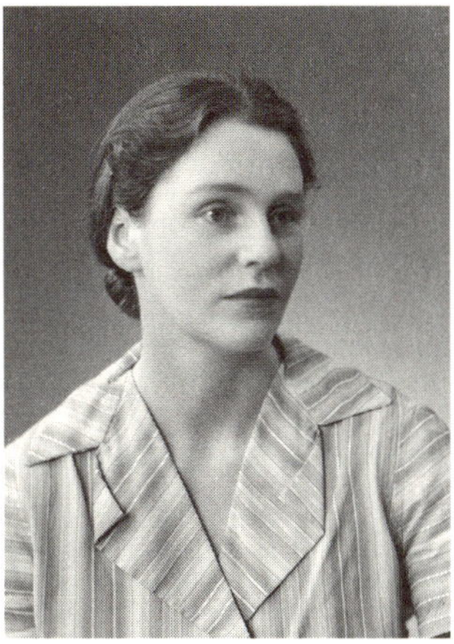
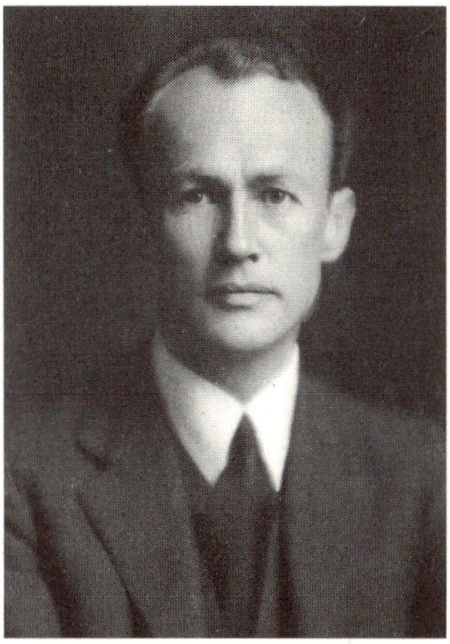
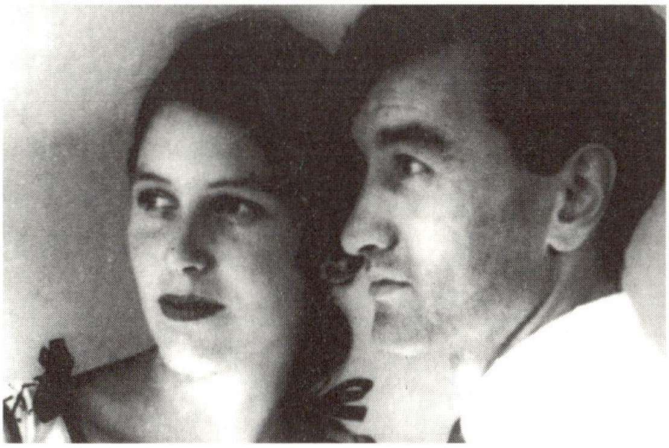

Clockwise from top left: Author James Courage; journalist and author Robin Hyde spent time at Queen Mary Hospital and Auckland Mental Hospital; Dr Ivan Sutherland was a patient at Ashburn Hall in 1951; poets Alistair Te Ariki Campbell and Meg Campbell both suffered from depression. Meg spent several periods at Porirua Hospital between 1958 and 1979.

farming for writing. 'He simply regarded me as no good, ineffective, a sissy — no proper son for him to have engendered.'[32]

Courage lived mostly in England, and began to suffer from depression while at Oxford University. On 13 July 1932, Courage wrote in his diary: 'Appalling depression — really rock bottom — everything in the world went black. This culminated in the evening when I burst into tears when Mrs M. came to see me, and wept for an hour and a half. I really think she saved me from suicide.' Courage's mood subsequently improved, and by 16 July he was 'feeling much stronger: despondency vanished'. These words may suggest a see-saw nature to his depression, or what doctors sometimes dismissed as hysteria or neuroticism. The depression was ongoing and linked to stress. He described the years during which he worked long hours in a bookshop and then wrote late at night as filled with 'depression, much anxiety, homosexual guilt, tension, stomach pains, inadequacy feelings'.[33]

The connection between stress and depression and personal, family and professional pressures was evident in the life of the academic Ivan Lorin George Sutherland, who was admitted as a voluntary patient to Ashburn Hall in Dunedin during October 1951. At his admission he was adamant: 'this cannot be happening to me — I lecture in philosophy and psychology — I cannot believe it — besides my mind is perfectly clear'.[34] Sutherland had recently returned to work after a year's sabbatical from Canterbury University College, a period during which he had planned to research and write a significant book on Māori, their welfare needs, social-psychology and race relations in Aotearoa.

The sabbatical should have been a relaxing but productive year, free from teaching and administrative responsibilities. However, while on leave Sutherland continued to work at an unrelenting pace: accepting several requests to lecture and present broadcasts, travelling extensively throughout the North Island to visit Māori communities and attend hui, accompanying Ernest Corbett, minister of Maori affairs, and senior government officials, as well as on his own research trips, and providing advice and writing reports for the university and then Department of Maori Affairs.

Like some high achievers, Sutherland found it hard to say no and, it seems, was consumed by a sense of duty, regardless of the impact on his mental health. Moreover, he considered that his goal of publishing his life's work was derailed when, during his sabbatical year, a former student,

Ernest Beaglehole, published on race relations in New Zealand in an international journal.[35]

Sutherland's academic anxiety was compounded by a difficult relationship with his colleague, the esteemed philosopher Karl Popper, a Jewish émigré from Austria. In 1936 Popper and Sutherland both applied for the chair in philosophy at Canterbury University College. Sutherland was appointed as professor, and Popper as a lecturer. Popper — who had an international reputation, whereas Sutherland did not — resented being Sutherland's junior.[36] Sutherland found Popper argumentative and uncooperative. He was also trying to juggle his academic and community commitments with his devotion to and love for his wife, Nancy, and five children, while also maintaining a large property at Cashmere, near Christchurch.

It is perhaps not surprising, then, that on 21 September 1951 Sutherland's doctor, D. E. Currie, began to treat him for a 'nervous disorder'. Sutherland was suicidal and, after initially refusing, he agreed to be admitted to Ashburn Hall. He was diagnosed with involutional melancholia — as we learnt earlier, a term in common use for 'middle-age' depression. In fact, Sutherland told Ashburn's medical superintendent, the psychiatrist Reginald Medlicott, he had suffered from depression much earlier, when living in London during 1922–1923 and trying to complete his doctorate from the University of Glasgow, and again in 1947 when serving as an honorary major lecturing to Jayforce, the New Zealand forces that were part of the British Commonwealth Occupation Force in post-war Japan.[37] Sutherland said that this depressive episode was precipitated by having to decide to purchase a home and large property in Christchurch.

Sutherland was treated with electroconvulsive therapy (ECT) at Ashburn Hall. Only nine days after admission, he left against Medlicott's advice. He told his wife that he would never return to a mental asylum, and that nobody was to know about his breakdown or time at Ashburn.[38] On 21 February 1952 Sutherland disappeared. Ten days after an extensive search by family, friends and associates throughout the country, his body was discovered by two schoolboys in a paddock at Sumner in Christchurch.

Sutherland was held in high esteem by Māori, especially Ngāti Porou, who had respectfully named him Paikea, after one of their legendary tīpuna. He had a close relationship with Ngāti Porou leader (and minister of native affairs from 1928 to 1934) Apirana Ngata. Sutherland wrote *The Maori Situation* in 1935, which was:

> a plea to his fellow-European for a more sympathetic, a more intelligent, understanding of the Maori point of view . . . By his writings, his spoken words, his personal dealings with Maori and Pakeha, Sutherland stood with a few others — some would say he was first in recapturing and strengthening mutual respect and understanding between the two races in New Zealand.[39]

A tribute in *The Journal of the Polynesian Society* testified to Sutherland's warm character and intellect. His friend John Beaglehole (Ernest Beaglehole's brother) wrote: 'There can have been few men in New Zealand who were so kind, or who took such an unforced, simple pleasure in being kind . . . I think second of his enthusiasm — for people, for things, for causes.'[40]

The educationalist and lecturer Arnold Campbell and public servant Dick Campbell jointly wrote of Sutherland: 'He always gave the impression of being intensely alive. There was a dramatic quality about him, which showed itself in his ways of thinking, his conversation, his teaching. Nothing he took up was done half-heartedly.' Ivan Sutherland was 54 when he ended his life.

We can see that many prominent sufferers of depression in Aotearoa have left a creative or academic legacy through which they communicated their pain but also their joy, enthusiasm and wonder, even when their lives ended in suicide. Many who live under the dark cloud of depression also experience periods of brightness; they have habits, work and relationships, culture, faith and convictions that provide meaning and structure to daily life, and ways to deal with bigger existential questions.

In 1981, the Kiwi band Blam Blam Blam released the song 'There is no depression in New Zealand', whose ironic lyrics highlighted the economic downturn in New Zealand and the civil and racial unrest brought by the impending national Springbok rugby tour. The song's title could also be said to evoke the Kiwi trait of avoiding, denying or silencing mental depression. Clichés, usually heavily gendered, such as 'She'll be right', 'Grin and bear it',

'Be a man', 'Don't be a wuss' have been incorporated into national narratives of stoicism, practicality and of not being emotionally flamboyant. Alistair Fox has explored how the novels of Maurice Gee, Stevan Eldred-Grigg, Witi Ihimaera and Alan Duff highlight how the gendered aspects of Pākehā and Māori cultures and the 'historically conditioned forces at work' have damaging psychic impacts on men.[41]

Denying depression is how many people in Aotearoa have lived under the dark cloud. This complicates distinguishing melancholia and depression as mental conditions or mental illness, as distinct from the more general experience of life's woes, sadness and worry. Again, the experiences of ex-servicemen reveal how depression, with the additional legacy of war trauma, could persist. Returned soldier Jack Marshall suffered from depression long after the Second World War, but suppressed his feelings. 'I'm very sensitive to my responsibilities with my wife and children. And so it was my sense of responsibility that just took me through the motions. I never really enjoyed my jobs. But I've just had to keep going,' he told Alison Parr in 1995.[42]

The weight of hiding depression could be too much for some. A graduate of the Otago Medical School who specialised in psychiatry at the Maudsley military hospital in London before the Second World War went on to become a veteran of that war. He attained the rank of major in the Royal Medical Corps, serving in a psychiatric unit on the front at Normandy, and at other psychiatric hospitals in Europe.[43] He treated soldiers with war trauma, including depression, and published an article on it. In 1946 he returned with his family to Aotearoa to take up a position as a medical officer at a psychiatric hospital. In 1948, aged 40, he committed suicide through barbiturate poisoning. He left a note stating:

> I bitterly regret it but cannot struggle on any longer. I know I can never get over this depression. I have struggled against it with varying success for so many years and I can't struggle any longer. Don't blame anyone but me — it's unfortunate I was just made so that I could not cope with things properly . . . I have been trying for half my life to conceal my depression and my general incompetency. I hope you and the children don't think too badly of me and do believe that at least up to now I have

> done my very best to carry on. I have reached the end of my resources and if I tried to keep going I would only pull you all down too.

The psychiatrist's obituary acknowledged that his death was a great loss to the profession, and that he was held in high esteem by colleagues and patients.

The denial of depression, the refusal or inability to discuss it, and the attempt to be seen as an 'independent man' features in many suicide reports. So, too, does worry over matters that others might let pass. Many wives had insights into the depression and worry their husbands may have concealed for years, but others were not aware of why their husbands killed themselves. The economic reforms of the late 1980s proved too much for some small business owners and farmers. The wife of one man said that he had been an independent person who had thought that he would be able to sort out his own problems, but always worried about things that other people just took for granted. His way of coping with his anxiety and depression was to work at his business for very long hours.[44]

As we saw in chapter 1, the distinction between sadness and depression was noted as early as 1898 by *The Auckland Star*, which reported on a lecture on melancholia delivered overseas by Dr Burnet of Kansas City Medical College.[45] 'In ordinary sadness there is a cause comprehensible to the individual, and he will seek to remove it. In melancholia there is no apparent cause.' Burnet's dichotomy was simplistic because sadness is not always easily traced to a cause, while reasons for melancholia were often given by sufferers and observers.

Much later, in a 1964 article in the *N.Z. Family Doctor*, Dr Hugh Freeman addressed the question of when sadness ceased to be normal and became an illness. One of his answers was that this depends on the usual personality of the person. Freeman wrote that when depression 'becomes a misery that fills a person's whole life and takes the pleasure out of everything that he usually likes, it has gone beyond the limits of normal feeling . . . Probably the best guide is the fact that the sadness is not relieved by distractions,

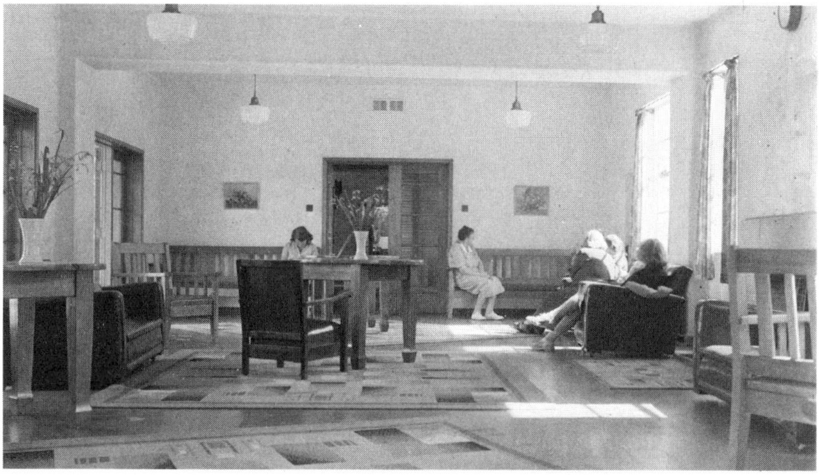

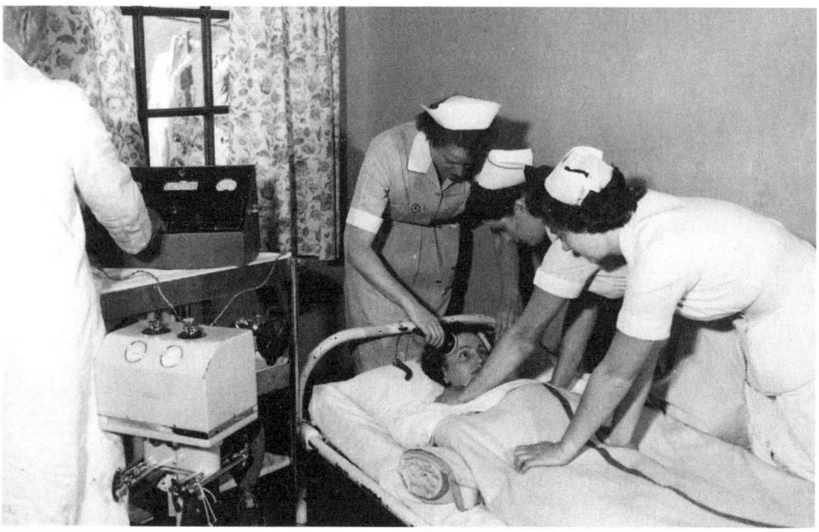

Above: A day room at Porirua Hospital in the 1950s. *Below:* A 'mock' electroconvulsive therapy training session at Porirua Hospital. In this unmodified-treatment scene the 'patient' (a nurse playing the role) is being restrained to prevent injury. In the early years of the treatment, anaesthetics and muscle relaxants were not used but these later became standard and were delivered by injection, given by an anaesthetist.

such as going out to an entertainment or having friends come in to visit.'[46]

During the 1960s an older woman who relocated from a city to a rural area felt that she had no friends and became lonely and depressed.[47] Her husband's attitude followed that of his parents, that mental and physical illness could be overcome through the power of positive thinking. She told student researcher H. M. Horton 'there was nothing wrong in her life, "so if you convinced yourself that this was so [that there was nothing wrong] you became well"'. The woman had several 'breakdowns', and felt suicidal, yet, despite consulting various doctors and spending periods in two different psychiatric hospitals, she explained to Horton that between these times of depression she was 'perfectly well'. Her Christian faith was strong during these times of wellness, but, as she told a clergyman, when having suicidal thoughts, 'you have no belief in anything'.

Debates about 'normal sadness' as distinct from a diagnosis of medicalised depression have persisted since the 1960s, mainly outside Aotearoa. The American academics Allan Horwitz and Jerome Wakefield argued in 2007 that the tick-boxes of symptoms used by many health professionals for diagnoses of depression subsumed and silenced the human condition of sadness and created depression as a disorder.[48]

In 2015 Francis O'Gorman, a professor of English literature at the University of Edinburgh, published a history of worrying that argued that the contemporary concept of worry was part of modernity: 'Worry is not a disease, not the same as saying, "I am dispirited" or "I am depressed": Worry is a form of fretfulness, of mental uncertainty and persistently tremulous bother . . . mostly, an everyday one; a habit of thinking that keeps falling out of any formal definition of "mental illness".'[49]

The British psychiatrist and academic Derek Summerfield has cautioned against relegating terms such as 'distress', 'sadness', 'despair', 'gloominess' and 'pessimism' to the hold-all of depression.[50] Alain Ehrenberg, a French sociologist, considered that depression 'had become a tool to define much of our woe and, through various means, to lighten our load'.[51] This assessment seems rather harsh, and I concur with Jonathan Sadowsky that depicting depression as 'fashionable' or due to life's woes can deny the profound despair with which people who are depressed or diagnosed with depression live.[52]

Through researching thousands of coronial inquest reports during the twentieth century in Aotearoa, historian John Weaver's team interrogated whether suicides were due to some form of 'mental health motive', which they estimated at between 25 and 40 per cent.[53] They suggest that this figure would have been higher if substance abuse was included. Other leading motives that they categorised for suicide were work or finance, marital or romantic, and physical ailments. These motives were considered against different historical contexts within eras of social and economic change in Aotearoa, categories that did not fall under mental illness, but perhaps could be considered as part of life's woes.

Weaver was not convinced that almost a quarter of all suicides from 1900 to 1950 were due to what doctors during the late twentieth century would diagnose as clinical depression.[54] Instead, he emphasised historical sources of stress such as war or economic depression as having a causal effect on suicide numbers. To my understanding, although suicide statistics may have fluctuated according to historical periods, this does not necessarily negate the fact that suicide victims may also have been depressed. Coroners' reports often concluded that a person died of self-inflicted injuries while in a state of mental depression. Weaver argues that the discourse of 'depression' — so often reported by witnesses and coroners — served the cultural function of explaining a suicide as irrational without suggesting madness.[55]

Otago medical student Conan Fowler wrote in 1972 that 'the diagnosis of depression involves distinguishing it from healthy unhappiness . . . In healthy unhappiness a person can seek advice and gain help from friends, relatives or from spiritual sources. A depressed person, however, is handicapped by a disturbance of primitive, central, regulating mechanisms with alteration of mood and outlook.'[56] This distinction infers that the barrier to seeking help comes from within, but looking for support is also difficult within a society where depression is not openly discussed or brings stigma, and where there may be few resources available for mental health.

The historical evidence that I examined — medical records, coroners' reports, newspapers and memoirs — indicates that there was a fine line between 'taking it on the chin', and coping with minor and major issues that were worrying, and when this worry fell into melancholia or depression.

John G. was diagnosed with melancholia while at Seacliff from 1915 until 1917.[57] He arrived after attempting suicide and came with a long list of 'life's woes'. His case notes suggest that he tended to 'blame himself for worrying in excess of what might have normally been caused by these reasons'. Those reasons included losing investments in a dredging boom in 1903, the death of at least three out of seven children born between 1901 and 1908, and, in 1910, the destruction of his rental house in a fire. His case records recorded a 'loss of emotional control', and his wife said he threatened her and failed to provide support.

John's depression worsened after he was fined because his children were not attending school, and after facing legal action when his pig uprooted a neighbour's garden. It was likely that he would lose his job because he had been before the court. Around 1921 he and his wife divorced, but he lived on for a further 21 years, until his death in 1942, aged 79. John certainly experienced his fair share of problems throughout his life (albeit some perhaps of his own making), but his melancholia was linked to excessive worry. Some people might have been able to shrug off these woes, but John worried so much that he was committed to a mental hospital.

Academics and medical professionals have debated the distinction between the burden of life's woes and depression, as most of us have. Being unable to cope with life's stresses when it appears that others can compounds the pain and denial of depression. A patient described in medical student J. B. Aubrey's 1973 research in Dunedin shrugged off her despair: 'Plenty of other people go through far worse troubles but then they cope quite well. I am an inadequate person, I suppose.'[58] Others in this study regarded their inability to cope with the 'normal stresses expected in life' as a failing, or that requiring medication for the 'maintenance of normality indicates some inadequacy'.

This contrasted with physical illness, which 'is something the patient has no control over but is obvious and readily explained'. These patients' self-assessments are illuminating — not only pinpointing guilt, anxiety and denial, but also raising the question of what constitutes 'normal' stress.

It may seem incongruous to discuss attempted suicide and suicide in a chapter that has promised to speak to how people have led complex lives while dealing with depression. Suicide and attempted suicide are threaded through our history of depression, along with other ways in which people have reacted to stress, whether stemming from personal relationships or caused by external factors such as war or work.

Attempted suicides were recorded when they came to the attention of medical and police authorities, but many more attempts (or thinking about suicide, as in 'suicide ideation') were never recorded. For example, when H. M. Horton examined suicide-related statistics for 1964 in Aotearoa, he ascertained that 207 people had died and another 900 had been admitted to hospital for attempted suicide; however, the actual number of attempted suicides would have been much higher, as many of those who tried to take their own lives did not ever come to the attention of authorities.[59]

I recall that as a young person during the 1970s in Dunedin there were times when depression and other factors precipitated some of my peers to attempt suicide through overdosing with prescribed drugs or slashing their wrists. We tried to make sure our friends purged the toxins, and we applied plasters and bandages to the cuts. Sometimes we knew someone who could stitch up cuts 'off the record'. These kinds of suicide attempts have never been notified, either to authorities, or often to families.

Sometimes it was only by chance that a fatality was averted. In 1914 a 'butcher's boy' in Denniston on the West Coast discovered 53-year-old Elizabeth T. hanging by a rope from the ceiling. He cut her down and she was admitted to Seaview mental hospital with melancholia.[60] This was not her first attempt to kill herself; earlier she had tried to throw herself onto a railway line. Elizabeth attributed her condition to the 'recent troubles' in Reefton, where there was an industrial strike and a lock-out of miners. Her 'troubles' were also as a mother who had seen too many of her children die — eight of 12. She became very low when she was alone.

Elizabeth was discharged from Seaview in 1923, but attempted suicide again. Early one morning she left her bed and was later found at the bottom of a cliff by a miner. She was bleeding heavily from the head and admitted to hospital.[61] But as Seaview's medical superintendent had remarked in 1914, she was also 'a cheerful looking woman, fond of a joke, and rational in conversation, in fact the last case one would expect to be suicidal'. She appeared to cheer up when she had people with her. Despite her depression and suicide attempts, Elizabeth lived until the age of 81, dying in 1942.

Annie S. lived a lonely life as a wife of a farmer on a large high-country sheep station in Canterbury.[62] In 1915, aged 50, she was admitted to Seacliff after throwing herself out of a window when she was in a state of 'extreme mental depression', although her first 'attack' had been when she was 26 years old. Annie had previously tried to drown herself and injure her children and others. Her husband told medical superintendent Truby King that her symptoms began when she was nursing her first child. Annie died in 1936 in Tīmaru, aged 71.

In 1967 Otago medical students H. M. Horton, S. D. R. Lang and R. T. Lienert completed dissertations on depression and attempted suicide.[63] Participants discussed strategies that helped them cope with their depression. One man who was admitted as a voluntary patient to a psychiatric hospital in Otago after a suicide attempt had become depressed, anxious, withdrawn and unable to sleep, and said that he was always lonely. A turning point came when he realised the kindness of neighbours, who provided transport to enable his wife to visit him in the psychiatric hospital. 'People were not against him.' He said that his main purpose in life 'is to give all to his children'.

In 1966, Lang interviewed 12 patients who had been admitted to Ward 10 at Auckland Public Hospital during a two-month period for attempting suicide with analgesics and/or soporific substances. Three-quarters reported insecure childhoods, with parental arguments, separation, absence, financial worry and frequent house shifts. One participant, who had overdosed on barbiturates, articulated how depression and suicidal thoughts could creep up: 'I am so sorry that I took them — I was saved, that's the main thing. It is better to be alive — there is hope . . . I was just so miserable. I have enjoyed my life. I certainly never thought about suicide. I don't know just when I started to be depressed.' Her husband's recent death was undoubtedly a significant contributing factor.

Lienert, who interviewed 14 patients at Cherry Farm Hospital who had attempted suicide, found that depression was a common factor. As noted earlier, though, precise figures for the links between depression and attempted suicide are elusive because attempts do not always come to the attention of medical or police personnel. Mr R., who had considered suicide, had been treated for depression since he was 22 years old, first by the family doctor, then at the psychiatric department at Dunedin Hospital, at Ashburn Hall, and several times at Seacliff, where he had shock and drug therapy during the 1960s.[64] He said he had no problems or worries, and thought it would be good to stay at Seacliff permanently. He returned to his clerical job, but rarely socialised.

Living under the dark cloud has been particularly challenging for specific sectors in Aotearoa, such as those within rural communities. As seen in chapters 2 and 3, the stresses faced within these environments have been present since colonial times. Māori were dispossessed of their whenua and resources. Arcadian dreams were never fulfilled for many immigrants. While the reality of rural life, and of being a farmer, has long displaced earlier bucolic fancies, there remain high rates of depression and suicide in rural communities, although not at especially higher rates than within other communities in Aotearoa. Pressures include economic and environmental challenges, and the denial of depression.

The historians John Weaver and Doug Munro have drawn attention to how the New Zealand rural dream and the vagaries of expansion and prosperity could, when a rural downturn set in, induce misery and suicide for some. As noted in chapter 4, the years of economic downturn during the 1920s and the Great Depression were especially felt by returned soldiers, who may have also suffered war-related mental and physical disabilities. Some may have been frustrated with the harsh, seemingly unending labour involved in clearing primary or secondary bush on land-settlement scheme blocks.

Weaver and Munro stress that the high rates of suicides in the rural sector between 1900 to 1950 were 'not caused by rural life *per se*. But a privileging of agriculture through a national myth obfuscated the challenges of farming in a market economy and passed over crises experienced by the exploited but essential rural labourers (including Māori) and the burdens of rural women.'[65] They suggest that 'rural men coped less successfully or felt the crises more intensely'.[66] For example, when a 51-year-old who had unsuccessfully tried to take his own life was asked why he had shot himself, he replied: 'There is no grass, the cows are starving. A cow kicked over a bucket this morning and that was the end of everything.'[67]

When research scientist and suicide expert Annette Beautrais researched rural suicides between 2007 and 2015, she found that mental illness — particularly, depression, anxiety and substance abuse — was common, along with other problems, such as the declining physical health of older farmers.[68] Relationships, legal, work and financial stress contributed to suicide risk, but these were also widespread in the general population.

The question remains as to when and why problems in daily life and general economic crises induce more than profound sadness, anger and interpersonal tension among rural people. Coroners' records are replete with reports of financial worry among farming families, along with mental depression and suicide. In 1940 at Selwyn, in Canterbury, an employee noted that his boss was 'worried about farm transactions and in a highly nervous condition', while his wife knew that he was very upset about selling his farm and being unable to acquire another suitable one.[69] This man committed suicide in 1945.

During the late 1950s another farmer's wife observed that for several years her husband had suffered periods of acute mental depression and threatened suicide. He was treated by a doctor specialising in 'nerves', who suggested treatment at Porirua Hospital after the farmer attempted suicide. He chose instead to return home, and soon after, over Christmas, shot himself. A tipping point was possibly a high mortgage, but he had also been seriously affected by the death of a son 11 years earlier.[70]

Mental depression may have been acute in rural areas during the Great Depression, and again since the 1980s, but all had not been not well down on the farm during much earlier times. As we saw in chapter 3, isolation and a harsh working environment could induce depression in the 'lonely land'. Jacob H. lived until he was 82, dying in 1943, but in 1914 he had been admitted to the Auckland Mental Hospital.[71] At the time he was a farmer in the Franklin district, leading a solitary life, and he became despondent and depressed because of a lack of income and being unable to find work. He told a doctor in the hospital that 'his thoughts were jumping through his head and that he was going to fly apart'.

In 1915 two farmers, Angus M. and Donald G., both in their early fifties, and both from Maungatua in Taieri, were admitted to Seacliff within two days of each other with melancholia caused by worry. Angus was unmarried and, according to his brother, a hotel keeper in Mosgiel, had 'been brooding much over the loss of a farm' that he had operated for 21 years.[72] Angus said 'that there is nothing left for him now and at times he would like to die . . . in one of these fits of depression he did try to shoot himself'. Angus's depression was especially marked in the morning. He had eight siblings, but had led a lonely life for many years and had hoarded his money. After his discharge from Seacliff in 1917 he later resumed farming near Tīmaru, and died in 1931, aged 68.

Donald's melancholia was also induced by 'life's woes' — in this instance, financial worry — but it seems that once he began to experience melancholia he was also troubled by his family's history of mental illness. It was an era when this was considered hereditary.[73] His uncle had been a patient at the Seacliff asylum for several years and had died there, and one of his sisters had also been admitted to Seacliff for three months. Another sister, a farmer's wife in Maungatua, hanged herself in her bedroom a year before Donald was committed to Seacliff. The inquest revealed that for many years she had been low, depressed and melancholic.[74] Donald spent five months in Seacliff, returning home to his wife. He died in 1933, aged 70.

It is not known what life had dealt Donald's sisters, but the story of Margaret H., a farmer's wife and also from Maungatua, indicates that it was not only men who experienced 'life's woes' in rural Aotearoa.[75] She married at 22, and 13 years later, in 1905, was admitted to Ashburn Hall for five months. By then she had given birth to six children, one of whom was stillborn. Margaret became worried when her husband decided to buy a farm in Southland, and she experienced melancholia and 'marked depression', considering herself unworthy and about to die and fearing that her children would be taken from her.

She was discharged after around four months in Seacliff, but although she returned to take care of her family she believed that her husband wanted to get rid of her. Her husband died 10 years later, and Margaret lived near Milton until 1941.

As we have seen throughout this chapter, while some lives, such as Robin Hyde's, are cut short, many people live long lives through which their depression is either intermittent or persistent. Depression does not necessarily lead to suicide, and nor does it mean unremitting sadness and apathy. People living under the black cloud can be creative, busy and caring, but their lives can also be mundane, or taken up with the daily business and crises of survival. Some come to terms with their depression, perhaps through personal insight, the support of loved ones, or with one of the treatments discussed in chapter 7.

How do those with depression, their families, communities and the medical profession consider depression? Is it a serious mental disorder, a mood, part of life's woes, or even — as a former patient described it — an 'untouchable disease'? 'It was as though I'd been in a leper colony . . . People would look at me with great concern and ask: "How are you?" I felt like saying: "I've done something you haven't done. I've been round the twist and back again."'[76] These words speak to survival, but they also show how so often this struggle has been against the denial and stigma of depression.

This chapter opened with words written by two of New Zealand's great writers, Alistair Te Ariki Campbell and Meg Campbell, who lived together with depression. But depression also tore them apart. When I read their letters to each other I was struck by their mutual love and passion, but also by the ordinariness of their lives as they raised a family and dealt with a range of problems, from paying the bills to infidelities. Their experiences shine through in their collection *It's Love, Isn't It?*, published the year after Meg's death and the year before Alistair's.[77]

Dreams of Porirua Hospital

You were on the far side of the lake,
dancing among the tall grasses,
smiling at your hands,
weaving before your face — like moths,
like white moths.

When you came to me,
you wore a white slip — nothing else.
You were cold and wet from the lake.
When *they* came in,
we were still embracing
and you were still shivering.

They came across the frosted grass
in their great policeman's boots,

cracking the moon
in the iced puddles.

I had to empty out my pockets
like a common criminal.
How could I explain the flowers
you gave me — the wild flowers —
your love letters,
the words worn smooth as pebbles?

I have your love words still,
so thin and transparent with neglect.
How could they give them back,
and laugh!
I will take them down to the beach,
I will call out your name —
please, listen —
I will send them skimming the waves
all the way to the open sea.

— *Alistair Te Ariki Campbell*

6.

Depression, ethnicity and culture

> It must be understood however that he is entirely away from his Countrymen and on that account feels isolated and dependent. If he had any companions who would come and see him occasionally and if he were in his own country, I think his condition would be more favourable . . . he has great difficulty in understanding our language and we have great difficulty in understanding him.[1]

In 1916 Dr James Beattie, medical superintendent of the Auckland Mental Hospital, wrote these words to Indar Singh, who lived in the Punjab, about his son, who was Beattie's patient. Some time before 1913, young Pheru Singh, the only son of Indar Singh, had bid farewell to his family in Karnana village, in the Punjab's Jalandhar District. Like many Punjabis and other Indians during the early twentieth century, he was in search of adventure and work overseas — in his case in Fiji and then New Zealand.[2]

In Fiji Pheru Singh worked for Jeanine and Fred Whittaker, who found him 'so faithful' that they brought him to Te Puke, in the Bay of Plenty, when they moved there in 1913.[3] In early 1915 Pheru Singh was informed that his brother-in-law had died while serving with the imperial army during the First World War. This induced a severe mental reaction; according to a constable at Te Puke, Pheru Singh became violent, restless, incoherent, noisy and then silent. He refused to speak or open his eyes and called on God to kill the Germans.

Pheru Singh was admitted to Auckland Mental Hospital on 3 March 1915, aged 26, and diagnosed with melancholia. This assessment changed to cataleptic stupor (an inability to react to the world) — a disorder rarely diagnosed. Indar Singh wrote to Beattie on 5 November 1915 asking for the 'proper name of disease'. Beattie responded that Pheru Singh 'suffered a severe form of melancholia with delusions'.

The term 'manic depression' (bipolar affective disorder) was not common in New Zealand's early psychiatric nosology, but with hindsight this possibly applied to Pheru Singh. Rather than trying to establish a diagnosis retrospectively, his story exemplifies the trauma and isolation that could induce melancholia and depression in many non-European migrants. When Kahan Singh, a Sikh living in Taumarunui, wrote to Beattie on 14 August 1916, to enquire about the cost of sending Pheru Singh back to India, there were only a few social networks among the 181 Indians recorded in the 1916 census in Aotearoa.[4] Pheru Singh was probably the only South Asian (and Sikh) in the Auckland hospital, which had 1216 patients in 1916.[5]

The difficulty of cross-cultural communication with those suffering from melancholia and depression runs as a theme through this chapter. Pheru Singh shut down communication with others, although his 'madman' look may have been performative when he was photographed.[6] Pheru Singh retained his long hair — possibly because Jeanine Whittaker asked Beattie on 18 March 1915 to not allow Pheru Singh's hair to be cut because as a 'high caste native of Punjab' he would be 'stoned' if he ever returned to India with his hair cut.[7] Mrs Whittaker also wrote to Pheru Singh, as 'it may cheer him up', but when Beattie suggested that she and her husband visit him she declined. She did inform Indar Singh about his son's incarceration.

Indar Singh's exchange of letters with Beattie reveals his love and concern for his son. When Singh tried to secure permission to travel to New Zealand to collect his son and take him back to India Beattie was sympathetic, but doubted that any shipping company would agree to accept a patient from a mental hospital who had not been discharged.

Pheru Singh remained in Auckland Mental Hospital until he died from phthisis (tuberculosis) on 8 August 1919. His tragic story remains remarkable because the available historical record contains few instances of non-Europeans suffering from depression or melancholia. As discussed in this chapter (and in chapter 2), the lack of source material is a major impediment to reconstructing a history of depression that is sensitive to culture and ethnicity. The writer Ingeborg Stuckenberg (see chapter 3) was one of only a few non-British Europeans to leave records that spoke to their despair, loneliness and disappointment after settling in New Zealand. There are very few written sources about the history of depression among immigrants who were not from Western Europe.

Despite the small pool of source material, this chapter explores melancholia and depression among selected groups of non-British migrants and their descendants and is written to ensure that the layers of ethnicity and depression are not swamped by Pākehā narratives of depression. The lack of primary research on the history of mental health among New Zealand's ethnic minorities makes it inevitable that those voices are often refracted through Pākehā and European lenses. This chapter does not refer to refugees and asylum seekers, many of whom have faced complex mental health issues, partly because of the lack of accessible data but also because mental health research on refugees and asylum seekers tends to fall outside the period this book covers.[8]

The role of culture and ethnicity in mental depression remains hugely under-documented and under-researched. Historically in Aotearoa this was even more the case,[9] partly because of minimal, biased or faulty sources. Asylum records, coroners' reports and newspaper sources contained limited documentation relating to Māori and ethnic minorities and the case notes of the accessible periods were sketchy.

Even when there was documentation, such as in the case of Pheru Singh, there could still be errors or misunderstanding between cultures and languages. Pheru Singh was variously referred to as Taru Singh, Faru Singh, and Pheroo Singh. His religion was recorded as a 'Hindoo', but he was a Sikh.

Chinese names were frequently changed, too. The clan name that precedes given names was transposed to become a surname, and there could be many misspellings. For example, Ah Foi Chang was the name recorded for a Chinese miner admitted to Seacliff hospital in 1906 with melancholia, but Reverend Alexander Don — a Presbyterian minister who could speak Cantonese and had close ties to the Chinese community, and who compiled the invaluable *Roll of Chinese in New Zealand, 1883–1913* — confirmed that his correct name was Tsui Cheung.[10] His admission papers recorded the 55-year-old as single and that he had been in Otago for 25 years. This recorded marital status may not be accurate; many early Chinese immigrants were married but as their families were unable to join them in Aotearoa this was often not noted on hospital records.

Restricted access to mental health archives in Aotearoa limit historical research into many non-British immigrants. Researchers are unable, for example, to view most mental health records relating to early Pacific migrants to Aotearoa because this migration took place predominately after the Second World War. Moreover, the records reflect only formal interactions, meaning we are only alerted to depressed immigrants when, such as in the case of Pheru Singh, they are committed to an asylum or other healthcare facility. Many immigrants during the surveyed era lived in rural or remote areas and were unlikely to access general medical treatment, let alone for mental conditions.

The extensive global literature on mental health and depression is also inadequate when applied cross-culturally to a historical study of depression. That literature is rooted in Western psychiatric concepts of depression against which other cultural understandings were set. With the spread of Western psychiatry, hegemonic diagnostic manuals and pharmaceuticals, this perspective has tended to become universal, forming what historian Jonathan Sadowsky calls the 'Empire of Depression'.[11] But the imposition of such foreign frameworks on others' lives is rarely informative, and can lead to misleading perspectives and conclusions.

Anthropological studies of mental illness have provided a counterpoint to this Western-centric model but, even then, usually cover only specific cultures.[12] And the various understandings of the causes and meaning of mental disturbance within different cultures also accounts for a lack of data. Generalisations about non-Western cultures are fruitless and ethnocentric. They also do not reflect the reality that cultures are not stuck in a time-warp. In addition, just as health practices have changed over the past hundred years so too have those within different ethnicities in Aotearoa as they became accustomed to state health practices.

The complexities of migration patterns are equally relevant; new migrants might have very different views to those within settled communities, and from those born and educated in Aotearoa. For example, some reports have highlighted the stigma and shame surrounding mental illness within Asian and Pasifika immigrants in Aotearoa,[13] but broad ethnic categories such as 'Asian' or 'Pasifika' homogenises cultures and do not account for the long history and the generations of settlement in Aotearoa. Some new immigrants may hold more traditional views about mental illness, whereas others are open to alternatives or prefer a biomedical approach.

Although the English terms 'melancholy' or 'depression' did not explicitly exist within many non-Western cultures, this does not mean that people did not suffer affective (emotional) states and somatic (bodily) conditions akin to depression.[14] However, the responses to this suffering were very different within societies where Western medicine was absent, under-resourced or avoided. Family, community and spiritual care and treatments prevailed.

Many colonial doctors under-diagnosed depression in patients who did not come from a similar cultural and linguistic background to themselves. In Aotearoa many doctors looked for identical symptoms to those found in British patients. Doctors could be culture-blind or hold preconceptions about the propensity of other cultures to exhibit specific mental disorders. For example, doctors in African colonies under-diagnosed melancholia and considered depression to be rare among Indigenous patients.[15] This bias carried to the United States, where Black Americans were more likely to be under-diagnosed with depression and over-diagnosed with schizophrenia.[16]

In Fiji, psychiatrists Henry Murphy and Ram Narayan wrote in 1979 that Indigenous Fijians were more prone to mania and Indo-Fijians to depression. Such assessment was based on physical, behavioural and racial stereotypes.

> It is commonly recognized that Fijians, as well as being the more robust, are the more likely to act out under stress, and this can give their mental disorder a manic character. The slighter Indians, in contrast, are more likely to withdraw into themselves under stress, and any turning of anger in on the self, as can easily happen during such withdrawal, is likely to show itself

> as depression or, in the extreme, as suicide, a condition which occurs much more often in the Indians than in the Fijians.[17]

In Papua New Guinea, the psychiatrist B. G. Burton-Bradley found depressive responses uncommon, although depression could appear as psychoneurosis or a shame reaction. 'It usually lacks the prolonged, gloomy, retarded character of some European depressions,'[18] he wrote in 1975.

As noted in chapter 2, during the nineteenth century depression was often erroneously seen as a 'white man's burden' or an outcome of civilisation that Indigenous people did not face. This thinking later became entwined with questions about the expectation of happiness, and whether that expectation was more the norm within Western culture than in other cultures.[19]

In September 1900, Jam Kim (Tang Chin Tsaan) escaped from the Benevolent Institution in Caversham and wandered around Dunedin's streets, sometimes brandishing a big stick. He was picked up by police, certified under the 1882 Lunatics Act and admitted to the Seacliff asylum.[20] Dr Paterson commented on Tsaan's strange appearance and dress. This was possibly the 'mad Hakka doctor', who was also a gold miner and poet living at Adams Flat near Milton.[21] Other Chinese called him 'three-quarters', which Reverend Alexander Don said meant 'cranky'.[22] Tsaan's name was translated by Don as 'Illustrious Envoy', but became misprinted in *The Outlook* as 'Illustrious Energy',[23] the title subsequently adopted for a film about two Chinese miners written and directed in 1987 by Leon Narbey.

Although the archival evidence is vague, the movie captures the despair, loneliness and unravelling of the mind that set in for many Chinese miners in Otago. In the movie, the younger key character, Chan, is shown continuously walking, not only because this was his main means of travel but also to transform movement into a metaphor depicting restlessness, mental torment and the unsettled migrant.

Reverend Alexander Don wrote in 1905–1906 that Seacliff's medical superintendent, Truby King, 'thinks that the number of Chinese in Seacliff Asylum — usually about 20 is proportionately excessive. But considering their loneliness, change of climate and surroundings, absence of their womankind, and so on — I think the number is small.'[24]

Don was referring to the migrant Chinese from Guangdong (Canton), most of whom worked in the Otago goldfields, and later on the West Coast. In 1869 there were over 2000 Chinese in Aotearoa; by 1881, the number was 5004.[25]

Don, who himself suffered from depression throughout his life, undoubtedly recognised how the black cloud could descend upon the mind when separated from family, living within an alien culture and in a harsh environment, and being disappointed about not realising life's goals. In his case, depression may have been brought on by living in Guangdong (1879–1881) or travelling in the back blocks of Otago, failing to convert many Chinese to Christianity. Don was never admitted to a mental asylum, but nor were most depressed Chinese immigrants.

Don had the privileged status of a white man, and in the above quotation neglected to mention the racism directed at Chinese immigrants as another potential cause of depression in Aotearoa. The 1881 Chinese Immigrants Act introduced a poll tax of £10 and a restriction of one Chinese passenger per 10 tons of cargo. In 1896 the tax was increased to £100 (about $20,000 today), and one Chinese passenger was permitted to board for 200 tons of cargo. Prolonged estrangement from kin would have affected the mental health of some, as the cargo restrictions made it extremely costly to return to China and prevented family from coming to New Zealand.

These restrictions were waived in 1934, but not abolished until 1944. So, after 1881, many Chinese immigrants faced the double stress of being indebted to their employers — who often were kin — for advancing the cost of their passage to Aotearoa, and of having to find more money to pay the poll tax. The despair at not returning to China with any of the anticipated wealth or the prospect of dying away from family in a foreign land became too much for some and led to depression.

As we have seen, at that time immigration restrictions and costs made it prohibitive for most wives to join their Chinese husbands. This meant that in nineteenth- and early twentieth-century Aotearoa, the Chinese community — like the Indian, Lebanese and Dalmatian communities — was predominately male, reflecting the intention of these early migrants to return and retire to their homelands. Regardless of their original preferences or intentions, there is no doubt that their final goals were shaped by New Zealand's racist immigration policies, such as the poll tax faced by Chinese, and the 1920 Immigration Restriction Amendment Act, which introduced racially based restrictions through an immigration permit system that favoured white British immigration.

Racial violence could also drive Chinese mad. In 1867 the *North Otago Times* reported that a Chinese miner who was seeking work as a gardener tried to introduce himself to the good people of Naseby in Central Otago. Instead,

> the poor fellow was subjected to what, in his opinion and that of his countrymen, is the last indignity, his pigtail was cut off, and not content with this, a crowd calling themselves Englishmen . . . cuffed and kicked him about with brutal violence, and finally placed him in a cask and rolled him about the town. The poor trembling Celestial at last escaped from his persecutors and was found a day or two afterwards wandering about in the open country in a half-demented state. He could speak scarcely any English but was taken care of by a constable . . . Since then, however, he has become a hopeless maniac and is now in Dunedin Lunatic Asylum.[26]

Despite this dreadful treatment and outcome, Thomas Sincock, a sub-inspector of police at Naseby, wrote to *The Otago Daily Times* that the matter was 'much exaggerated. The Chinaman was a great liar, and I am strongly of opinion a good deal of his conduct was assumed, for purposes of his own.'[27]

Alcohol abuse was rarely associated with mental illness in Chinese in nineteenth-century Aotearoa, but there was a link between opium use and depression, especially when opium became unavailable. Opium use and dependency was easily — and often lazily — attributed to Chinese who suffered mental illness or committed suicide. In 1880 Ah Yow, 'a great opium eater', as *The Otago Witness* put it, hanged himself in Lawrence's gaol.[28] He had been sentenced for stealing from Weatherstones Cement Goldmining Company's tailrace, but opium withdrawal, considered to lead to mental depression, was cited as the cause of his suicide.

Chow Chow, a miner from Beaumont aged around 50, told an interpreter (whom he had known for several years) that he would cut his throat or in some way 'shuffle off this mortal coil', as apparently he was 'sick of life'.[29] When he was admitted to Seacliff in 1887, his mental despair was attributed to opium. He refused to speak, would not come indoors, and lay on the ground.

Ah Ben spent 20 years in the Hokitika asylum until he died there in 1932, aged 84.[30] Opium was cited as inducing his melancholia, as were the skull injuries that he had sustained during a fight with Lue Soo, with whom he had shared a hut at Reefton.[31] After Ah Ben was admitted to the Seaview asylum in 1912, he became withdrawn, sitting in a 'cramped position, never smiles never speaks when attempt is made to rouse him, he becomes infuriated. His fellow countrymen avoid him and will not speak to him.' He could possibly have been discharged, given that he initially showed 'few or no mental symptoms'. However, Ah Ben lacked community support and was unable to work.

Many years later, in 1940, opium smoking was implicated as the cause of a Chinese immigrant's suicide. He had immigrated to Aotearoa in 1930, leaving his wife in China, but he had not been able to find work for the preceding two years.

> 'He has kept poor health for the past two years and has done no work during that time' (uncle); smoked a 'good deal' of opium; 'I do not know what sickness he suffered from'; very sick on day of death (friend with whom deceased was staying); 'He had no money and no property' (uncle); only property was his clothes; 'Chinese Association, tried to get him to go back to China, as he had no money and had been unable to earn a living for a considerable time. He refused to leave New Zealand, as his native town is now under Japanese control' (friend). Eighteen months in public hospital. Sergeant C. R. Duke, who conducted the inquest, said that opium was now difficult to get, according to other Chinese, and lack of it made habitual smokers depressed.[32]

'Did you ever see a mad Chinaman?' This appalling question, first posed in a letter to the editor of the Dunedin *Guardian* in 1873, was reproduced by other newspapers circulated in the Otago goldfields.[33] After the anonymous writer had visited the Dunedin Lunatic Asylum, the following was penned:

> There are six of them in the Lunatic Asylum, who are said to be mad . . . How does anyone know that they are mad? Who made the medical examination? It is no joke to talk to a Chinaman at any time, even through the medium of an interpreter, but to question him as to his madness I regard as nearly impossible. As for their own doctors or interpreters pronouncing them mad, that I look upon as sheer nonsense. Anyone who was in Victoria ten years ago will bear me out in this. Chinamen, as a rule, are peaceful, industrious fellows, who will work ground on which Europeans would starve, and whose pertinacity in growing cabbages amongst paving stones by the aid of liquid manure is beyond praise, as is indeed their ingenuity in robbing hen roosts and cleaning out puddling machines; but as for their going mad I do not believe it.

Putting aside the diatribe, this letter points to stereotypes Europeans had about madness in other cultures, and highlights issues with cross-cultural communication and diagnosis within the colony's asylums. Remarks about Chinese patients were usually based on their appearance or behaviour, and often no diagnosis was given. What can be made of a doctor's stereotypes when he observed that Chow Chow's appearance is typical of his race? Chow Chow may have understood very little English, but how did this enable the doctor to conclude that Chow Chow 'appears to be of feeble intellect'?[34]

'Delusional insanity' was a common diagnosis for Chinese, but this broad term made assumptions about different cultural and spiritual beliefs, and about signs of madness. In the winter of 1893, a 51-year-old Chinese miner from Cardrona took to the nearby ranges to climb the highest hill so that he could be a king and reach the sky with the aid of a piece of white paper.[35] He was found by a policeman and then committed to Seacliff mental asylum, where he was diagnosed with melancholia. Truby King dismissed him as 'depressed and stupid looking, sullen, vacant. Takes no interest in anything.'

The signs of depression among Chinese in colonial Aotearoa were usually overlooked. When we talk about the denial of depression, we must look backwards as to how this has been part of our culture — not just in the mainstream, but for many diverse cultures. In the case of the Chinese, it could be difficult to obtain family evidence of a patient's changes in moods or behaviour because of language difficulties and cultural miscommunication, or because family lived overseas, or there was familial silence.

This may have been an issue in 1888 in determining whether Tu Wong, a 30-year-old gold miner from Reefton, was really insane.[36] He was found guilty of assault, and sentenced to gaol, but refused to work or speak and 'behaved in a strange fashion'. His father and several brothers lived in Greymouth, but communication problems apparently made it impossible to obtain his history. Tu Wong was discharged from Seaview asylum as 'not insane'. Another Chinese miner admitted to Seaview talked nonsense. His Chinese friends were afraid of him, which made it difficult for doctors to find out more about his past. He had, it was recorded, an intense dread about something evil.[37]

Tu Wong's facial expression was 'morose' when he was admitted to Seaview asylum. Doctors seemed surprised that many melancholic Chinese patients like Tu Wong would not talk, not even with other Chinese. Yet withdrawal among melancholic fluent-English speakers in the asylum was a 'normal' symptom; their lack of communication with others was rarely commented upon. Some Chinese patients may have been reluctant to communicate because of former tensions with other Chinese. Ah Yew, for example, had attempted to burn a neighbour's hut at Waikaia.[38] He was considered a nuisance in his community, and insane; sleeping all day, not working, but at night trying to set the grass on fire, yelling and blowing to scare away the devil. Ah Yew told an interpreter that he had lost money due to the 'knavery of his partner'. In Seacliff he talked 'to no one, not even his fellows'.

Dr James Ng, a general practitioner in Dunedin during the second half of the twentieth century and a historian, reminds us of the long history of Chinese doctors who treated Chinese, as well as patients of other ethnicities, in rural and later in urban centres.[39] Many Chinese were suspicious and avoided Western medicine. Some Chinese herbalists became well known, such as Wallingford Chan (Chan Ting Ming) of Christchurch, who treated 'nervous depression' during the first half of the twentieth century.[40] His father, William Yau-kum Chan, had migrated to Dunedin in 1892, and worked as a market gardener before joining his father, Chan Tsung-fu, in his herbalist shop. After William died in 1934, Wallingford took over the family's herbalist business and advertised his services around the country.

Most of the early accounts of melancholia and depression among Chinese relate to gold mining communities. But, as seen in Wallingford Chan's family history, and that of other Chinese in Aotearoa,[41] as mining dried up by the turn of the century many had already moved to urban areas, where they faced other challenging living and working conditions. In 1914 doctors pinpointed the environment that Sue H. Y. lived in as the cause of his melancholia and extreme depression.[42] Like many Chinese and Indians at the time, he worked as a fruit hawker. He lived in Dunedin's Walker (later Carroll) Street, a neighbourhood notoriously known as the 'devil's half acre' because of crime, prostitution, slum housing and gambling. It was also called 'outcast Dunedin' because ethnic minorities, especially Chinese and Lebanese, settled there.[43] After Sue was admitted to Seacliff hospital he refused to eat and was suicidal. He also suffered from nephritis, an inflammation of the kidneys.

Some early immigrants to Aotearoa from Dalmatia had similar experiences of melancholia and depression to the Chinese miners. They, too, experienced racism, although not as a colour bar. Dalmatians were considered 'white', but not British, because Dalmatia was a part of the Austro-Hungarian empire before the First World War.[44] Some Dalmatians were diggers on the South Island goldfields during the 1860s, but by the 1880s most had shifted to dig kauri gum in the upper North Island. Word of the possible riches in 'Nova Zelanda' filtered back to villages in Dalmatia. It is doubtful that those alluring stories included descriptions of the harsh environmental conditions gumdiggers endured, or the loneliness and estrangement from family and culture.

Auckland's early asylum records reveal that among a small number of Dalmatian patients admitted with melancholia and depression, separation from family was heart-breaking. Within the sample, most of the patients were young, aged from 18 to 23. Two young gumdiggers, aged 20 and 18, admitted to the asylum from 'Babylon' in Northern Wairoa (Hawke's Bay)

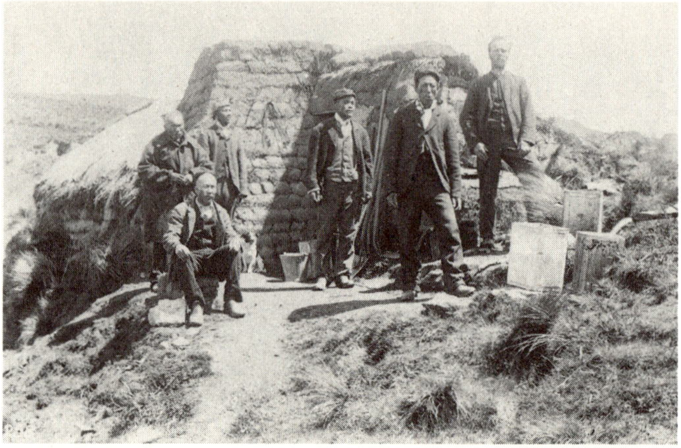

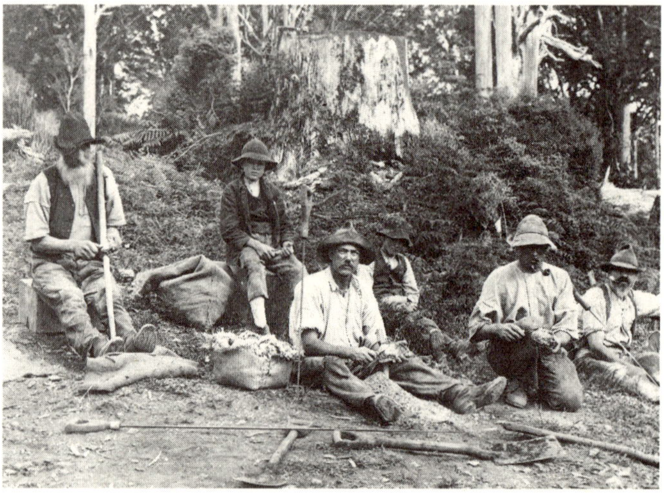

Clockwise from top left: Chinese gold miners and Reverend Alexander Don in Tuapeka, Otago, c. 1900; Chinese 'doctor' Jam Kim (Tang Chin Tsaan), known as the 'mad Hakka doctor'; an advertisement by the herbalist Wallingford Chan; early Pacific immigrants, such as these women taking a break in a factory, and Anna Carlson (above), worked hard and provided mutual support but still could become despondent; many gumdiggers were young men from Dalmatia.

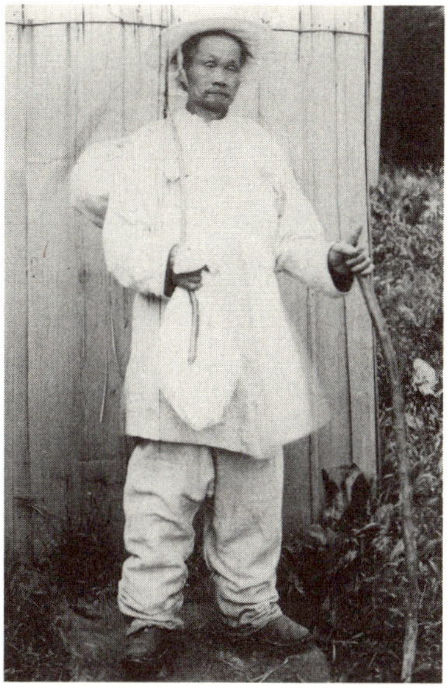

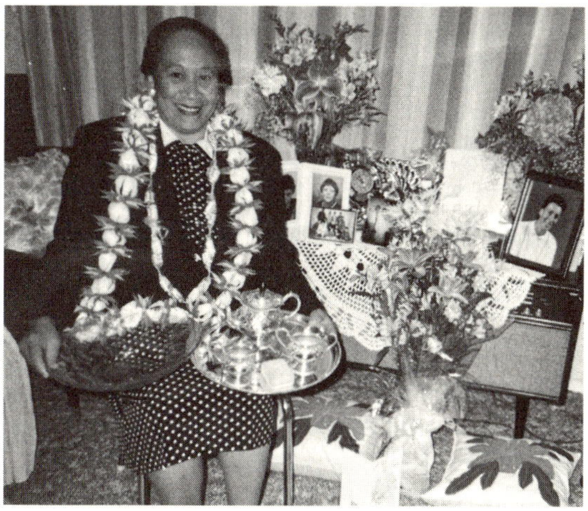

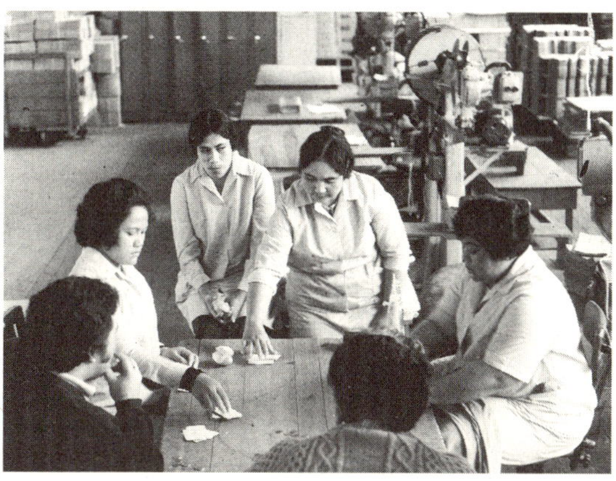

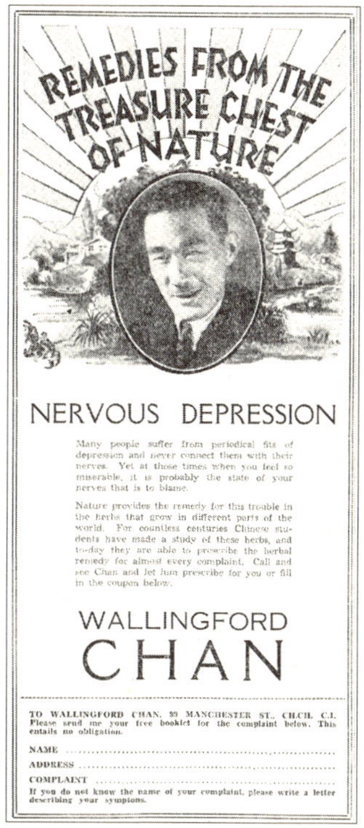
REMEDIES FROM THE TREASURE CHEST OF NATURE
NERVOUS DEPRESSION
Many people suffer from periodical fits of depression and never connect them with their nerves. Yet at those times when you feel so miserable, it is probably the state of your nerves that is to blame.
Nature provides the remedy for this trouble in the herbs that grow in different parts of the world. For countless centuries Chinese students have made a study of these herbs, and to-day they are able to prescribe the herbal remedy for almost every complaint. Call and see Chan and let him prescribe for you or fill in the coupon below.
WALLINGFORD
CHAN
TO WALLINGFORD CHAN, 33 MANCHESTER ST., CH.CH. C.1.
Please send me your free booklet for the complaint below. This entails no obligation.
NAME
ADDRESS
COMPLAINT
If you do not know the name of your complaint, please write a letter describing your symptons.

and Whitianga (Coromandel) in 1911 and 1912 were only 14 and 17 years old when they had arrived in Aotearoa.[45] Nineteen-year-old Slavo P.'s despair shows in his case notes from the Auckland asylum.[46] A gumdigger, he was admitted from Mercury Bay (Coromandel) in 1900 in a very thin and weak condition. Slavo was delusional and regarded the interpreter as his father — which is possibly indicative of Slavo's loss of family. Anton V., aged 23, clung to a constable, wanting his protection.[47] Anton told a doctor through an interpreter that he was melancholy because he had not seen his people for nine months.

As with other non-English-speaking immigrants, language and cross-cultural communication impeded others' understanding of the mental health problems experienced by many Dalmatians. The absence of others within the asylum who spoke the same language made isolation and depression worse. When Nicholel M. was visited by 'Austrian friends' they did not see anything wrong with him and found his conversation rational. Apparently Nicholel's melancholia and problems developed when 'stranded away', presumably from other Dalmatians. Hospital attendants reported that there had been no active sign of insanity since he was admitted.[48]

The act and meaning of suicide are also culturally defined. This does not mean that it is not tragic for both the sufferers and those who mourn them. As we saw in chapter 2, in the past suicide has been simplistically represented by many Europeans as a cultural or impulsive response within many non-Western cultures, and not attributable to sustained mental depression.[49] Some British and European doctors even regarded suicide as a marker of civilisation. Most doctors in colonial New Zealand clearly did not include non-white ancient civilisations, such as that of China, in their definition of 'civilised'.

It seems that there were several suicides and attempted suicides among Chinese pioneers in Aotearoa, many who were depressed. James Ng's study of *The Tuapeka Times* revealed reports of 10 Chinese suicides during the 1870s and 1880s.[50] The reasons reported were unexpected debt, bad news from home requiring money, shame of arrest, sickness (such as leprosy, partial paralysis, insanity) and destitution.

In 1876, 22-year-old Kum Gee, a gold miner at Macetown in Otago, became intensely melancholic after family deaths. He tried to burn down the hut he shared with another miner, and cut his own throat.[51] Kum Gee was saved by two European miners, who staunched the wound with tow (coarse fibre) and took him to the hospital at Frankton. When he appeared in the Queenstown court, charged with trying to commit self-murder, he had a listless expression and was despondent. He was acquitted on the grounds of insanity and sent to the Dunedin Lunatic Asylum. The following year he was discharged and was to be sent back to China in the care of his 'countrymen'.

In 1877, Ah Quee, a 28-year-old miner from Kumara on the West Coast, was also discharged from Seaview asylum (probably suffering from melancholia) so that he could return to China.[52] It is not clear whether he did, but in 1883 a person named Ah Quee drowned himself at Roxburgh in Otago. Like Kum Gee, Ah Quee had become 'despondent' after his cousin Ah Chin was murdered at Shingle Creek.

> He was to have been taken to Dunedin today on account of his unusual and peculiar action of late, but while his mate was preparing breakfast for him he went outside, sallied down to the river took off his hat, boots and coat, and jumped off a projecting ledge of rock into the river. The current at this point is very strong, and he must immediately have been carried into midstream and down the river, as the spot has been dragged without discovering any signs of the body. He seemed never to have recovered from the shock of the death of his relative.[53]

There are many other tragic stories. A young gold miner, Ah Chew, aged 21, fatally hanged himself from a rafter of his hut at Six Mile Creek, near Cardrona, while considered to be under 'temporary insanity'.[54] In 1885 Sew Wing's employer, Sew Shew, told him that he was unfit for work, but he lent him £1 towards returning to China. Sew Wing had been working as a cook in a Chinese boarding-house in Stafford Street in Dunedin for only about a fortnight when he found the cooking fire too painful to his eye, which had been injured in a dynamite explosion when he was working as a railway labourer.

He became 'depressed in spirits' and threatened to end his life. Sew Shew had thought Sew Wing was slightly out of his mind, as he used to talk frequently in a nonsensical manner and was often low-spirited. Sew Wing left Sew Shew's employment, apparently to go to Kyeburn in the Maniototo. Instead, his body was brought up in the buckets of a dredge near the Rattray Street wharf extension in Dunedin.[55]

Sew Wing's wife and family were far away in China. His depression and suicide were likely also due to the despair and shame he felt about returning home empty-handed after three years in Aotearoa. The historian Daniel Davy suggests that suicide may have been chosen by some Chinese as a means of returning home after death to be 'reunited with family members both living and dead'.[56] The ability to fulfil this wish depended on clan members or friends undertaking the rituals for the deceased's bones to be sent home, and paying for the passage to China.

Many years later, in 1938, a Chinese greengrocer who had immigrated to Aotearoa in 1908 hanged himself in the back of his shop in Wellington because of shame at losing his money.[57] He left a suicide note that was translated:

> Last year, one evening in August or September, while I was away listening to a radio broadcast of the Sino-Japanese war news, some fiendish and heartless thief came and stole my money. I dared not say anything. I could but grieve in silence. It was like losing things behind locked doors for who would have believed the theft. I have no means of replacing the sum, and now before me there is only the Road of Death. My shame is so great that I came [could not] face my friends, so I have decided to commit suicide. In my death I wish my brother and friends continuous and unlimited success and prosperity so that even in my grave my heart could yet expand with happiness. My grief cannot be fully conveyed, nor my bitterness expressible. Alas! Alas! To think that it should end like this! This is my farewell-note, written with tears.

This suicide note indicates the shame felt by some immigrants when they could not realise their dreams or remit money home to support kin.

Feelings of depression, loneliness, disappointment and isolation from their families have persisted among more recent migrants, including those from other ethnic minorities. For example, in the late twentieth century there were suicides among Indian immigrants who became depressed. For some women, the excitement of starting a new marriage in a new land did not always compensate for the disappointment of life there and being profoundly lonely and homesick.[58] These feelings could be compounded if they lived in an isolated geographical and social environment, such as a farm or in the suburbs, where there was possibly limited transport.

The ability or confidence to speak English was another pressure earlier Indian immigrant women faced. Some women became vulnerable during pregnancy and when caring for a baby or young children if they were separated from female kin by thousands of kilometres. Family and religious tensions also induced some Indian immigrants to despair: for example, when one partner was Hindu and the other Muslim. Failed business and employment aspirations also thread through these tragic stories, especially for young Indian men.

Although there are common themes among all immigrants that can precipitate depression, the vulnerability and fear for those of ethnic minorities who held precarious visas or were in dependent domestic situations could induce depression and suicide. New Zealand began to open its borders from the late 1980s to enable visas for international students, but some still felt isolated, depressed and suicidal, such as one young Indian man who hanged himself when his visa was due to expire. He did not want to return to India, possibly in fear of shaming his parents.

In 2022, over 8 per cent of New Zealand's population traces heritage to Pacific cultures, and most government and non-government agencies use the term 'Pasifika'. However, this term is not accepted by all Pacific peoples in Aotearoa: some people from Melanesian cultures consider the term to not include them. Many Pacific peoples have other ancestral roots, too, especially from Europe and Asia. In this book, the terms 'Pasifika' and 'Pacific peoples' are used.

Just as it is difficult to demarcate ethnic names or boundaries, so it is not easy to quantify depression and mental health statistics for Pasifika, but studies indicate a marked increase in depression rates among Pasifika in recent decades.[59] By 2006, compared to other ethnicities, Pacific peoples, especially those who are younger and New Zealand-born, had a higher prevalence of mental disorders and high rates of suicide. How do these disturbing trends fit into a longer history of depression in Aotearoa and the Pacific diaspora?

Sustained migration from the Pacific Islands to Aotearoa began after the Second World War. By then New Zealand had a 'Pacific empire'.[60] The Cook Islands and Niue had been annexed by New Zealand in 1901; self-government and a relationship of free association with New Zealand came to the Cook Islands in 1965, and for Niue in 1974. Britain had annexed the Tokelau atolls in 1916, and transferred administration to New Zealand in 1926. Tokelau is still administered by New Zealand, and Tokelauans are New Zealand citizens. When the First World War broke out, New Zealand seized control of Western Sāmoa (a German protectorate since 1900), and from 1920 until its independence in 1962 administered the territory as a mandate for the League of Nations, and then as a trust territory for the United Nations.

New Zealand's spheres of influence and historical ties were also through trade, church, education and health in Fiji, Tonga, Solomon Islands and the New Hebrides (Vanuatu). Female domestic workers from the Cook Islands were at the vanguard of Pacific migration to Aotearoa, although, as we saw with Alistair Te Ariki Campbell, there had been earlier movement between the islands and Aotearoa. As with most immigrants, those from the Pacific were attracted to Aotearoa by economic and employment opportunities that were not available in their homelands.

During the 1960s and early 1970s, many Pasifika were low-waged workers in city and suburban factories, or employed, often part-time, as cleaners or domestic workers. Kinship and church ties were significant in Pasifika migration, as well as the prospect of a better life and education for children.

It has been suggested that the first generation of Pacific migrants did not suffer mental health problems to the same extent as the Aotearoa-born.[61] In 2020 about two-thirds of Pasifika were born in Aotearoa, with more than half aged under 25.[62] While research plots an alarming rise in reported mental health issues and depression among Pasifika, there were probably always psychological conditions within Pacific cultures that led to depression. Mental health disorders have long existed within Pacific cultures,[63] but the explanations and the terms used were not explicitly melancholia or depression. In 2018 the Tongan Methodist minister Reverend Tevita Finau told Radio New Zealand journalist Indira Stewart that 'When I grew up in Tonga there were no talks of depression. There was talk of people exhausted, fatigued, but there was no word for depression that I could think of or could recall. Except people just saying that people have overworked or stress themselves out and not depressed.'[64]

Indigenous terms, concepts and treatments referring to similar states of mood to melancholia and depression were present within Pacific cultures, yet attempts to pin down a depression lexicon within Pacific cultures must be qualified. Translation from Pacific languages into English psychiatric terminology is problematic. The cultural and spiritual contexts of language are paramount. Some words are sacred and should not be publicly spoken. Indigenous ontologies and practices were not static and became entangled with the external, through colonialism, Christianity and Western medicine.

Western medical and psychiatric nosology has also changed. The words listed in the table on the following page can be equated with depression even though a biomedical meaning is not directly expressed. For example, in Tokelauan fakenoanoa means 'having sadness', but can refer to depression.

As Tokelauan research participants in Aotearoa have reported, difficulties even revealing sadness to others inhibits the recognition of depression. 'I just can't say to anybody oh I feel sad today . . . they don't even know that I am sad. In my own self I just keep it to myself. That's why it is so hard for us to see the sign of somebody being depressed because they hide their feelings most of the time.'[65] Family or community members may only be alerted to a problem when the depressed person physically or emotionally withdraws.

Lexicon: Depression, worry within selected Pacific cultures[66]

Māori	pōkē, pōuritanga, tiwhatiwha, whakapōuri, pōururu, rāwakiwaki, taumaha hārukiruki
Samoan	ma'i popole, ma'i manutu
Fijian	yakaloloku, yalolailai
Cook Islands Rarotongan	maromaroā
Niuean	fakaagitau
Tokelauan	popole, fakaatu, fakenoanoa
Tongan	loto ta'ota'omia, loto mafiasia, te'ia
Vanuatu (Bislama)	wota fol blo aes (water falls from your eyes), hart blong mi i hevi (a heavy heart)

Language is only part of Pacific understandings of mental health and illness. The holistic approach, outlined with Māori in chapter 2, also applies to Pasifika; ontology is relational and spiritual, stressing balance between spiritual, mental and physical health.[67] Mental health starts from wellness, as in the Samoan expression 'soifua malōlōina o le māfaufau' (mental wellbeing, or a mind that is healthy).

As discussed in chapter 2, mental illness within Māori cultures could be linked to social and spiritual violations. The restoration of mental health within many Pacific cultures lies within a cultural framework, where Indigenous healers are key to restoring individual and community wellness. Ancestors may have been offended, and if balance was not restored, ill health could pass through generations. According to Kiwi Tamasese and other Samoan experts on the fa'a Sāmoa, a curse (malaaumatua) could condemn 'the person to a life outside of family and village relationships, and hence a life without purpose . . . sometimes mental illness results from an inability to fulfil responsibilities and obligations to their families, villages and districts of belonging'.[68]

In 1965 in Aotearoa Auckland psychiatrist Laurie Gluckman treated Salote, a Fijian patient who was suffering from anxiety and depression and who considered she had been subjected to draunikau (a curse or witchcraft) by a woman she had offended in 1948 in Fiji. Gluckman observed that draunikau victims who suffered a minor physical illness often developed an emotional reaction, with depression, weight loss and a sense of hopelessness.[69]

In 1990 the New Zealand anthropologist Wendy Cowling emphasised that in Tonga the blame for negative mental conditions was projected to the spirits and away from the patient.[70] However, within many Pacific societies stigma towards 'madness' (or blame from a curse) sometimes harmed individuals, who might be shunned or blamed for negative events within the community.

In 2021, Rachael Lemalie Umaga testified to the Royal Commission of Inquiry into Abuse in Care about the shame and stigma she experienced as a Pasifika woman. She had been a patient since 1992 in psychiatric units in Wellington with diagnoses including postnatal depression, bipolar affective disorder and, incorrectly, epilepsy. Equally, she stressed the social and economic issues common to many Pasifika:

> The feeling of shame is very real. For people that have been in these units, they carry the stigma of shame. We feel shame. Shame stops us from making friends. The stigma makes us untrustworthy of people, always insecure and cautious of people all the time . . . The use of the word 'mental' carries negative connotations. I feel that it doesn't take into account the fact that there are many issues that make someone unwell and behave the way I behaved. These are issues like social issues, housing issues and socio-economic issues . . . domestic violence . . . Many Pacific people still do not fully understand mental health and respond negatively to people such as myself who have been in psychiatric wards.[71]

The stigma and shame of mental illness also links to the 'masking' of mental distress within Pacific cultures.[72] Smiling, associated with politeness and courtesy, can hide underlying emotions, making it difficult to recognise depression. Like many people, Pacific peoples are uncomfortable with the

English words 'insanity' and 'madness', but also with similar Indigenous terms. Humour or avoidance within Pacific cultures can both deal with uncomfortable issues and deflect from publicly acknowledging or addressing the private pain of mental illness.[73]

It is important to look to the past as well as to contemporary Indigenous cultures to consider mental depression among Pasifika in Aotearoa, but historical pressures and changes caused by migration are equally relevant. Most immigrants from the Pacific Islands were optimistic about their future lives, but the reality could be brutal, lonely and depressing, even when Pacific migrants had the support of kin and church.

I first met Anna Tuakanakore Carlson in Newtown, Wellington, in 1992, when she warmly shared her life story with me.[74] Tears and laughter followed. I did not expect Anna's story to reveal depression because my research had focused on her being a happily settled immigrant from Cook Islands. Anna was very open about where our discussion led. She told me that she had arrived in Auckland in 1948, when she was 16 years old, but although she was with her parents she was lonely and nostalgic for Rarotonga's Takuvaine valley, where her wider family and friends lived. Anna missed her great-aunt, aged in her nineties, who had told Anna before she departed for New Zealand that she would never see her again. That prophecy came true.

Anna felt sad, especially for 'our old people left behind'. Sadness and longing soon became more enduring — the psychological isolation common to many immigrant women[75] — especially for a young woman alone in a suburban house while her parents were at work. Like many immigrants who looked to the 'land of opportunity', Anna was disappointed by her first impressions of Auckland — the cold and rain, the ramshackle houses in which many papa'ā (Europeans) lived — so different from a young woman's dreams in Rarotonga of a better future in Aotearoa.

Things looked brighter when Anna got a job as a domestic worker in a role similar to a nurse aide and moved into the nurses' hostel at Auckland hospital with other Pasifika women. She spent her time off enjoying netball, church, shopping, movies and dances. She fell in love with an immigrant from England and became pregnant. He proposed and wanted Anna to join him in England, but her heart remained in the Pacific.

Anna faced her pregnancy alone, but had her parents' support. After the birth Anna came to 'really love' her daughter. But her parents decided to foster their granddaughter, and when she was six months old they took her to live with them in Rarotonga. Anna now suffered the profound loss a mother experiences with adoption, even with tamariki 'āngai — open adoption involving close family and culturally endorsed.[76] Anna became seriously ill and depressed.

She resumed paid work but was homesick and, most of all, missed her baby. Anna eventually returned to Rarotonga and, she says, 'my illness lifted as soon as I was on the boat. Life became good, really happy.' Not only was she reunited with her daughter, but in Rarotonga she also met Charlie, whom she eventually married. They settled in Wellington, where they became elders of the Cook Islands community.

Anna faced considerable personal challenges and, although deeply depressed at times, she lived an active, rewarding and loving life until she died in 2012.

Anna was among the early waves of Pasifika immigrants with fewer immigration problems. But later Pasifika migrants and their families experienced economic and family pressures, and the anxiety over their immigration status, especially during the Dawn Raids of the 1970s,[77] and faced great mental strain. This was a time when police and immigration officials invaded Pasifika homes during the early-morning hours to 'round up' alleged overstayers, regardless of their citizenship status. Those who were prosecuted were deported, often along with their families, to the Pacific Islands. The shame, stress and depression for Pasifika who had vulnerable immigration status did not ease during subsequent decades, and this could lead to depression and suicide.[78]

Other factors in such tragedies were economic precarity, poverty, and substandard and crowded — albeit often supportive — housing. Faith and church fellowship might mitigate loneliness and depression, but for one older Tongan woman that was not enough. She especially missed her children, who lived outside Aotearoa, but the stress of being an overstayer probably was the final straw, leading to her ending her life.[79]

Loneliness, estrangement from family, culture and environment, economic problems, harsh working conditions, shame at not being successful migrants, stigma, and the impact of discrimination have all contributed to depression among migrant communities. However, only a small number of non-British and non-Irish immigrants were admitted to mental institutions in colonial Aotearoa, and the numbers suffering from depression were, and remain, much higher than reported. Studies continue to reveal the lower utilisation of health services and diagnosis, especially for mental illness, among ethnic minorities in contemporary Aotearoa.

Although the 2014–2015 New Zealand Health Survey reported Pacific and Asian New Zealanders to have the lowest rate (5 per cent) for a mood disorder diagnosis, other researchers have pointed out that this contradicts findings that Pasifika report higher psychological distress than non-Pasifika — which is no doubt indicative of Pacific peoples' mental distress not being 'picked up' by mental health professionals, or of the avoidance of this issue among many Pacific people.

Māori, Pacific and Asian New Zealanders are more likely to be under-diagnosed with depression compared to European New Zealanders. This 'inequality may reflect ethnic group differences in access to, expectations from and style of communication with medical professionals'.[80] In 1977 a meeting of community groups in Ōtara, South Auckland, heard of the serious difficulties that local people — many of whom were Pasifika — had in accessing a doctor.

> When people are sick they usually feel depressed, miserable and worried. The idea of seeking medical help is to have the depression, misery and worry removed by the healing arts of a doctor. Most people in New Zealand are able to get medical attention quite easily. Not so the people of Otara. Instead of a visit to a doctor being easy and comforting, for the Otara patient it can be a hideous nightmare, filled with hassles and frustrations . . . For most patients in Otara, they are faced with long waits, confusion, inconveniences, expense and wasted

> time . . . The hard struck people are those with children who are unable to communicate properly in English.[81]

This book's epilogue outlines some initiatives and culturally appropriate measures to address gaps in mental health delivery and in the recognition and treatment of depression among our ethnic minorities. Clearly there is still much historical research required on mental health, specifically depression, within New Zealand's ethnic communities.

7·

'Quacks', shocks, docs and drugs

In 1873 Thomas Aicken, the superintendant of the Auckland asylum, praised opiates in the treatment of 'some of the worst and apparently most hopeless cases of melancholia'.[1] Medical practitioners in colonial New Zealand commonly offered opiates such as opium, morphine, laudanum and codeine, taken either by themselves or within prepared mixtures like Daffy's Elixir, Godfrey's Cordial and Dover's Powder. During the late nineteenth and early twentieth centuries, New Zealand's asylums used opioids as sedatives, along with chloral, sulfonyl, bromides, trional and paraldehyde.

In 1904 *The New Zealand Herald* reported that 'sleeplessness and melancholia' were due to the 'seductive influence of such hypnotics', although the same article cited a neurologist who recommended adding small amounts of sulfonyl hourly to a hot drink until sleep was induced to treat simple melancholia.[2] In contrast, Aicken's successor Dr Beattie advised nurses in 1911 against administering opium for melancholia because the patient may have already established a drug or alcoholic habit.[3]

Aicken and Beattie held these conflicting views on the early use of drugs to relieve depression during a time when there was limited pharmacological relief for the condition. It was not until the late 1950s that antidepressants, which at the time were considered not to be toxic, addictive or highly sedative, were introduced. But, as this chapter explains, modern drugs had many side effects, which could lead to unintended consequences.

Between the mid-nineteenth century and the 1980s people with depression underwent a plethora of treatments, including compulsory and voluntary hospitalisation, outpatient treatment, psychotherapy, and shock and drug therapies. Throughout these changes in treatments — many of which were experimental or of short-lived efficacy — most people with depression could hopefully rely on the care and support of whānau, family, friends or the church and, significantly, their family doctor.

In the past, just like today, many sufferers and their families bypassed doctors and sought affordable (and not-so-affordable) alternative treatments for depression. In the nineteenth century European immigrants often relied on herbalists or apothecaries (chemists). Like chemists, some herbalists operated shops, but many sold their products through newspaper advertisements or as mobile vendors. As noted in the previous chapter, Chinese immigrants had their own medicines and doctors, although Chinese doctors also treated clients from other cultures. In nineteenth-century Britain, nerve treatments and tonics that often contained iron, quinine and strychnine were prescribed by doctors to treat mental collapse. According to the historian Janet Oppenheim, these tonics aimed to restore 'firmness to the patient's collapsed nerves and to stimulate the production of nerve force'.[4] In Aotearoa, tonics were widely advertised and people in remote communities purchased patent medicines through mobile vendors and treated themselves.

Nevertheless, patent medicines were controversial in Aotearoa, even in the nineteenth century. In 1885, picking up the pen for the positive side, the lead writer (presumably Edward Ball, the publisher) of the *South Canterbury Times* advocated that 'the prevalence of suicidal mania in these colonies' could be reversed if individuals treated themselves:

> This would allow them to throw off gloom and regain their normal spring and vigor . . . It is a great matter this regulation of the mind, this looking after its health as we should look after the health of the body. The one depends upon the other, and a

> diseased mind will give warning through some bodily channel . . . Who shall minister to a mind diseased? Therein must the patient minister to himself.[5]

But Frank Gifford, editor of *The Evening Post*, dismissed this claim as thinly veiled advertising for patent medicines,[6] which included Mother Seigel's Curative Syrup, Mrs Winslow's Soothing Syrup, Holloway's Pills and Dr Williams' Pink Pills. Dr E. C. West's Nerve and Brain Treatment, advertised during the 1880s and 1890s, was guaranteed to treat 'Hysteria, Dizziness, Convulsions, Fits, Nervous Neuralgia, Headache, Nervous Prostration caused by use of alcohol or tobacco, Wakefulness, Mental Depression, Softening of the Brain resulting in insanity and leading to misery, decay, and death'.[7]

Several tonics evoked the humoral theories of disease, which persisted in Western medicine from antiquity through to the nineteenth century. According to this school of thought, the body contains four humours — black bile (known as melancholy), yellow or red bile, blood and phlegm — and any imbalance of the humours results in disease. This included a connection between melancholia, depression, digestion and the liver.[8] Widely available tonics and treatments for indigestion and diarrhoea, in which the active ingredient was often bismuth subsalicylate, purported to cure depression. 'Pearson's Peptochlor will absolutely cure you. Peptochlor dispels depression, which in most cases can be traced to indigestion,'[9] declared one advertisement. Eccles' Phosphorton was touted as a cure for nervous headaches and other neuralgic affections: 'It creates new Nervous Fluid and Brain Matter by supplying the Blood with its Electric life Element, Phosphorus — the very core and centre of the brain itself,' an advertisement for it declared in 1913.[10]

During the Great Depression of the 1930s, advertisements for Marshall's Fospherine claimed that it could 'Get rid of jumpiness, fear and mental depression. Reinvigorate your nervous system . . . The mighty tonic that never fails.'[11] As the economic situation deteriorated, workers who 'cracked up . . . when their nerves refused to work overtime or showed signs of mental depression' read advertisements recommending this tonic.[12] Even Eno's Fruit Salt, which in 2023 is sold as an antacid, was once marketed as allaying 'nervous excitement, depression, and restores the nervous system to its proper condition'.[13]

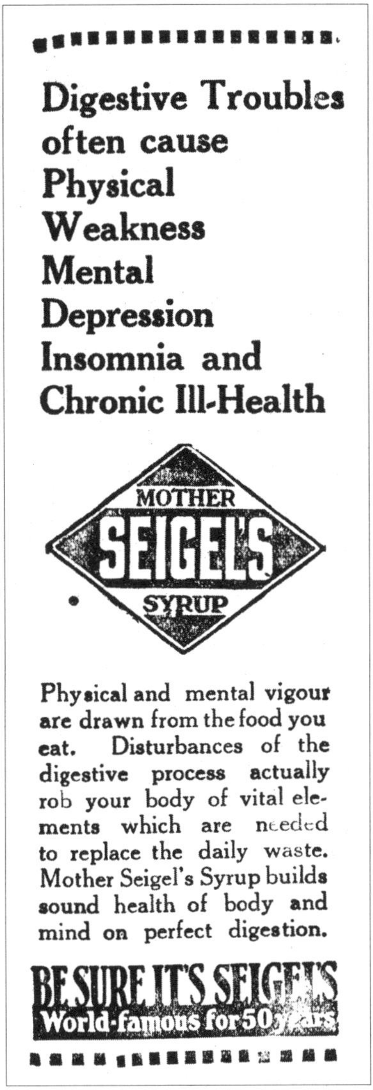

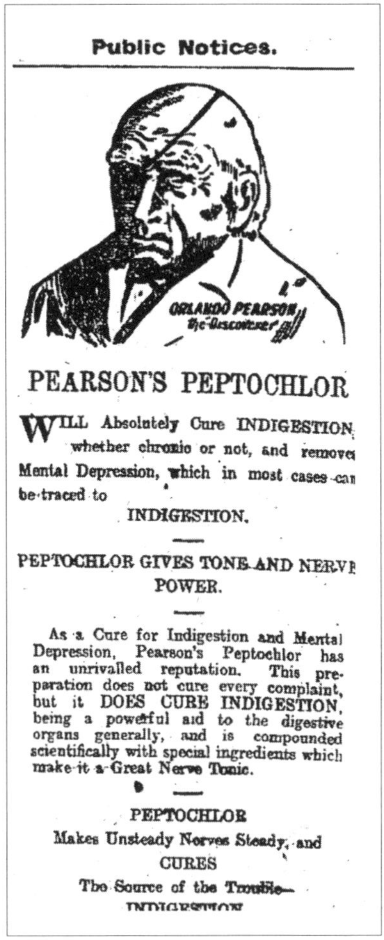

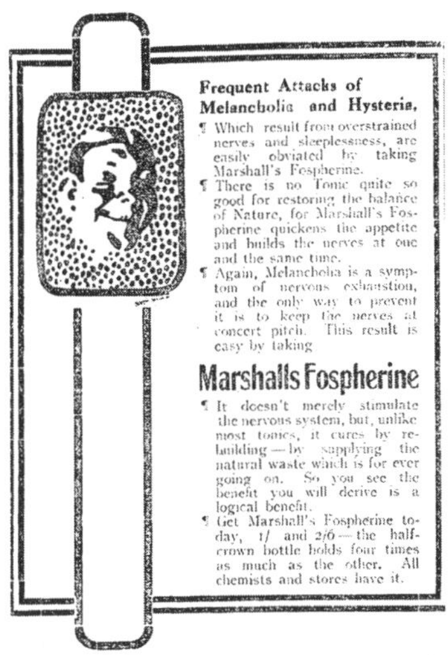
Frequent Attacks of Melancholia and Hysteria,
¶ Which result from overstrained nerves and sleeplessness, are easily obviated by taking Marshall's Fospherine.
¶ There is no Tonic quite so good for restoring the balance of Nature, for Marshall's Fospherine quickens the appetite and builds the nerves at one and the same time.
¶ Again, Melancholia is a symptom of nervous exhaustion, and the only way to prevent it is to keep the nerves at concert pitch. This result is easy by taking
Marshalls Fospherine
¶ It doesn't merely stimulate the nervous system, but, unlike most tonics, it cures by re-building—by supplying the natural waste which is for ever going on. So you see the benefit you will derive is a logical benefit.
¶ Get Marshall's Fospherine to-day, 1/ and 2/6—the half-crown bottle holds four times as much as the other. All chemists and stores have it.

Advertisements for late nineteenth- and early twentieth-century over-the-counter cures for depression.

Highly potent alcoholic spirits, notably Wolfe's Schnapps, were advertised from 1863 until 1950 as a medicine for mental depression, although in later years a doctor's prescription was needed to purchase these from a liquor retailer. The appeal of foreign beverages was used to market Emile Frese's Hamburg Tea; George Barclay of Woollahra, Australia, said in an advertisement that it relieved his severe attacks of biliousness and depression. Hamburg Tea could be purchased from Neil's Botanic Dispensaries, which had branches in Dunedin, Invercargill and Tīmaru, while Neil's Botanic Influenza Mixture was advertised as being able to alleviate muscular pains, headaches and depression, all symptoms of flu.[14]

Impey's May Apple was advertised in several newspapers between 1901 and 1925 with this compelling explanation:

> Did you ever feel 'anyhow'? That feeling of miserable depression, of moroseness, a disinclination to work or even to talk. Some people suffer constantly from this 'anyhow' feeling, and don't know how it comes about. It arises from the inability of the liver to do its ordinary work. The functions of the liver are extremely important, so much so that impairment arising from any organic cause quickly disturbs the harmony and health of the whole system. Its office is to eliminate the carbon from the blood, and when the liver goes on strike you feel 'anyhow.' This is when you should reach out for Impey's May Apple.[15]

While merchants and herbalists touted patent medicines and tonics, other practitioners known as 'quacks' practised therapies throughout the country.[16] Even after the Quackery Prevention Act, aimed at preventing the sale of sham medical remedies, was passed in 1908,[17] several 'doctors' continued to provide alternative treatments.

One was Henry Victor, an English clairvoyant, psychic reader and healer who promoted himself as being able to relieve melancholia, rheumatism, nervous and stomach troubles, and paralysis, among other things.[18] Victor advertised in several newspapers, offering therapies such as homoeopathy, hypnosis, botanical medicine, hydropathy and electrotherapy to alleviate depression. He travelled extensively throughout New Zealand, including Otago, Southland, the West Coast and Canterbury, claiming to treat melancholia and other mental and physical conditions, including epilepsy, using a variety of methods. In 1906 he called himself a psychologist, but by 1911 he was declaring himself to be a metaphysician.[19] By then he had added magnetic and electric treatment to his medical repertoire. Victor also gave lectures on these conditions and treatments.

Electrotherapy as a treatment for nervous disorders was employed in Victorian and Edwardian Britain, and by the early twentieth century it was being practised in New Zealand.[20] In 1905 a 'Dr McLaughlin', whose services were available in Wellington's Willis Street, claimed in an advertisement in *The New Zealand Times* that 'Electricity will cure you.'[21] He applied 'electric belts' to treat obesity, nervousness and sexual ailments. Nearby, Mr and Mrs Goodman offered massage and what they called psychotherapy as a 'remedy for drink and drug habit, insomnia, neuralgia, nervous prostration, mental depression, worry, and all diseases which lead to physical, nervous and mental breakdown'.[22]

Further south, in Invercargill, in 1915 Minnie C. was treated by P. B. Macdonald, a metaphysician.[23] She had been feeling weak in body and mind because all of the 'electricity has gone out of her body'. She was depressed, restless and, according to her husband, slept only a few hours each night. Macdonald offered the 'most scientific methods of relieving suffering', including magnetic healing. Minnie, who was later diagnosed with melancholia and committed to Seacliff Mental Hospital, where she stayed for almost two years, told a doctor there that Macdonald's influence was 'of a bad nature and puts bad thoughts into her mind . . . of a sexual character'. These thoughts centred around guilt about not having more than four children and about the contraceptive methods that she practised with her husband, as well as breast-feeding her babies for at least 16 months.

Seacliff's medical superintendent Truby King dismissed the metaphysician's treatment because, 'as usual in such cases' of those who consulted people he probably dismissed as 'quacks', Minnie had 'acquired various pseudo psychological catchphrases' such as 'I feel that my nerves are overheated. I think my upper brain is dead and that all my thoughts are carried on by a lower brain.' Despite Minnie's longing for more children, and her feelings of guilt over practising contraception, Truby King recorded that she 'has absolutely no insight into her true condition and cannot be brought to understand that she is mentally abnormal'. Despite her 'abnormality', Minnie lived a long life, dying in 1961, aged 89.

For a minority of people, self-help through a combination of psychology and spiritualism was another alternative to medical intervention for 'conquering moods of depression'.[24] In 1925 Practical Psychology Clubs were formally founded in Auckland, Wellington, Christchurch and Dunedin, although practical psychology had been advocated by spiritualists in Aotearoa since the late nineteenth century.[25] Practical psychology aimed to popularise psychological thought and practice, rather than relying on professional medical experts, or a Freudian or psychoanalytic approach. These psychology clubs emphasised the interrelationship between mind, body and spirit through 'practical' advice literature.[26] The clubs often hosted speakers from Britain. In 1938, the Dunedin Practical Psychology Club held a discussion on depression:

> The underlying cause of one's depression was ill health, although the mental attitude was mainly the controlling factor. One could not separate, however, the three forces — the spiritual, the mental, and the physical. Only through the harmonious working of these three could poise be acquired. Fear was a destructive element which was also a root cause of depression. It was sometimes a reaction from some episode in childhood, and made itself felt at unexpected moments in an inferiority complex or self-pity . . . environment and uncongenial surroundings, and also the reactions to others with whom one came in contact, led to depression which was difficult to surmount. One could overcome the uncongenial vibrations from another by being so busy radiating good that it could not touch them.
>
> A writer had said, 'Within yourself is the cause of whatever comes into your life,' therefore, by reconstructing his mental outlook man could change his life. The road was not easy, but through constant facing up and mental discipline the pathway

> became clear. All that was needed was a spiritually awakened consciousness, together with determination, perseverance, and a realisation that all life was something to be tuned into.[27]

In addition to alternative therapies or self-help, by the early twentieth century self-medication to relieve depression, anxiety, insomnia or physical pain included commercially available barbiturates (sedatives), the first of which was Medinal (a salt) and Veronal (an acid). Unfortunately, these drugs could be addictive, and rather than providing relief could instead exacerbate depression and anxiety in long-term users, as Dr E. Solkind wrote in a research article published in the British medical journal *The Lancet* in 1926.[28] Veronal and Medinal were readily available in Aotearoa; the writer Robin Hyde reported in *The New Zealand Observer* in 1932 that these drugs were implicated in several deaths in Auckland.[29]

Hyde could draw upon personal experience. The side effects of her addictive self-medicating with paraldehyde and high doses of Medinal to relieve her physical and mental pain may have also contributed to the stammering, low weight, difficulty concentrating and auditory hallucinations that were recorded in her patient notes at Auckland Mental Hospital between June 1933 and December 1935.[30]

Inquest reports also revealed how depression could lead some sufferers to overdose on barbiturates, or how the drugs themselves could induce despondency. A 29-year-old chemist's messenger with a 'morbid disposition' told a doctor at the Trentham Racecourse that he had swallowed 36 Medinal tablets because he was 'tired of life'.[31] On this fourth suicide attempt he asked to be saved, but it was too late.

Family doctors have long treated patients with melancholia and depression outside of institutions, but they were also often the first to refer patients to a mental hospital. An ongoing problem was whether these patients should be treated separately from chronic or severely disturbed patients within a mental hospital.[32] Another issue within general hospitals was the provision of facilities for those with mild depression that were separate from the facilities provided for those who were mentally unwell.

In 1937, after a patient committed suicide on his farm, Dr J. G. Campbell advocated the need for specially equipped wards in Whangārei hospital for the treatment of melancholia.[33] 'I discussed his going into hospital, but I always had to agree with him that the hospital treatment was not suitable for his particular case . . . Cases of this type require treatment in specially equipped wards, and these are lacking at the present time. This is not peculiar to the Whangarei Hospital.'

As discussed in chapter 4, more therapeutic and less restrictive facilities were available in selected psychiatric hospitals to treat soldiers with war trauma following the First World War. A few of these depressed patients were treated in low-security and more 'homely' facilities, such as Wolfe Home and, from 1931, the Lodge at Auckland Mental Hospital, where writer Robin Hyde lived and where she had the attic as her study.[34] The Lodge's medical superintendent, Henry Buchanan, aimed to 'prevent long-period recoverable cases (such as mild melancholia, of whom we have many) being sent into main building wards'.[35]

> [W]hat we want in our ordinary asylums is gentleness, capacity for extending sympathy, and restoring self-respect to all. Sunny, bright houses we want for the mentally distressed, with everything like restraint carefully in the background. We want, by the harmony of civilization and concord, to tranquilize the nervous systems of the functionally insane. We want to preserve to society all those people who, in an old country, would never have gone mad. We want, in fact, discrimination, and must bear in mind that dozens who are put in lunatic asylums in this Colony would be kept in their own houses in more domestic England, and that we are daily ruining the intellects of citizens by crowding all classes together in hopeless confusion, and ministering to their wants by the rudest tools our rough-hewn civilization places in our hands.[36]

At Sunnyside in 1949, the artist Rita Angus was housed away from the more seriously disturbed long-term residents and encouraged by staff to resume her creativity.

In 1952 Cherry Farm Hospital, 50 kilometres north of Dunedin, opened as a therapeutic psychiatric community, designed for patients to live within villas and with more freedom (although this did not always occur in practice) than in the old asylums such as Seacliff.[37] Cherry Farm closed in 1992 as outpatient treatment and community care for depressed patients became standard throughout the country. Such deinstitutionalisation was partly in response to patient advocacy groups and partly a cost-cutting measure, even if the transition from institutional to community care remained inadequately resourced.[38] As we have seen throughout this book, families and friends had long provided much of the care for depressed people in Aotearoa, many of whom had never required institutionalisation.

Poet Meg Campbell, 'desperately depressed', recalled that her first impression of Porirua Hospital 'was that I'd arrived at the Mad Hatters' Tea Party'.[39] By 1979, she found on her final admission to Porirua Hospital that it was a place of 'refuge':

> [S]taff were better trained than they used to be — more liberal-minded — There was swimming, psychodrama, occupational therapy and physiotherapy . . . I think many people left that and went back into the community. Ward 10 wasn't locked. You were there on trust. It became a place where I longed to go if I was in strife and depressed. People need a refuge.[40]

Psychiatric hospitals may have provided refuge, but they could also be sites of lifelong confinement. Theresa H. was admitted to Seaview Asylum in 1905, possibly with puerperal melancholia. Her house and 'seven or eight' children were in a 'filthy neglected state . . . She is depressed and listless, and very reluctant to speak and reply to questions, speaking almost in a whisper, and originating no conversation. She appears to avoid notice, and keeps head covered with an apron,' her notes recorded.[41] Theresa died in Seaview Psychiatric Hospital in 1942 aged 72.

Theresa H. was married, unlike Agnes F., who was admitted to Seacliff Mental Hospital in 1913 shortly after giving birth.[42] Truby King assessed Agnes's condition as 'melancholy combined with a marked lack of moral sense'. She was discharged, but readmitted in 1914 after a miscarriage. Again, Truby King stressed her 'moral insanity' and unsuitability to care for her child. The child remained with Agnes in the hospital, but was sometimes taken to another ward when things got 'unreasonable'. It is unclear whether Agnes, who died at Cherry Farm in 1969 aged 83, ever had time away from institutions.

There were only a few residential alternatives to the large psychiatric institutions. Some non-military patients could be treated at Queen Mary Hospital at Hanmer Springs after the hospital was transferred from the Department of Defence to the Department of Health in 1922. Ashburn Hall, which now operates as Ashburn Clinic in Dunedin, has been the country's oldest private mental asylum.[43] By the Second World War most of Ashburn's patients were voluntary, a situation which, during the following decades, became increasingly more common within state mental hospitals as well. The historian Warwick Brunton suggests that this may have been because as 'more effective treatments for mental illness were introduced, patients became more willing to enter mental hospitals voluntarily'.[44]

Admission procedures for hospitals became somewhat more relaxed, too, and few people wanted the stigma of compulsory committal. Private clinics had more facilities and staff, and could offer a variety of occupational and recreational therapies such as art, crafts and drama; this increasingly became the practice in many public hospitals. When Dr Reginald Medlicott was appointed as Ashburn's medical superintendent in 1947, he introduced therapeutic community principles (a participative group-based approach for residents and staff) and some psychotherapy, but he also supported convulsive therapies (outlined below). However, as a private clinic, attending Ashburn Hall was far beyond the financial resources of most people who suffered depression.

Private patients were transferred to public psychiatric facilities from time to time; it might be considered that the patient required the more secure and coercive facilities available in public institutions, or they might be moved when their family could no longer afford private care. Ann G., who suffered from melancholia with delusions, was admitted to Seacliff in 1877 and in 1884.[45] Then, from 1885 until 1887, she was a patient at the private Ashburn Hall, after which, because her friends were unable to pay the fees, she was returned to Seacliff.

Isabel M., aged 21 and from Invercargill, was treated at Ashburn in 1898 for melancholia and depression, and as a voluntary patient from 1912 to 1913. In 1914 she spent a year in Seacliff, where she was described by

Truby King as a 'neurotic degenerate, victim of foolish fears of delusions, lacking in self confidence, subject to fits of depression during which she becomes suicidal'.[46] Isabel was later a patient at Sunnyside from 1916 until 1917. Her body was found in the sea near Ōamaru in 1921.[47]

Charles G., a school teacher originally from Wellington, was diagnosed with severe melancholia, and he was also moved around: he was originally a patient at Ashburn (1895–1898 and 1905–1909), and was then transferred to Sunnyside Hospital, where he was assessed as depressed and agitated. He then spent 1910–1913 in Seacliff.[48] He died in 1932 in Wellington.

The historian Jonathan Sadowsky has suggested that psychoanalysis, and its role in defining and treating twentieth-century depression, has been underestimated by historians, despite psychoanalytic hegemony being 'roughly concurrent' with the rising rates of depression in the United States.[49] This hardly applied to New Zealand, where commanding figures in early twentieth-century psychiatry such as Truby King and the director general of mental hospitals Theodore Gray dismissed the 'talking cure'. As late as 1924 Truby King rejected this 'latest professional shibboleth', instead advocating the curative properties of country life, 'which provides the most natural, healthful, and enjoyable forms of occupation and recreation — besides being the best of sedatives for restoring rest and sleep'.[50]

Dr Patrick Savage, medical superintendent of Sunnyside Hospital, was also sceptical about the value of psychotherapy. 'The depth of exploration of a patient's mind varies with the necessity of the case. Deep exploration is not always necessary and is often inadvisable,' he said in 1961.[51]

We have seen in chapter 4 how historians have suggested that the success of psychoanalysis with soldiers from the First World War contributed to a tolerance for psychoanalysis and psychotherapy within the wider medical community. The evidence for this is limited, however. While talking therapy was used to treat war neurosis cases from the First World War at Hanmer Springs, doctors Percy Chisholm and Sydney Rhind considered this as superficial psychoanalysis.[52] They recognised the therapeutic value of uncovering the subconscious mind, but did not go so far as exploring Freudian therapy.

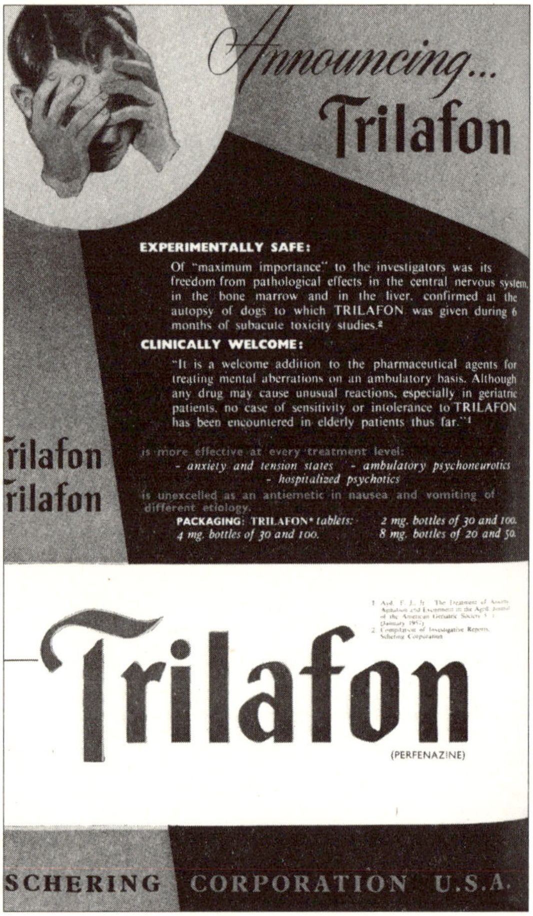

Mid-twentieth-century advertisements in *The New Zealand Medical Journal* for prescribed medicines for depression and anxiety.

PREPARATIONS OF INTERNATIONAL REPUTE

RIKER

NOW AVAILABLE IN NEW ZEALAND

RAUWILOID*

brand alkaloid hydrochlorides of Rauwolfia serpentina

Rauwolfia in its optimal form and the preparation of choice in essential hypertension, 'Rauwiloid' contains the hypotensive alkaloids, reserpine and rescinnamine, as well as other desirable alkaloids, but not those of the yohimbine group, which are rejected in the extraction process. Moreover, 'Rauwiloid' is biologically tested and standardized.

2 mg. tablets in bottles of 20, 60 and 500

DOSE: 2 tablets nightly

RESERPINE

'Serpiloid'* brand

The chief sedative alkaloid of Rauwolfia serpentina, for those clinicians who prefer to treat hypertension with a single alkaloid. Reserpine is now finding an ever-increasing use in psychiatry, where its greater calming effect is of considerable value.

0.25 and 0.5 mg. tablets in bottles of 25, 100 and 1,000

1, 3 and 5 mg. tablets in bottles of 100

Ampoules 5 mg. in 2 c.c.; boxes of 6

Rauwiloid and Reserpine are accepted as a charge under the Social Security Fund.

Other Riker products available in New Zealand are Veriloid,* Rauwiloid + Veriloid, Rauwiloid + Hexamethonium and Theodrox,* the most satisfactory form of oral aminophylline.

New Zealand Agent: Miss K. I. White, MPS., P.O. Box 469, Wellington, C.I.

* *Registered Trade Mark. Regd. users:*

RIKER LABORATORIES LTD. LOUGHBOROUGH LEICS. ENGLAND

LOS ANGELES TORONTO PORT ELIZABETH

Among the pioneering professionals in Aotearoa who treated depression with psychoanalysis and psychotherapy were Dr Stuart Moore in Dunedin,[53] Dr I. M. Allen in Wellington, Dr Kathleen Mary Todd and Dr Gilbert Tothill at Auckland Mental Hospital, and Dr Charles Maurice Bevan-Brown and Dr Enid Cook, who worked in private practice in Canterbury. Bevan-Brown and Cook were instrumental in establishing a clinic for medical psychology in Christchurch and the New Zealand Association of Psychotherapists (NZAP) in 1947.[54] NZAP's foundational meeting included refugees from Europe such as psychoanalysts Eva Fischman (from Auckland) and Mario Fleischl (from Wellington).

From 1923 to 1939, Bevan-Brown had worked as a psychiatrist and psychotherapist at the Tavistock Clinic in London. After his return to Aotearoa in 1940 'he found most of the medical profession, and the public generally, were ignorant, unreceptive and often hostile to the teaching of the principles of psychotherapy and mental health'.[55]

According to Dr J. C. McKenzie, who was the medical superintendent of Timaru Hospital from 1927 to 1963, most doctors in Aotearoa regarded psychotherapy 'with great suspicion as having theories and techniques smacking of charlatanism. The medical student of that day got no glimmering whatever of the vast amount of neurotic illness in the community most of it misdiagnosed as organic in origin and demanding prolonged medication or worse still, drastic surgery.'[56] An emphasis on individual responsibility in treating depression — rather than addressing the socio-cultural context — became common in therapeutic circles and was advocated by some psychiatrists. In 1957 Christchurch psychiatrist Dr David Livingstone suggested that

> It is perhaps too easy to convey to a patient the impression that he has been the victim of circumstances as an infant. To succeed in therapy patients should take increasing responsibility for their treatment procedure and current behaviour in society. The patient should take an active part in his own cure as soon as he is strong enough to do so.[57]

However, only a minority of psychiatrists and psychologists were drawn to treatment through talking; physical and pharmaceutical treatments for depression remained dominant during the twentieth century.

In 1935 António Egas Moniz, a Portuguese neurologist, popularised lobotomy (more commonly called 'leucotomy' in New Zealand) as a treatment for mental illness. It involved cutting connections in the brain's prefrontal cortex from the thalamus to disconnect thoughts and affect.[58] This drastic operation attracted international attention, especially after Walter Freeman and James Watts finessed the technique in the United States after 1942.

In September 1942, visiting military neurosurgeon Lieutenant-Commander W. J. Gardiner of Cleveland Clinic, Ohio, performed leucotomies on two women at Porirua Hospital; 'pitiable unhappy beings who showed no sign of spontaneous recovery'[59] but who, it was reported, were 'rescued . . . from complete insanity' after Gardiner inserted a surgical instrument into their skulls and cut their prefrontal nerve fibres.

One of these women, aged 65, was a patient at Porirua Hospital between 1936 and January 1943.[60] In 1936, she had been treated for over three months at Queen Mary Hospital in Hanmer Springs after becoming very depressed and apprehensive. Her depression returned when she went home, and she was admitted to Porirua Hospital, depressed, very introspective and complaining of 'various hypochondriacal ideas'. In March 1937 she attempted suicide by puncturing her neck and trachea with a knitting needle. Medical superintendent Reginald Medlicott published details of her lobotomy in 1942 and post-operative state in *The New Zealand Medical Journal*:

> On inserting the hollow calibrated needle on the right side the anterior horn of the lateral ventricle was entered and cerebrospinal fluid escaped; on reinserting it slightly anteriorly no fluid escaped and section was made on this level . . . The brain appeared somewhat shrunken and on inserting the exploring needle fluid again escaped. On reinsertion anteriorly the anterior horn was entered again and the surgeon . . . cut through the tip of the anterior horn of the lateral ventricle . . .
>
> The patient slept quietly for about twelve hours after the operation . . . She answered simple questions with yes and no

> and obeyed nursing instructions. Later in the day, however, she became mildly restless, muttered to herself if left alone and would attempt to remove the dressing from her head. She was occasionally incontinent during the first few days; and her temperature was 100°F. for two days. Her restlessness decreased rapidly and she remained clearly orientated for time, place and person and showed no gross memory defect . . .
>
> Gradual diminution of the intensity of her depression with an increasing interest in her surroundings: she was showing an interest in books within a few days of the operation, took a pleasure in her meals, and would make a few spontaneous remarks such as 'That was lovely!' when she had been given a cup of tea. This stage lasted over two months and during it she retained the appearance and motor habits of her previous agitated melancholic state and would restate her former depressive ideas. These ideas did not, however, have the same paralysing effect upon her conduct as formerly and her external contacts gradually developed.
>
> She became very careful of her dress and bodily cleanliness, reliable in conduct, and worked satisfactorily in the laundry. Slowly her depressive ideas disappeared; she stated that she felt really well, wrote asking her daughter to give her a home and displayed full insight into her condition . . . only remnants left on discharge were a rather uneven agitated way of speaking, and a slightly stooped posture . . . put on 35 lbs. in weight . . . discharged in January, 1943, to live with a married daughter.[61]

In the same article, Medlicott provided details of 'case 2', a former nurse aged 62, who was also subjected to a lobotomy by Gardiner. She had been a patient at Queen Mary Hospital, and in 1933, when she was depressed and introspective, at Sunnyside. She believed that her relatives had died because of her masturbation, and that she was suffering from cancer. This woman was diagnosed with agitated melancholia and became self-destructive, including attempting suicide. She was difficult to feed, required observation and needed individual nursing. Case 2 was transferred to Porirua, where the depressive symptoms became overshadowed by a 'growing detachment from reality, gross introversion, losing contact with the real world and sinking into a world of her own', her notes recorded. She remained 'restless, abusive, and obscene' after the lobotomy and Medlicott did not anticipate recovery.

Despite this gloomy outcome, Medlicott advocated lobotomy for those with longstanding depression that had not responded to convulsive therapy, to break 'faulty emotional patterns'; if successful, 'a repatterning occurs along more normal lines so that the patient is no longer dominated by morbid preoccupations and is able to readjust to normal life again'.[62] The 'prefrontal lobotomy used with discretion is a real advance in psychiatric treatment', he wrote in *The New Zealand Medical Journal* in 1942.[63]

By 1946 about eight leucotomies had been performed throughout Aotearoa.[64] Dunedin Hospital, linked to the Otago Medical School, aimed to be the country's centre for neurosurgery and from April 1944 to March 1950, 65 leucotomies were carried out by specialists Murray Falconer and Anthony James.[65] Among the 14 classified as melancholics, 11 apparently benefitted from the procedure, but only one was discharged. Two patients died.

These operations enabled the Dunedin neurosurgeons — 'guided by their impressions of the gravity of the patient's illness into making a "major" or a "restricted" cut' — to compare the methods of the American psychiatrists and neurosurgeons John Scarff and Lothar Kalinowsky with those of the pioneers of lobotomy, Freeman and Watts. According to the Dunedin surgeons, with the major cut the surgeon could 'make a more thorough section; and consequently one more satisfying to his surgical prowess'.[66] However, the outcome of the more dramatic operation, or any lobotomy, rarely benefitted patients.

In 1945 Malcolm Brown, medical superintendent of Seacliff, agreed to three patients with 'grave depression' having leucotomies. There was no dramatic recovery, and they 'required a long spell of careful psychiatric nursing and re-education'.[67] Between 7 August 1946 and 20 November 1952, 154 patients (24 depressives) had leucotomies in Auckland. Eight died, five within the hospital.[68]

Given the low rates of long-term improvement to patients' mental states, the risks involved in this kind of surgery and the strain that post-operative care put on limited mental health staff, it was not surprising that scepticism emerged about leucotomy as a treatment for severe mental illness, let alone depression. Theodore Gray regarded neurosurgical procedures as a treatment of last resort. It was not a cure, although it could stabilise a patient's mental condition at a 'lower level than normal'.[69]

One young woman, who suffered from severe depression with bipolar disorder, had two leucotomies during the late 1950s. They were ineffectual — as were the over 1300 electroshocks she had received since her admission to a mental hospital in 1952, when she was aged 15, until she was transferred to another mental hospital during the 1980s. She committed suicide in 1990.[70]

The treatment of melancholia and depression in New Zealand, as globally, radically changed with the introduction of shock and pharmacological therapies: the 'magic bullets' of modern psychiatry.[71] By 1954 Reginald Medlicott, one of New Zealand's most ardent proponents of convulsive therapy, had treated 900 patients (over 16,000 treatments) with various forms of it, including electroconvulsive, electronarcosis and non-convulsive stimulatory treatments, insulin coma and subcoma, and prolonged narcosis.[72]

Both medical and lay discourse and representation in Aotearoa lauded the 'dramatic' results of shock therapy — whether insulin coma, metrazol or electroshock. By the 1940s, the heroic doctor who cured insane patients through modern therapies had become part of New Zealand popular culture. Movie-goers were guaranteed laughs if they watched *Bedside Manner*, which referred to shock treatment, and the romantic drama *Dr. Kildare's Strange Case* offered:

> the first picturisation of the use of insulin shock treatment to rouse a person out of insanity and bring him back to mental normalcy. Dramatic highlights of the feature include the actual administration of the insulin shock treatment, and reactions of the patient following the treatment and a bird's-eye view of a delicate brain surgery.[73]

After insulin coma therapy was pioneered in 1933, it was seen by Medlicott as the 'treatment of choice for schizophrenics'.[74] Dr John Plinez, a San Francisco physician who visited Auckland in 1938, also considered insulin coma therapy as 'particularly successful' in treating minor forms of insanity, which included depression.[75] Insulin treatment commenced at Seacliff in 1938, and by 1939 a special ward was designated because the therapy involved intensive nursing.[76]

Insulin coma therapy at high doses (100–150 daily units or more) was largely discontinued in Aotearoa by 1961, but therapy with lower doses (30–50 units) continued in some hospitals.[77] It has been suggested that if insulin coma therapy worked it was because patients tended to be chosen for their good prognosis and were given special treatment.[78]

In 1934 Ladislas Joseph von Meduna injected camphor oil into a catatonic patient in Budapest and developed a convulsive agent, pentylenetetrazol or metrazol (Cardiazol). Five years later, Cardiazol treatment was first administered at Porirua Mental Hospital, and then 'extensively' to over 150 patients there. A chronic melancholic patient who had spent five and a half years in Porirua in a depressed state made a rapid improvement with Cardiazol injections and subsequently returned home.[79] In 1943 Auckland psychiatrist Kenneth Stallworthy praised the profound effect of Cardiozol therapy in depressive illnesses. A 63-year-old retired school teacher who was being treated for depression wrote in 1941:

> I became unaccountably bored and tired, I began to suffer from depression in the morning, I found difficulty in concentrating as my brain seemed addled and unresponsive. The depression began to be continuous and thoughts of suicide intruded; I grew steadily worse. In the mental hospital I could see no way out of the difficulties but by way of self-destruction . . . I hated the whole world . . . When the first injection was given I had no fears even though I thought it meant death, I bore the preliminary pain calmly because it was fully deserved, but I woke up, and especially after the third or fourth treatment woke up as from a deep sleep feeling calm, fresh and clear-headed. The turmoil of the mind died down to calm my mind then became orderly and logical for periods which gradually became longer as the treatment continued.[80]

Stallworthy observed: 'Within a fortnight this man was transformed from an incontinent, agitated, severely depressed and pitiable object to a state of normal mental health. He maintained this for six months; then relapsed and convulsive treatment was repeated with similar remission.'

But clearly the promise of cure from depression through convulsive therapies was not always borne out. There could be a brief respite, but it was not always permanent. Moreover, Cardiazol treatment was terrifying to many patients.[81] After the injection, convulsion started before the patients lost consciousness, which American psychiatrist Lothar Kalinowsky reported as 'a very unpleasant feeling of impending death . . . the fear derived therefrom is a severe setback for subsequent treatments . . . Failure to obtain a convulsion makes the patient very apprehensive and uncomfortable.' Alternatively, Reginald Medlicott observed that there could be spontaneous fits within a few hours after the induced fit.[82]

The undesirable features of Cardiazol therapy spurred Christchurch businessman Tracy Thomas Gough to try to make something better.[83] His interest was piqued in 1941, when he learned of Ugo Cerletti and Lucio Bini's 1937 experiments with electric shock treatment in Italy. Gough studied electric shock treatment in medical journals, and unsuccessfully tried to import an apparatus or its components. In 1943, using Kiwi ingenuity, he and Leonard Johns, an electrical engineer on his staff, built a machine that they developed from a rough sketch of the circuit followed by experimentation.

In his 2021 family memoir *Come Back to Mona Vale,* Gough's great -grandson, Alexander McKinnon, shed further light on how Gough's entrepreneurial foray into medical equipment intersected with his daughters' experiences of mental illness.[84] It is quite possible that Gough was spurred to find a replacement for Cardiozol therapy after the death of his 29-year-old daughter Alison in 1942 from cardiac failure. She had been committed to Sunnyside Hospital in 1941 (there had been an earlier admission in 1939), following the death of her mother, Julia. The coroner stated that Alison suffered from schizophrenia, while her hospital notes recorded depression, as well as mania and psychosis. She was administered the sedative drugs phenobarbitone and paraldehyde, as well as being shocked with Cardiozol. Gough's other daughter, Beryl, also diagnosed with schizophrenia, was admitted as a mental patient after ECT became available. She was subjected to several ECT treatments between 1945 and 1948 when she was a 'voluntary boarder' at the private Hornby Lodge in Christchurch.

Electric shock treatment using Gough's machine was administered to patients at Sunnyside Hospital with 'highly successful results', especially for involutional melancholics — those first showing depression later in life.[85] Yet a spat broke out over who could claim glory for introducing ECT to Aotearoa: Gough and an engineer from the private sector, or Gray, the government's director of the Mental Health Department. In spite of these 'turf wars', by the mid-1940s several patients were being administered ECT.[86]

Reports from Auckland, Seacliff, Kingseat and Tokanui mental hospitals noted 'striking' results for patients with melancholia and depression. At Porirua Hospital, Reginald Medlicott found 'little fear shown by patients toward the electric treatment'.[87] This was hardly Meg Campbell's recollection of the fear she experienced 'when hearing the hum of the "machine"'.[88]

In 1945 Medlicott recounted in detail in *The New Zealand Nursing Journal* the procedure followed for ECT at Porirua Mental Hospital.

> The electrodes are applied one on each temporal region and a current of a known voltage is allowed to pass for a known period of time. If the first shock fails to produce a convulsion the voltage and time are increased by steps until a convulsion is produced.
>
> In elderly and very frail patients or those with any orthopaedic disability in whom it is felt that the full violence of the convulsion might carry unnecessary risk, shocks are preceded by an intravenous injection of a drug known as curare. This drug produces a generalised paresis [weakness] of skeletal musculature within two minutes and when the shock is given the violence of the resulting seizure is greatly diminished. The risk attached to the use of this drug is that if too great a paresis of muscles of respiration is produced, breathing ceases. The influence of curare, however, is quickly counteracted by giving an injection of prostigmine and artificial respiration is carried on till normal breathing resumes.

> The nursing technique of convulsive therapy and the management of complications is important. The patient remains in bed on treatment mornings, has no breakfast and should be persuaded to empty his bowels and bladder prior to treatment . . . on a hard mattress under which is placed a fracture board. A bolster, easily made by rolling blankets, is placed under the mid-thoracic spine and, during the convulsion the patient is held by several nurses; one nurse holds the shoulders firmly down on the bed, another holds the hips down, while another restrains the arms. A gag is placed in the mouth at the commencement of the seizure and the lower jaw supported to prevent dislocation.
>
> At the completion of the convulsion the senior nurse feels the pulse, watches the return of normal respiration and reports any abnormality to the doctor. Respiration should commence immediately after the convulsion but in electro-shock therapy there is sometimes a protracted cessation of respiration and artificial respiration may be necessary . . . The patient resumes consciousness in anything from a few minutes to half an hour and it is the usual practice in this hospital to return the patients after treatment to an observation dormitory . . . until full consciousness is resumed, when they are given a late breakfast.
>
> . . . Patients often complain of some memory loss during treatment, but they can be reassured that their memory will return to normal within a few months. Episodes of confusion and temporary aggravation of symptoms which sometimes occur are short and seldom serious . . . Convulsive therapy is the treatment of choice in those mental states in which there are gross changes in mood either in the direction of depression or elation. Melancholics, particularly those of the involutional period respond dramatically to this treatment.[89]

Medlicott acknowledged that many long-term patients did not recover: 'after years of illness their personality deteriorates, and their final picture may resemble schizophrenic regression more than melancholia'.[90] This assessment differed from that of Malcolm Brown, Seacliff's medical superintendent, who found that ECT could modify behaviour disorders among patients with long-term illnesses, allowing many 'to lead happier and more useful institutional lives'.[91]

Variations of ECT also came to Aotearoa. Reginald Medlicott claimed to be the first psychiatrist to use electronarcosis outside the United States, employing it at Porirua in 1942.[92] Between 1945 and mid-1953 Medlicott oversaw 8118 treatments of electrotherapy that led to narcosis lasting from 6 to 12 minutes, which was induced through injecting thiopentone anaesthesia, although sometimes insulin subcoma was used. Patients subjected to electronarcosis tended to be those who had been diagnosed with schizophrenia and affective psychoses.

Doctors in Aotearoa were convinced that electroshock could alleviate depression. Medlicott even approached an engineer in Wellington to design a machine to trial brief stimuli electroconvulsive therapy, but found that this induced more fear among patients than standard ECT.[93]

ECT was inflicted on patients in Aotearoa in more extreme ways. In 1957 Dr Rina Moore described 'therapeutic dissociation' by ECT treatment in a paper delivered in 1957 in Dunedin to the Australasian Association of Psychiatrists. Moore (Te Whānau-ā-Apanui, Ngāti Kahungunu, Rangitāne) was New Zealand's first female Māori doctor, graduating in 1949.

Moore practised psychiatry at Nelson's Ngawhatu Hospital until 1963. Here, over the course of eight years, 'therapeutic dissociation' by ECT was administered to 25 women who had not responded to other treatments. These women, many with severe depression, were subjected to an extreme therapy that aimed to erase their delusions and hallucinations and reinvent them. If a patient remained in a state of confusion for a lengthy period, then a rest from delusions supposedly assisted in recovery. Patients were treated daily, until temporary dementia resulted. In an article published in *The New Zealand Medical Journal* in 1958, Moore wrote:

> As the daily treatment progresses there is a loss of initiative and narrowing of interests, and a general lack of concern. Gradually, after a week or more, mental confusion and imperception

> occur, so that the patient does not recognise objects, persons and places. There is complete poverty of imagination, so that while at first some effort may be made to get out of bed to the toilet, the patient eventually becomes incontinent of urine and faeces unless regularly toiletted. Eventually complete aphasia and agnosia occur, and finally there is a breaking up of the personality organisation. It is important at this stage that the treatment be continued until there is complete loss of personality. The patient may show gross regression until she curls up into the antenatal position . . . Towards the end of the treatment the patient loses all touch with the environment except response to those conditioned reflexes which are so habitual that they have become automatic and probably require little cortical response to carry out. For instance, the patient responds to regular toileting, and if a spoon is presented to the patient, her mouth will open. Eventually, especially with a younger person in the age groups between 20 and 30 years, this is all lost.[94]

The women subjected to this treatment under Moore's watch included those with severe depression who had tried various treatments, including narcoanalysis, prolonged narcosis, ECT and sometimes psychotherapy. Moore reported some success, such as a woman admitted with neurotic depressive reaction: 'After her recovery from the therapeutic dissociation by ECT she had no memory of how she felt prior to treatment and did not realise subjectively the complete change that had taken place, with her social adjustment to other people. A month after treatment her memory had completely returned, and she decided she would like to get married, which she did three months after her discharge.'[95]

Another woman diagnosed with recurrent neurotic depression had, since the age of 31, been a chronic invalid with several periods in hospitals. She had not benefitted from psychotherapy. Short courses of ECT relieved her tensions but not permanently. She had also been given prolonged narcosis, again with only temporary relief. She was discharged, but was readmitted to the hospital suffering from depression, sleep disturbance and headaches. Following a course of therapeutic dissociation by ECT, she returned to her job as a florist.

ECT's success was widely acclaimed in New Zealand despite later criticism. Former Porirua nurse Peter Sanders recalled in 1989 that it was 'really magnificent' in severe depressive cases, and a student researcher suggested it could abort a depressive episode for many patients.[96] Brian Barraclough, an assistant medical officer at Sunnyside Hospital during 1956 and 1957, recalled how ECT was administered to patients with the machine, an anaesthetic trolley, and nurses moving from bed to bed. He said that Patrick Savage, Sunnyside Hospital's medical superintendent, described them as 'like a well-trained gun crew'.[97] Savage, who would later become Oakley Hospital's medical superintendent, enthused in *The Press* in 1961 that ECT had once brought happiness to patients more than any other therapy:

> It was one of medicine's major therapeutic advances for the first half of this century. Shock treatment is quite painless. The patient has no memory afterwards of the treatment, since unconsciousness is immediate. Very often, as he sits up after the treatment, a patient will ask when it is going to start. This treatment is used only in selected cases and is often combined with relaxant or anaesthetic drugs as necessary. It is given about three times a week until the doctors feel there is sufficient improvements for the treatment to be discontinued . . . A few patients complain of fear, but we find that what they're frightened of is an imaginary picture of horrors which they've made up for themselves. Such a picture is built on misinformation.[98]

One patient from Sunnyside found relief: 'You feel as though the cobwebs have been blown away . . . After three weeks in hospital, I was completely cured and lecturing by the end of the year.'[99] Another former patient told journalist Jennifer Hamilton in 1977 that doctors had tried almost everything for her depression, but ECT was the only treatment that stopped her feeling suicidal.[100] Christchurch psychiatrist John Dobson, then chair of the New Zealand Committee of the Australian and New Zealand College of Psychiatrists, spoke of a woman who became very depressed during her three pregnancies, but after ECT treatment during her last pregnancy was 'completely cured'.[101]

Age was no impediment for shock treatment according to Dobson. In 1950, R. Presland and Harold Palmer of Dunedin Hospital's Department of Psychiatry declared that convulsion therapy was 'indicated in all states of depression, whatever age the patient'[102] — an assessment that was to be challenged in years to come.

Shock therapies, enthusiastically transferred to Aotearoa from overseas during experimental phases, were highly controversial.[103] The renowned writer Janet Frame brought its negative effects to local attention when her book *Faces in the Water* was published in 1961. The protagonist Istina

> perceives the bed she must lie on to receive treatment as a 'coffin'; the electric current induces in her sensations of disembodiment and dropping into darkness; ECT causes the loss of cognitive perception (the sense of time, space, and self) and arouses feelings of grief the narrator cannot name; finally, ECT impairs Istina's capacity to reconstruct any sense of self . . . ECT causes her madness.[104]

Frame wrote in her autobiography, *An Angel at My Table*, that a 'Mrs R.' had urged her to voluntarily admit herself to Sunnyside in 1948 to receive the 'new electric treatment'. Mrs R. had also helped arrange for Frame to have her decaying teeth extracted (considered advantageous at the time given that ECT had no muscle relaxants). 'I was given the new electric treatment, and suddenly my life was thrown out of focus. I could not remember. I was terrified. I behaved as others around me behaved. I who had learned the language, spoke and acted that language. I felt utterly alone.'[105] Frame had been diagnosed with schizophrenia, a diagnosis that later proved to be incorrect. It seems clear from her autobiography that hospitalisation at various institutions after 200 unmodified ECT treatments induced 'madness', including intense times of aloneness and depression.

In a 1995 oral history interview about women living in Waihī, Estelle McInnes recalled that when she was a child in the 1950s her mother, who had postnatal depression, was sent from Inangahua on the West Coast to Sunnyside Hospital. 'They gave her ECT until she was totally not with us and became a non-person,' she told the interviewer. When nine-year-old Estelle was reunited with her mother, she found her a 'very shadowy person'.[106]

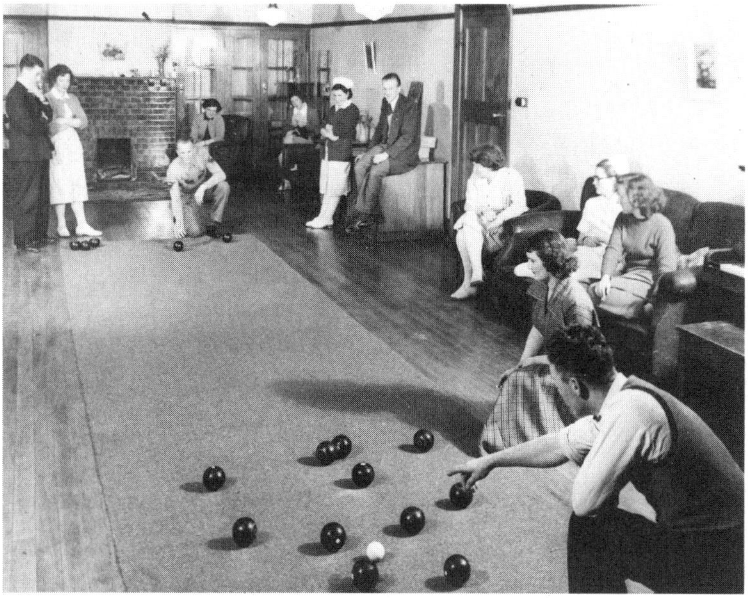

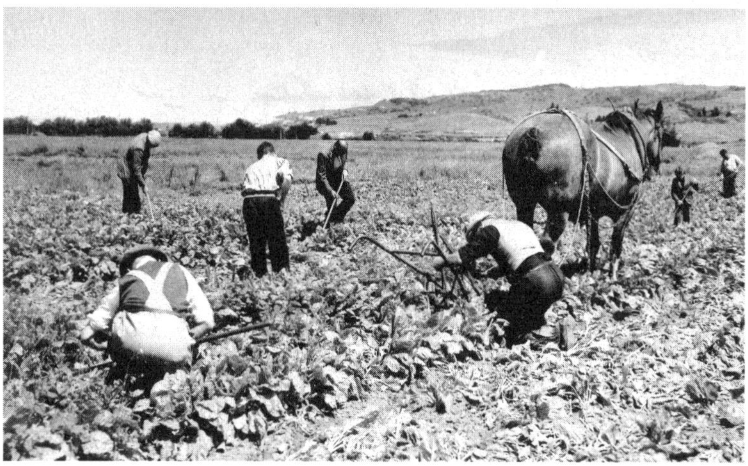

Work, creativity and recreation were considered therapeutic for patients with depression in New Zealand's psychiatric hospitals, but by the 1950s shock treatments and medication became the norm. *Above:* A staged image of recreation at Porirua Hospital, c. 1956. *Below:* Working in the Cherry Farm market gardens, c. 1960.

Dr Sanford Meyer, a visiting psychiatrist from the Pennsylvania Hospital for Mental and Nervous Diseases,[107] told reporters in 1958 that Sunnyside Hospital was behind the times, with too many patients having shock treatment instead of modern psychotherapy. Looking back during an oral history project about psychiatric nurses in 1989, former nurse Peter Sanders agreed that ECT had been overused at Porirua in the past.[108]

In 1958 Dr R. G. T. Lewis, director of New Zealand's Division of Mental Hygiene, disputed claims that convulsive therapy was overused in New Zealand, and argued that it could be most useful along with other forms of treatment.[109] As late as 1982, Professor Basil James, director general of mental health, was recommending ECT as an effective treatment in severe depressive illness, especially the 'endogenous type' (supposedly when depression was genetic, biological or had a physiological basis).[110] In 1985 a former trainee nurse at Sunnyside recalled that it was standard practice for patients to be administered ECT. After 'several bouts', ECT could lead to disorientation and a marked loss of their previous personality; 'severe loss of affect and appeared to be a zombie . . . They seemed like shells where people used to live but lived no longer.'[111] 'Loss of affect' is a common phrase in mental health discourse, usually referring to an inability to express emotion or empathy.

Electroshock could also be used as a punishment. Damning evidence was given to the Royal Commission of Inquiry into Historical Abuse in State Care, established in 2018, by surviving patients at psychiatric hospitals, including children who spent time at Lake Alice Hospital, near Bulls in the Rangitīkei, during the 1970s and who were punished with ECT.[112] Meg Campbell recalled such punishment even for singing at inappropriate times, which was considered at Porirua Hospital to be as 'causing a disturbance; a symptom of being deranged'.[113] She depicted the terror of electroshock in one of her poems:

Hole in the Head

I have sung every song I know this night —
my fourth in isolation. By morning
I am hoarse, and no one hears me
but the ladies who kick the door. 'You're
down for treatment and serves you right —

> making a disturbance!' But now they come,
> nurses who are warders, who are nurses,
> with hard, frightening hands. I plead
> and fight and pull off my clothes in a corner.
> Here is the doctor, nightmare eyes bulging,
> master of the machine which glides to the bed
> where I'm held, temples bared, teeth
> clamped on a rubber gag. 'How are you, Mrs Jones?'
> he says, just as the magistrate did.
> There is a smell of meths and then
> no air — no time to breathe . . . I leave them
> through a hole drilled by fire in my temples,
> escaping the explosion that ends all worlds.[114]

A common side effect of ECT was short-term memory loss, especially when electrodes were placed bilaterally (on both sides of the head).[115] Memory blank could last much longer for patients put under electronarcosis, who might also endure amnesic confusional states.[116] A woman who had several ECT treatments at Dunedin's Orokonui, Cherry Farm and Wakari hospitals during the 1960s told medical student researcher J. Guthrie that she could not remember her marriage, although she may have also blocked this out because it was an abusive relationship.[117] She often failed to recognise people she passed on the street. The woman refused further shock therapy, but agreed to take antidepressants and Valium. She was able to keep working as a clerk.

Narcoanalysis was trialled by some psychiatrists in New Zealand during the 1940s. Reginald Medlicott, medical superintendent at Porirua, explained in *The New Zealand Nursing Journal* in 1945 that barbiturate narcosis (intravenous sodium pentothal or sodium amytal) was administered so 'the patient loses his inhibitions and is able to recall and discuss experiences too painful or unpleasant to express otherwise'.

> [I]t may be possible to alleviate some of the stresses to which he [the patient] has been subjected, but the prime importance lies not with the stresses of life but the patient's faulty way of reacting to them. He must be shown how and why he is adjusting in a faulty manner and then re-educated so that he can replace his faulty actions by mature and more successful ways of living.[118]

Henry Buchanan, the medical superintendent of Auckland Mental Hospital, wrote in his annual report in 1946 that pentothal narcosis was utilised 'to a great and useful extent'.[119] The new therapy found its way into local popular culture:

> The first motion picture presentation of the new narcohypnosis method used by the army in rehabilitating psychoneurotic patients will be made in a military hospital sequence of the Rosalind Russell picture, 'Some Call It Love.' The method involves use of the drug sodium pentothal as a short cut to psychoanalysis and cure of mental patients.[120]

Narcoanalysis or narcohypnosis did not put patients completely to sleep. But deep sleep therapy, continuous narcosis, or deep sedation therapy, albeit with modifications, in which patients were put to sleep for several weeks, was used in Aotearoa to treat severe depression and other mental conditions. The method followed was modified narcosis, promoted by the controversial British psychiatrist William Sargant. These techniques were extremely dangerous and traumatic; alarmingly, from 1962 to 1979 at least 24 patients died at Chelmsford hospital in Sydney, and more were severely mentally and physically impaired by deep sleep therapy. In 1980 the Royal Australian and New Zealand College of Psychiatrists denounced the therapy.[121]

In New Zealand it seems that modified narcosis aimed for 12 to 20 hours of light sleep per day, during which the patient was nursed, was woken to eat three meals a day and was given fluids. During narcosis, the antipsychotic chlorpromazine might be injected, along with other drugs, anticonvulsants and vitamins. ECT was sometimes given while the patient was asleep.

The full extent of modified narcosis in New Zealand's hospitals, deaths (if any) and effects on patients is unknown, one reason being the appalling lack of record-keeping within state hospitals, especially at Cherry Farm.[122] The silence over modified narcosis also reflects the vulnerability and the lack of voice for patients, many of whom were young or prisoners. In 1991 the Department of Health commissioned a report by psychiatrist Professor Graham Mellsop and lawyer Michael Radford which identified an absence of written patient consent, although this had not been unusual medical practice in mental health during the 1970s — the period Mellsop and Radford reviewed. Mellsop and Radford also found a range of imprecise diagnoses for those who underwent modified narcosis, and questioned the reliability and recall of patient affidavits, which were mostly scripted by the Citizens Commission on Human Rights (which was aligned with the Church of Scientology).

The silence over the extent of modified narcosis used in Aotearoa speaks volumes about medical hierarchy and culture. In 2015 journalist Fran O'Sullivan, who in her twenties was a trainee nurse at Cherry Farm in the 1970s, spilled the beans in *The New Zealand Herald* on the 'Zombie Ward', a locked mental-health facility where women prisoners were treated with prolonged sleep therapy. O'Sullivan referred to a 'voguish new treatment by a foreign doctor (Dr X) at a time when it was starting to be roundly condemned elsewhere'.[123] That doctor headed the experimental narcosis unit during the 1970s, 'the domain of Dr X'.[124]

Mellsop and Radford's report identified three wards under Dr X where modified narcosis was administered between 1973 and 1978 for periods of around six weeks; in one year, at least 52 patients were subjected to this treatment.[125] The report was concerned with the inappropriate amount and type of drugs used by Dr X, including barbiturates and benzodiazepines, which are known to produce dependency.[126]

Many of the affidavits submitted by former patients at Cherry Farm to Mellsop and Radford's inquiry outlined their depression, along with other symptoms and diagnoses. Among the case notes of those receiving modified narcosis at Cherry Farm were those of an 18-year-old who had been diagnosed with schizophrenia, non-agitated depression, reactive depressive psychosis and antisocial personality disorder. A man who was a patient in 1973 testified that his life changed drastically for the worse after modified narcosis, ECT, and the drugs on which he became 'somewhat dependent'.

> I became unable to speak and I was totally restrained due to the amount of drugs that I was taking . . . left me with body spasms, it also left me emotionally unstable, I had mood swings, my concentration was gone which left me unfit for work, I lacked self confidence . . . I was at breaking point. I had no control over my bladder, which I felt was degrading. I was unable to show my affection for people.

Another patient, initially treated at Ashburn Hall for depression and an eating disorder, was sent to Cherry Farm, where she became severely depressed after narcosis treatment and a high level of medication. There were no 'positive effects from the narcosis treatment,' she said. 'It was the worst period of my entire life. I kept waiting for the miracle cure. I was desperate to have relief and persisted with my treatment for this reason.' In 2021 similar testimonies about the abuse and ineffectualness of deep sleep, and other psychiatric therapies were presented to the Royal Commission of Inquiry into Historical Abuse in Care.[127]

According to Patrick Savage, the term 'anti-depressive' was little known before 1958, when these drugs began to be used 'freely' at Sunnyside Hospital and were being prescribed by general practitioners.[128] Savage reported that anti-depressives raise to normal the depressed mood-level of affected persons without making them 'dopey'. He also lauded a new generation of tranquillisers, probably meprobamate (Equanil or Miltown), introduced around 1953. By the early 1960s these were replaced by the benzodiazepines (Librium, Valium, Serepax).[129] Savage cautioned that tranquillisers were not a replacement for electrical treatment.

Modern neuro-pharmacological offerings enabled many sufferers of depression to be treated as outpatients.[130] By the early 1970s some patients with severe depression were also prescribed phenothiazines or antipsychotics such as chlorpromazine, Trifluoperazine, Haloperidol and Perphenazine. Lithium carbonate, a mood stabiliser, designed to decrease the frequency and symptoms of manic episodes, was used to treat manic depression.

The anti-depressives that Savage praised were the 'tricyclics' and the monoamine oxidase inhibitors (MAOIs), which were developed by global pharmaceutical companies during the 1950s.[131] By 1951, some depressed patients in New Zealand were prescribed the tricyclic imipramine (Tofranil) and later, even in some cases before approval by the US Food and Drug Administration (FDA), tricyclics such as amitriptyline (Amirol, Arrow-Amitriptyline), nortriptyline, desipramine (Norpramin), doxepin (Anten), protriptyline (Concordin), and trimipramine. MAOIs offered in Aotearoa during the late 1950s included tranylcypromine (Parnate), phenelzine (Nardil), isocarboxazid (Marplan) and pargyline.

Many patients did not share the same enthusiasm as health practitioners for the new pharmaceuticals. Some patients resisted taking these medications, feeling guilt in 'relying on a drug to maintain normality'.[132] It could take at least two weeks for anti-depressive medication to kick in. Side effects might be significant: dry mouth, blurred vision, constipation, dizziness, weight gain, heart rhythm problems, sexual dysfunction and excessive drowsiness. These side effects were often the reason that many patients ceased taking their medication.[133]

MAOIs could cause either insomnia or drowsiness, and could be fatal in interaction with certain foods such those containing tyramine, which include hard cheese, aged meat and fish, home-brewed beer, wine, yeast extracts, soy sauce, soy products and avocado. Certain medications such as those that elevate blood pressure also had to be avoided. Several other risks are associated with MAOIs.[134]

These attitudes persisted when a different class of antidepressants, the selective serotonin reuptake inhibitors (SSRIs), became available in New Zealand during the 1980s. SSRIs are said to work by increasing the amount of serotonin, a neurotransmitter which is a natural substance in the brain that helps maintain mental balance. SSRIs prescribed in Aotearoa include fluoxetine (Prozac), sertraline (Zoloft), escitalopram (Lexapro), paroxetine (Paxil) and citalopram (Celexa), to name but a few. Many newer-generation antidepressants also promote the production of the neurotransmitter dopamine in order to restore concentration, motivation and positive feelings. However, recent research questions the role of serotonin in depression.[135]

Another side effect of using medication was that patients living outside of institutions might stockpile medication. Hoarding sedatives and psycho-reactive drugs was one route to suicide, as outlined in chapter 5, when Ivan Sutherland was prescribed a large quantity of sodium amytal.[136] Some depressed people overdosed on a combination of drugs and alcohol. In 1973 Dr Ronald Trubuhovich, a critical care specialist at Auckland Hospital, warned that tricyclic antidepressant drugs with a high toxic content were being prescribed by general practitioners to patients for 'reactive depression, failure to cope, or an inadequate personality state', and that they were at risk of taking an overdose.[137]

Trubuhovich advised that antidepressants (which he called a 'poison') should be used only to treat endogenous depression (considered long-term, biological and physiological). An example of his warning was a woman who had been prescribed a tricyclic anti-depressive and had swallowed several tablets during an argument with her husband. She told him that the drugs would only put her sleep. She began to have seizures and hallucinations, but because she lived in a rural area there was a delay in reaching a hospital, where she died.[138] She may have acted on impulse, but the availability of drugs that might induce oblivion were enticing for many people who suffered depression.[139]

Despite such tragic outcomes with medications prescribed for depression, as in former times the recovery and endurance of many people depended on family, friends and whānau. Historical evidence of this most essential support and treatments, especially after the 1920s, is slight, largely because of archival privacy restrictions. Dissertations written between the 1950s and 1970s by fifth-year students in preventative medicine at Dunedin's School of Medicine include patient testimonies about the role of their families and friends, rather than their limited contact with medical professionals, and offer valuable insights.

For example, one woman hospitalised for depression explained to Peter Dunn in 1968 that contact with doctors was mainly when they prescribed medication, but that her recovery depended on daily visits from family and friends. Another student researcher, Judy Herd, pointed out that some of the depressed women she interviewed in 1969 needed no medical treatment and could function adequately if supported by their husbands and family.[140]

But as we have seen, whānau, family and friends were not always supportive of those who were depressed. Embarrassment, shame and stigma have been evident in families and wider communities, even when melancholia and depression did not manifest as madness. Depression was often kept within the family, perpetuating the silence around the illness and the interfamilial dynamics that could reinforce tensions. Both could prevent individuals and families seeking external support, perhaps leading to intergenerational depression.

In 1971 Otago medical student J. M. Berryman spoke to a woman who was lonely, and afraid to cry in front of her husband or to ask him to help with the children when she was tired. Her husband claimed that he could not help her if she was unable to cope on her own. Another participant told Berryman that when she was alone with her husband, she had to leave the room to escape the intolerable silence.[141]

General practitioners have been at the forefront of recognising and treating depression in New Zealand. They could often recognise stress and provide appropriate relief and advice.[142] Patients in their waiting rooms from the late 1950s to the 1960s possibly flicked through copies of *N.Z. Family Doctor*, a magazine that featured articles on nerves and depression, accompanied by alarming images.[143] Students at the Dunedin School of Medicine researched patients with depression who were treated by the family doctor rather than attending psychiatric units.[144] Even when psychiatric patients were admitted to hospital, general practitioners have played a major part in long-term rehabilitation, such as checking on patients once they returned home and seeing whether the prescribed medication was effective or being taken.[145]

But a general practitioner's long-term care could not always alleviate depression or prevent suicide, even when a patient had long periods free of depressive symptoms. Before computers and the internet, it was difficult for health professionals to monitor patients' use of prescribed drugs. As many people started to feel better, or experienced the side effects, they may have stopped taking prescribed medicines. In the past it was easier to obtain prescriptions from different doctors, which might be filled at various pharmacies.

Until more rigorous pharmaceutical research was conducted and published during the late twentieth century, many general practitioners were unaware of the interactions between the drugs they were prescribing for depression and other conditions such as anxiety (such as diazepam, a benzodiazepine first marketed as Valium) and insomnia (such as triazolam, marketed as Halcion and commonly prescribed in Aotearoa during the 1980s), and for physical pain such as diclofenac (Voltaren).

Depressed patients sometimes hoarded medication: among the complex reasons for this could be a plan to commit suicide through taking an overdose. General practitioners sometimes referred depressed patients to counsellors, but options were limited. Outpatient services at hospitals sometimes provided counselling, and there were also self-help options, such as Alcoholics Anonymous, but these did not target depression. Those with severe depression might be referred to a psychiatrist by general practitioners, but it could be a long time before they secured an appointment. The other option, private health care, was unaffordable for most, while most private health insurance programmes offered very limited coverage for psychiatric care.

Several of the other treatments for depression outlined in this chapter have persisted, even if there have been significant changes in their application. Lobotomies, deep sleep, insulin coma and Cardiozol therapies may be confined to the past, but ECT is still advocated by some psychiatrists for severe depression or bipolar disorder that is considered resistant to other treatments. To date there is no solid research on patients and their families' views on how effective usage of ECT is within contemporary Aotearoa. There may be temporary 'relief' from severe depression but how long-term is this? Do some patients still feel pressured by some psychiatrists in agreeing to a course of ECT? The fear of undergoing ECT also continues to haunt some patients in our psychiatric units.[146]

Very few people diagnosed with depression today will ever see the inside of a psychiatric hospital, but they are likely to be prescribed medication and be urged to see a counsellor. Most depressed people remain in their homes and active at work, although far more now than in the past will consult a general practitioner about their mental pain. But there has also not been any slowing up of 'self-help' remedies and advice, especially with the advent, and escalation, of social media.

Epilogue: Bursting the black cloud?

'A nation that truly values and includes people with mental illness' was a goal of the Like Minds, Like Mine mental health campaign launched in Aotearoa in 1997 by the Ministry of Health.[1] Like Minds, Like Mine took a bold step towards promoting awareness of mental health and tackling discrimination against those with mental illness, through showing that ordinary and functioning people could suffer from many mental health issues, including depression. But ordinary New Zealanders were not initially at the campaign's forefront; instead high-profile Kiwis such as former rugby player and All Black Sir John Kirwan and musicians Mahinaarangi Tocker and Mike Chunn, who had 'done the walk', were engaged to 'do the talk'.[2]

Like Minds was initiated and funded by the ministry following the 1996 Mason Inquiry into mental health services in New Zealand, one of whose key recommendations was a public awareness campaign about mental illness.[3] Like Minds was lauded globally as an innovative and successful campaign, supported by local celebrities whose experience of mental distress connected with the public and related to the lived experience of depression and anxiety in what might be seen as a Kiwi way. Similarly, in 2009 the comedian Mike King set up The Nutters Club to encourage ownership of 'our own mental health'.[4]

The ongoing need for campaigns to raise awareness of depression and other mental health issues would suggest that, despite the many treatments for depression covered in the previous chapter — most notably new-generation antidepressants, the SSRIs (selective serotonin reuptake inhibitors) — the black cloud persists, with markedly increased rates of depression among Māori, Pasifika, Asians and other cultures reported. It is possible that awareness campaigns may have promoted this increase, by encouraging acceptance and the seeking of professional help, although this is unlikely to be the only factor.

The world's first online self-management programme for what was termed 'mild to moderate depression' was launched in Aotearoa in 2010. A part of this campaign featured Kirwan coaching sufferers to complete a daily task via video clips. The aim was to encourage individuals to self-manage depression through 'staying positive, better nutrition and physical activity, and finding creative solutions to problems'.[5]

Kirwan knew all about depression. He called depression and anxiety his 'black monster' in his 2010 book *All Blacks Don't Cry: A Story of Hope.*[6] 'I was clinically depressed, but I like to call it freaking out, because depression is such a word that people say, "Snap out of it." . . . What gets you through? Love, family, communication's a big one. You've got to talk it through. It's terrible when you're in there. But it's no big deal, it's pretty normal,' he wrote. Four years later he teamed up with clinical psychologists Elliot Bell and Kirsty Louden-Bell, and writer Margie Thomson, to produce *Stand By Me: Helping Your Teen Through Tough Times*, a book that explores teenage mental health through their lived experiences and tries to give whānau the tools and understanding to support their young ones.[7]

Kirwan went on to head the Sir John Kirwan Foundation, which offers young people skills and knowledge about mental health. A recent campaign, Mitey: Building the Mightiest Kids in the World, teaches mental health management strategies for school children in years one to eight, and includes processes for taming a balloon dog — the 'black dog' being a well-known metaphor for depression.[8]

The Mental Health Foundation has been at the forefront of depression awareness and advocacy in contemporary Aotearoa.[9] One of its key campaigns, Out of the Blue/Kia Mārama ('Let there be light'), launched in 2005[10] with the aim of helping people recognise when either they, or someone close to them, are depressed. The following year a partnership was formed between the foundation and the Auckland regional Māori public health provider Hāpai Te Hauora.

Since 1993 the foundation has coordinated an annual Mental Health Awareness Week, and since 1998 it has secured contracts to deliver programmes under Like Minds. The foundation has provided many other services for people with mental health issues, their support-persons and others interested in mental health and wellbeing, including comprehensive suicide prevention resources and providing information on ways to obtain help.

═══

Nationwide advocacy and awareness of mental health and depression in Aotearoa emerged during the 1980s, when mental distress among women, Māori, youth and those living in poverty became more evident. As neoliberal economic and social policies and practices were introduced, and the fallout set in, suicide rates increased. According to the historian John Weaver, during the years 1976–1998 suicide rates rose from 10 to 14 within 100,000 and the youth suicide rate was unprecedented.[11]

Neoliberal policies resulted in greater poverty and social isolation, but the spin was that you could get out of the black hole of poverty through personal endeavour, an approach that carried over into mental health campaigns. For while Like Minds promoted a sense of commonality among survivors and sufferers of depression through the message that they were not alone, the contradiction was that a sense of aloneness was part of the individualistic zeitgeist of the time.

Like Minds also reflected the prevailing mood of focusing on individual self-help over any causative environmental factors, through its highlighting of successful individuals who had pulled themselves through, glossing over those who faced economic as well as cultural pressures. As Weaver put it: ‘Mental illness entered popular discourse with greater frequency and honesty in the 1980s and 1990s, but that also favoured a misleading focus on the mental state rather than on factors that brought on the all-too-evident mental distress.’[12]

People with depression have been advised to consult family doctors and/or telephone health-line services, and, in the twenty-first century, to access internet resources. But this well-meaning advice is based on assumptions of access and privilege that are beyond the reality of many people's lives. For example, not everyone in Aotearoa can afford doctors' fees or has internet connectivity. Lack of confidence in the English language can be another constraint.[13] Still, today many general practitioners offer empathetic, practical and supportive advice about how to live with and treat depression.

Almost all prescribe antidepressants, usually the SSRIs and other 'new-generation' antidepressants. For some patients, though, there remain the obstacles, discussed earlier, of getting the time off work, having the resources to travel to a doctor's surgery and paying for the consultation and for filling prescriptions. Not to mention the issue for some within certain ethnic or community groups of visibility/invisibility in seeking such care.

Radically different psychedelic treatments for depression are now being explored globally, such as micro-dosing with psilocybin or using ketamine. Safe use in Aotearoa remains inhibited by legality, availability and access to appropriate therapists at a level most can afford to pay.[14] There are parallels with the constraints that have impeded the uptake of psychotherapy in the past: a lack of trained specialists, high costs and resistance from the medical establishment.

Today, although most general practitioners are reluctant to consider experimental and radical treatments for depression, they tend to be far more receptive to referring patients to therapists for talking and behavioural therapy, such as cognitive behavioural therapy (CBT), which by the late twentieth century was widely advocated in treating depression, either alongside medication or on its own.[15] However, doctors also know that these services are almost impossible to freely or immediately access, putting them out of reach for the majority of patients. There are also very few therapists conversant in New Zealand's many languages or who are aware of cultural nuances. For many general practitioners, prescribing medication often remains the main option.

In the twenty-first century, institutionalisation is highly unlikely for people who suffer depression, unless there are other serious mental conditions. Convulsive therapies for depression have been shunned by most — but not all — psychiatrists in Aotearoa.[16] Fortunately, most people with depression live in the community, pay their taxes, care for others, and their brains are not sliced, shocked, sedated or put to sleep as were the brains of some sufferers in the past. Today, people with depression may rely on medication, which is presumably safer and less disruptive than that administered to depressed people 50 years ago. There is also the option of counselling, for those who can afford and access it. And rather than consulting quacks, they can search the internet.

Public campaigns to tackle mental health and depression did not develop in a vacuum, but were part of the shift to deinstitutionalise and reform New Zealand's mental health services. Advocacy for change came from mental health survivors (later termed 'consumers') and mental health advocacy groups such as the Citizens Commission on Human Rights. In the late 1980s and early 1990s, the government commissioned Judge Ken Mason to head two inquiries into the country's mental health services that would prove ground-breaking: the first, submitted in 1988, examined aspects of psychiatric care and treatment in prisons, hospitals and the community; and the second, in 1995–1996, scrutinised the availability and delivery of mental health services in New Zealand.[17] Mason's second report recommended the establishment of an independent Mental Health Commission, which began as a ministerial committee in August 1996, and in 1998 became a Crown entity under the Mental Health Commission Act.[18]

Several other surveys, inquiries and reports concerning the nation's mental health followed, including the Confidential Forum for Former In-Patients of Psychiatric Hospitals (2005–2007).[19] The results of Te Rau Hinengaro, New Zealand's first large mental health study, were published in 2006, followed in 2015, 2016 and 2018 by the New Zealand Mental Health and Wellbeing Survey, which was conducted in people's homes to gauge views and experiences of mental health and wellbeing.[20]

In 2018 the Government Inquiry into Mental Health and Addiction recommended destigmatising attitudes and environments to end prejudice and discrimination, and more inclusion for people with experience of mental distress, especially Pasifika, disabled people, those with diverse sexual and gender identities, the prison population, refugees and migrants. The inquiry described Māori mental health outcomes as far 'worse than the overall population'.[21] Following this inquiry, Te Hiringa Mahara (the Mental

Health and Wellbeing Commission) was established in 2022.[22] But has this state investment in mental health surveys and reports in contemporary Aotearoa been enough to burst the black cloud?

Despite Mason's second report identifying the lack of Māori-based mental health services, a trenchant criticism of mental health campaigns in contemporary Aotearoa has been the lack of awareness and capacity to embrace cultural diversity. When in 2002 the government launched Te Puāwaitanga: Māori Mental Health National Strategic Framework,[23] the intention was to 'provide District Health Boards with a nationally consistent framework for planning and delivery of services for tāngata whaiora and their whānau, so they can meet the government's mental health policy objectives for Māori over the next five years'. However, further research revealed that the mental health needs of Māori and Pacific peoples had not been addressed.[24]

In 2019, the *Māori Mental Health Report* was released as part two of the Waitangi Tribunal's Health Services and Outcomes Kaupapa Inquiry (Wai 2575), urging that 'to understand the ultimate causes of mental ill health amongst Māori, a much broader lens must be adopted' across a range of government social and economic policies that affect determinants of mental health.[25] Following Mason Durie's seminal 2001 publication *Mauri Ora* there has clearly been an upswell in advocacy for a holistic and kaupapa Māori perspective to tackle depression, not just on marae or in rural settings but also within a range of contemporary urban lifestyles.

In 2020 clinical psychologist Rebecca Wirihana (Ngarauru kii tahi, Ngāti Maniapoto, Tainui, Te Rarawa, Te Aupōuri, Ngāpuhi Nui Tonu), researcher and Māori health advocate Cherryl Waerea-i-te-Rangi Smith (Ngāti Apa, Whanganui, Te Aitanga a Hauiti, Ngāi Tūmapūhiarangi) and Maori knowledge expert and master carver Tākirirangi Smith (Ngāi Tūmapūhiarangi) wrote a fictional vignette about a 22-year-old Māori woman, 'Teina', based upon their experience of working within both kaupapa Māori and mainstream mental health and addictions services in Aotearoa. Teina was experiencing major depressive episodes with psychotic features when she encountered mental health services. Their

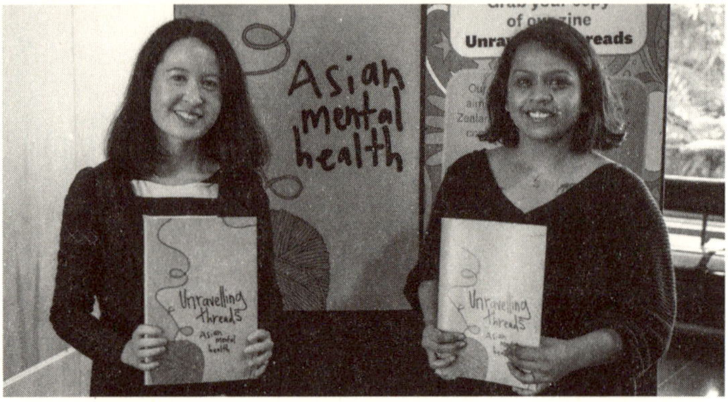

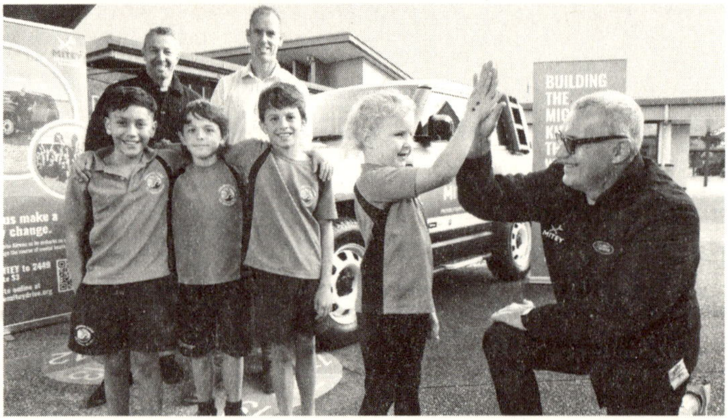

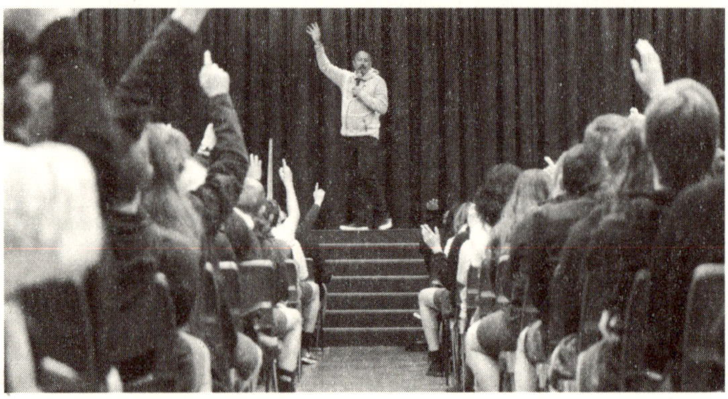

From top: Grace Gassin and Mehwish Mughal launch Te Papa's Asian Mental Health Project in 2022; Sir John Kirwan introduces the Mitey mental health education programme to children at Endeavour School in 2022; Mike King during a presentation at Matamata College, 2018.

vignette (which retains patient and practitioner confidentiality) illustrates how some of actual practices of kaupapa Māori involved:

> [a] Māori psychiatrist, a Māori psychiatric nurse and a kaiārahi Māori (kaupapa Māori practitioner) within the kaupapa Māori mental health service. Mihi whakatau (formal welcoming ceremony) and a karakia (prayer) were provided in te reo Māori by the kaiārahi Māori before the assessment began . . .
>
> The kaupapa Māori mental health team offered regular contact with the kaiārahi Māori and support to attend the kaupapa Māori therapy programmes provided within their service. Medication treatments for her depression and psychoses were discussed by the psychiatrist and monitored by the psychiatric nurse who visited Teina in her home with the kaiārahi Māori on a weekly basis initially.
>
> Once her symptoms of depression, suicide and psychoses reduced, a referral to the Māori psychologist on the team (who based his practice on kaupapa Māori interventions) was encouraged to provide individual therapy. Whānau sessions and support were also provided by the kaiārahi Māori . . . Teina remained under the care of the kaupapa Māori service for approximately three years until she was discharged back to her general practitioner for ongoing primary health care follow up.[26]

As this book went to press, the strongest critique of the limitations of contemporary mental health campaigns and publications to offer a kaupapa Māori approach is *Nōku te Ao: Sovereignty of the Māori Mind*,[27] compiled for Te Whatu Ora, New Zealand's national health service, in 2022. The report offers a Māori worldview of the factors that discriminate against Māori who experience mental distress, asserting that mental health interventions in Aotearoa have reflected non-Māori worldviews. The anthropologist Pounamu Jade Aikman stated in another report for Te Whatu Ora that Like Minds was 'built on a Western worldview, unable to adequately or appropriately support Māori or Pasifika people',[28] and lacked 'framing of Māori experiences within colonial contexts'.[29]

In 2021, Like Minds, Like Mine was re-branded as Nōku te Ao Like

Minds. It has partnered with Māori-led health organisations such as Te Rau Ora and Hāpai te Hauora (jointly with Te Kete Pounamu, the Mental Health Foundation and Ngā Hau e Whā), and Te Whare Wānanga o Awanuiārangi.

There has been a genuine effort to embrace kaupapa Māori within the health reforms rolled out nationally by the government during 2021–2022. But will recent Māori-centred mental health initiatives lift the black cloud? *Nōku te Ao* rightly emphasises how mental health cannot be isolated from structural and historical issues. Discrimination against Māori mental health sufferers remains entwined with racial and cultural discrimination.

Pacific peoples have been absent from most of the mental health and depression awareness campaigns in recent times. A report in 2006 found very few mental health resources for Pasifika;[30] even fewer designed for specific Pacific Islands cultures. Pacific cultures are not culturally homogenous, nor are their attitudes about depression or their access to mental health services all alike. For example, a clinical audit of a depression programme in Ōtara between 31 March 2009 and 30 September 2010 showed greater participation rates by Cook Island Māori than from Samoan and Tongan clients, although the reasons for these cultural differences were not given.[31] Mental health services that take a more culturally nuanced and holistic approach remain crucial to addressing depression.

Chapter 6 noted that although earlier surveys indicated that Pacific peoples had lower rates of reported mental distress than the general population, this did not necessarily mean an absence of depression or worry. In 2006 Pacific peoples with serious mental health disorders were far less likely (25 per cent) than the general population (58 per cent) to visit a health provider because of mental health.[32] Yet in contemporary Aotearoa, Pasifika, often more than other minorities, have faced marked stress from poverty, low incomes, unemployment, inadequate housing, high rents and the high cost of living, all while many were expected to donate money to kin, community and church in Aotearoa and in the Islands.[33]

Recent analysis, such as in *Te Kaveinga: Mental Health and Wellbeing of Pacific Peoples* — which is based upon the findings of the New Zealand Mental Health Monitor and Health and Lifestyles Survey — has found that

Pacific peoples, like Māori, are reporting higher levels of psychological distress and depressive symptoms than Pākehā and other ethnic groups.[34]

Resources for Pasifika have become more prominent on several websites addressing depression, but are still only available in a few Pacific languages.[35] The Ministry of Health now funds Le Va as a national centre for Pacific mental health and addiction workforce development. While depression has become more evident among Pasifika people, it is unclear whether this is a consequence of a greater willingness and ability to seek help, or whether rates are actually rising because of economic and social pressures, such as housing issues, unemployment or underemployment, and the disconnection from community or identity issues that have troubled many younger Pasifika and those born in Aotearoa.[36]

One of the most disturbing investigations into the treatment of patients in psychiatric institutions has been the mammoth Royal Commission of Inquiry into Abuse in Care, which commenced in 2018 and has heard the testimony of thousands of individuals who were in state or faith-based care between 1950 and 1999. It is set to deliver its final report in 2024. The commission is investigating why people were taken into care, what abuse happened and why, and the effects of the abuse. It is focusing on Māori, Pacific peoples and those with disabilities in care, because the numbers from these communities were disproportionately represented in care in that time period. Some of Rachael Lemalie Umaga's testimony was recounted in chapter 6. She considered that she had been labelled with various depressive conditions:

> that gave medical professionals a licence to pump me with more drugs. I believe they were just experimenting with their drugs on me. There was no thought or talk about therapy or alternative ways of healing, only drug therapy . . . mental health hospitals are not well places or conducive to healing. I don't have any faith in these hospitals whether they are inpatient or community. My biggest issue with any mental health service is that they are unwilling to consider other alternative treatments.[37]

During an informal admission in 2003 to Te Whare Ahuru (an acute inpatient unit at Hutt Hospital), Rachael's parents organised for a Samoan fofō (healer) to fly from Sāmoa to Wellington to treat their daughter.

Rachael's psychiatrist supported this care. Rachael found the experience positive.

> I remained well which I believe was attributed to the Samoan fofo. The fofo was not only healing, but the process was spiritual and natural. I was wrapped in leaves, plants and a sheet to help get rid of any toxins in my body by sweating it out. I was then showered with natural scents and leaves from rose bushes and was blessed at the end by the fofo.

Rachael had repeat admissions to Te Whare Ahuru:

> It was robotic. You were given medication on a regular basis and that was expected to make you well. There was no creative outlet, just some walks around the hospital grounds. I believe that options such as Samoan fofo or Māori massages should be readily available because they worked well for me . . . For me, medications should only be a last resort.

Rachael concluded her testimony with the questions: 'Who are going to be the reformers and who are going to make sure that there are big changes for the future of care? I believe that survivors are a good start to consult with.'

Mental health campaigns and resources for depression specifically for Asians in Aotearoa have been almost non-existent. A report written in 2006 found no mental health epidemiological data on Asian groups in New Zealand, and only one translated resource on depression.[38] This paucity of information speaks volumes about the current state of ignorance regarding the diversity of Asian communities and languages in Aotearoa, and the silence over the extent of depression within these cultures.

Cultural stigma about mental illness,[39] and assumptions that depression constitutes madness, are further factors. So, too, are loneliness and isolation. Depression among Asian immigrants has been associated with language problems, unemployment, separation from family and community, and, especially for refugees, traumatic experiences prior to migration.[40]

Depression among older migrants can be exacerbated by suburban isolation, especially when family members are working, and if seniors do not feel useful.[41] Before a widowed elderly Chinese woman aged in her eighties hanged herself during the late 1980s, she had told her doctor that she had become depressed because she felt she was getting old and was feeling useless.[42]

The loneliness of the migrant, described in chapters 3 and 6, continues. Today the face of racism may be somewhat different from the examples given in chapter 6, but the fear and anxiety caused by contemporary racism towards Asians remain key contributors to depression and feelings of exclusion.[43]

There is still a long way to go in addressing depression and the provision of culturally sensitive services within Asian cultures.[44] This unmet need is pertinent, given the significantly increasing proportion of New Zealanders who identify with an Asian culture; around 15 per cent in the 2018 census.[45] Many Asian people remain reluctant to seek professional help for mental health,[46] although there have been initiatives to provide culturally appropriate services and support by district health boards and within communities.[47] As in its earlier history, depressive disorders among Asians continue to be under-diagnosed in Aotearoa.[48]

In 2022 the Museum of New Zealand Te Papa Tongarewa launched a project on Asian mental health in Aotearoa.[49] At its launch project leader Mehwish Mughal explained:

> We need to move beyond looking at mental health issues from a western psychiatric lens. We need to recognise the plethora of ways people from Asian and other minority communities conceptualise and respond to mental health and mental health issues. We need to honour these pieces of knowledge and practices. We need to move beyond the stereotypical representations of Asian communities in the mental health space. We need to move beyond changing attitudes and behaviours of individuals and question the structures and systems which influence these attitudes and behaviours.[50]

I have ended this book by looking at recent efforts in Aotearoa to lift the black cloud for Māori, Pasifika and Asian communities. Other programmes have emerged to address the high rates of depression among vulnerable, traumatised and isolated groups, such as refugees, rural people, the elderly, physically disabled people, and those who identify as sexually and gender diverse (LGBTQIA+).[51]

The internet has played a key role in raising awareness, providing support and tackling the stigma of depression, but is this enough when public health provision faces serious shortcomings and criticism? And does social media reach those target groups who have alarmingly high rates of depression? In spite of the shortcomings of social media, and although it has been identified as a contributor to the accelerating rates of depression and anxiety among youth,[52] the same technology can be a positive and effective channel for tackling depression, and several mental health websites specifically target young people.

Identifying such inadequacies and shortfalls, as well as what is working, indicates that more historical research on depression among diverse groups in Aotearoa is clearly needed[53] if we are to be a 'nation that truly values and includes people with mental illness'. Looking at how past generations in Aotearoa understood and experienced depression opens us to greater awareness of the intergenerational impact of mental distress. This does not necessarily imply a predetermined outcome, but rather can offer more understanding into how people have lived under the black cloud.

We need to examine contributing factors, practices and behaviours and, most importantly, how these are nuanced by culture, if we are to effectively address current problems and prevent or minimise future issues. In doing this, not only should the concept of depression as an illness be questioned, but, as therapist Maria Milmine has advocated, a mental health system designed as one size fits all, for the largest group in mind, also needs to 'extend equally well to all'.[54]

This book has traced how depression and melancholia were part of the old black cloud hovering over some in Aotearoa, and has shown how these mental conditions have been experienced, articulated, understood and treated here. Just as there was concern in New Zealand's early days about the burgeoning number of the mentally ill, today we hear about an epidemic of depression. In part, this may be attributed to a greater recognition and acceptance of depression rather than an increase in the actual number of those in our population who experience depression. What is clear, though, is that for many in Aotearoa a dark cloud that casts a shadow over how they live and experience their lives remains.

Although the contributory factors for this darkness are individual, varied and complex, we as a community need to acknowledge the wider contexts — familial, social, economic and ethnic, among others — that bring these into play, and try to mitigate these factors if we are to effectively support those with depression, and prevent or minimise future suffering.

In undertaking this task, questions remain about whether we are a nation that values and embraces mental wellbeing for all of the diverse minds, bodies and cultures that live in our challenging physical, social, economic and political environments. If we are, then we can move from being the land of the old black cloud to an Aotearoa with brighter and more colourful clouds.

Notes

Abbreviations

AJHR *Appendix to the Journals of the House of Representative*
AS *Auckland Star*
ANZ Archives New Zealand
ANZJP *Australian and New Zealand Journal of Psychiatry*
AR Auckland Repository
ATL Alexander Turnbull Library Collections
CR Christchurch Repository
DR Dunedin Repository
DSC *Daily Southern Cross*
EP *Evening Post*
ES *Evening Star*
HC Hocken Collections Uare Taoka o Hākena
JPS *Journal of the Polynesian Society*
NEM *Nelson Evening Mail*
NZH *New Zealand Herald*
NZJH *New Zealand Journal of History*
NZMJ *New Zealand Medical Journal*
NZT *New Zealand Times*
ODT *Otago Daily Times*
RNZ *Radio New Zealand*
WR Wellington Repository

Introduction

1 Åsa Jansson, *From Melancholia to Depression: Disordered Mood in Nineteenth-Century Psychiatry* (Cham: Palgrave MacMillan, 2021), ix, offers a different perspective to mine: 'I didn't come to this topic because of an interest in melancholy as a feeling or a personal experience with depression.'

2 See Jacqueline Leckie, 'Serendipity or Working with Circumstances,' in *Serendipity: Experience of Pacific Historians*, ed. Brig V. Lal (Honolulu: University of Hawai'i Press, 2024), 258–77.

3 ACGS 16231/1637, COR1961/1178, R23863898 (ANZ WR).

4 Michelle Walker is completing a PhD thesis, 'Exploring Mental Distress Related to Childbirth in New Zealand, 1860–1980,' at the University of Otago.

5 Eleanor de Jong, 'Kind of Blue,' *New Zealand Listener*, 10–16 July 2021, 16–25. The cover of this issue asked 'Down Time. Are our ordinary issues being wrongly diagnosed as mental illness?' The article highlighted Lucy Foulkes, *Losing Our Minds: What Mental Illness Really Is — and What It Isn't* (London: The Bodley House, 2021). See also: Jonathan Sadowsky, *The Empire of Depression: A New History* (Cambridge; MA: Polity Books, 2021); Gary Greenberg, *Manufacturing Depression: The Secret History of a Modern Disease* (New York: Simon & Schuster, 2011).

6 Alistair's letters to mostly Meg part 1, 20 October 1963, ATL, 91-046-1/05.

7 Wendy Parkins, *Every Morning, So Far, I'm Alive: A Memoir* (Dunedin: Otago University Press, 2019), 46–47.

8 See Warwick Brunton, 'Mental Health Services,' *Te Ara — the Encyclopedia of New Zealand* (2011, revised 2022), accessed 13 July 2023, www.teara.govt.nz/en/mental-health-services

9 On the contradictions of access to mental health archives in Aotearoa, see Barbara Brookes, 'Mental Health Records: Who Controls the Past?,' *Archifacts* (April 2015): 8–16.

10 In 1960 Auckland Mental Hospital was renamed as Oakley Hospital, and in 1973 as Carrington Hospital.

11 For an analysis of how different doctors diagnosed patients at Ashburn Hall, see Elspeth M. Knewstubb, 'Respectability, Religion and Psychiatry in New Zealand: A Case Study of Ashburn Hall, Dunedin, 1882–1910' (MA thesis, University of Otago, 2011), http://hdl.handle.net/10523/1734. Ashburn Hall was first established as a private mental asylum in Dunedin in 1882 by Dr Edward William Alexander and James Hume. It catered to more affluent or middle-class patients than those in the public psychiatric hospitals.

12 Jonathan Sadowsky, 'Before and After Prozac: Psychiatry as Medicine, and the Historiography of Depression,' *Culture, Medicine and Psychiatry* 45, no. 3 (2021): 487.

13 ADCB 16174, p. 45, #22846 R8674018 (ANZ WR). Listed as Jane Sampson Dick.

14 Digital sources include Papers Past (https://paperspast.natlib.govt.nz), Online Cenotaph (www.aucklandmuseum.com/war-memorial/online-cenotaph) and Ancestry.com

15 John C. Weaver, *Sorrows of a Century: Interpreting Suicide in New Zealand, 1900–2000.* (Montreal: McGill-Queen's University Press / Wellington: Bridget Williams Books, 2014).

16 William Pember Reeves, *The Long White Cloud: Ao Tea Roa* (London: Horace Marshall & Son, 1898). Reeves' mental distress and loneliness is taken up in chapter 3. The name 'Aotearoa' was first used by Māori and referred only to the North Island of New Zealand. The whole country was called 'Aotearoa me Te Waipounamu'. By the 1850s the term 'Aotearoa' appeared in Māori language newspapers. Thomas Bracken's New Zealand anthem of 1878 was translated into Māori by T. H. Smith, who called New Zealand 'Aotearoa'.

17 Erena Wikaire et al., *Nōku te Ao: Sovereignty of the Māori Mind* (Wellington: Te Whatu Ora, 2022), 21, www.nokuteao.org.nz/noku-te-ao-sovereignty-of-the-maori-min

18 Sadowsky, *The Empire of Depression*; Sadowsky, 'Before and After Prozac.'

1. Discourse and diagnosis

1 'Highly Contagious. Depression and Gloom. Need for Optimism,' *The Poverty Bay Herald*, 27 December 1930, 15, https://paperspast.natlib.govt.nz/newspapers/PBH19301227.2.126

2 *White Ribbon*, 18 August 1931, 6, https://paperspast.natlib.govt.nz/periodicals/WHIRIB19310818.2.17

3 *ES*, 16 April 1932, 9, https://paperspast.natlib.govt.nz/newspapers/ESD19320416.2.34.1

4 Jonathan Sadowsky, *The Empire of Depression* (Cambridge, MA: Polity Books, 2021), 28.

5 See German E. Berrios, 'Mood Disorders: Clinical Section,' in *A History of Clinical Psychiatry: The Origin and History of Psychiatric Disorders*, eds German E. Berrios and Roy Porter (New York: New York University Press, 1995), 384–408; Roy Porter, 'Mood Disorders: Social Section,' in *A History of Clinical Psychiatry*, 409–20.

6 CAHW 27346/88, #358 R18946511 (ANZ CR).

7 CAUY 12251 #4630 R20127941; CBDB, 23547/12, #496 (4630), R22858048 (ANZ CR).

8 'Gisborne Suicide,' *The Northern Advocate*, 15 October 1947, 5, https://paperspast.natlib.govt.nz/newspapers/NA19471015.2.68

9 Sadowsky, 'Before and After Prozac,' 494–95. I do not retrace the global history of depression, as this has been well documented and debated, especially by Sadowsky, *The Empire of Depression*. See also Clark Lawlor, *From Melancholia to Prozac: A History of Depression* (Oxford: Oxford University Press, 2012).

10 Daniel Hack Tuke, ed., *A Dictionary of Psychological Medicine. Giving the Definition, Etymology and Synonyms of the Terms Used in Medical Psychology with the Symptoms, Treatment, and Pathology of Insanity and the Law of Lunacy in Great Britain and Ireland* (Philadelphia, PA: P. Blakiston, Son & Co., 1892), 1, 354.

11 Janet Oppenheim, *Shattered Nerves: Doctors, Patients, and Depression in Victorian England* (New York: Oxford University Press, 1991).

12 Ibid., 3.

13 Nancy C. Andreasen, *The Broken Brain: The Biological Revolution in Psychiatry* (New York: Harper and Row, 1984).

14 Stanley W. Jackson, 'A History of Melancholia and Depression,' in *History of Psychiatry and Medical Psychology*, eds E. R. Wallace and J. Gach (Boston, MA: Springer, 2008), 443.

15 Jackson, ibid., 444.

16 Sadowsky, 'Before and After Prozac,' 495.

17 I am indebted to Jackson's summary, 'A History of Melancholia and Depression.'

18 Sadowsky, *The Empire of Depression*, 165–66; Sadowsky, 'Before and After Prozac,' 492. Sadowsky cites Edward Shorter, *How Everyone Became Depressed: The Rise and Fall of the Nervous Breakdown* (Oxford: Oxford University Press, 2013).

19 Jansson, *From Melancholia to Depression*, 3.

20 Greenberg, *Manufacturing Depression*.

21 Dan G. Blazer, *The Age of Melancholy: Major Depression and Its Social Origins* (New York: Routledge, 2005). Cited in Sadowsky, 'Before and After Prozac,' 491.

22 Matthew Philp, 'Scientific Pastors: The Professionalisation of Psychiatry in New Zealand 1877–1920,' in *'Unfortunate Folk': Essays on Mental Health Treatment 1863–1992*, eds Barbara Brookes and Jane Thompson (Dunedin: Otago University Press, 2002), 195.

23 Dorothy Page, *Anatomy of a Medical School: A History of Medicine at the University of Otago, 1875–2000* (Dunedin: Otago University Press, 2008), 138.

24 Keith Sinclair and Trudie McNaughton, *A History of the University of Auckland, 1883–1983* (Auckland: Auckland University Press / Oxford University Press, 1983), 283.

25 German E. Berrios, *The History of Mental Symptoms: Descriptive Psychopathology Since the Nineteenth Century* (Cambridge, Cambridge University Press, 1996), 314.

26 'Incipient Melancholia,' *AS*, 30 May 1898, 3, https://paperspast.natlib.govt.nz/newspapers/AS18980530.2.14

27 'The Asylum Suicide,' *EP*, 27 November 1897, 5, https://paperspast.natlib.govt.nz/newspapers/EP18971127.2.55

28 John King, Inspector of Asylums, 'Reports on Lunatic Asylums in New Zealand', *AJHR*, 1870, D-29, 5.

29 AG-447-6/06 Ashburn Hall, Case book, vol. 4, 1898–1900, folio 156, #261 (alternate #236), 'Intermediate Case Book' (HC).

30 YCAA 1048/15, folio 354, #5250, R1481810 (ANZ AR).

31 It is not clear how long this was for, but according to Ancestry.com Frederick died in 1921 in Auckland.

32 YCAA 1048/12, folio 304, #4399, R1481806 (ANZ AR).

33 YCAA 1048/15, folio 78, #4974, R1481810; box 13, #4578, R1481807 (ANZ AR).

34 'Not Guilty', *Press*, 6 February 1930, 3, https://paperspast.natlib.govt.nz/newspapers/CHP19300206.2.9

35 For example, I. M. Allen, 'Neurasthenia with Depression,' *NZMJ* 13 (1933): 122–33; Oppenheim, *Shattered Nerves*, 79–109. Neurasthenia is discussed in chapter 4.

36 CAUY 12251/30, #4606, R20127941 (ANZ CR).

37 CAHW 27346/91 #662, R18946514 (ANZ CR).

38 The family member or friend signing this bond agreed to provide proper care and to prevent the person from doing injury to themselves or others, subject to a penalty of £50.

39 DAHI 19956/73, #5563, R6670183 (ANZ DR).

40 YCAA 1048/17, folio 94, #4590, R1481809 (ANZ AR).

41 DAHI 19956/73, #5452, R6670183 (ANZ DR).

42 Berrios, *The History of Mental Symptoms*, 311–12.

43 Mental hospitals of the Dominion (report on) for 1935, *AJHR*, 1936 Session I, H-07, 2, 5.

44 E. P. Brasted, 'The Female Division of a Mental Hospital: Porirua Mental Hospital, Wellington' (PM diss., University of Otago, 1945), 21.

45 Gordon Short, 'Case of Mental Depression,' *NZMJ* 34, no. 83 (1935): 342–43.

46 ACGS 16231, COR1942/1350, R23744683 (ANZ WR).

47 Medical Statistics Branch, Department of Health, *Census of Mental Hospital Patients, 1961 New Zealand*, Special Report Series no. 9 (Wellington: Government Printer, 1963).

48 Conan Fowler, 'A Study of Depression in Middle-aged Housewives' (PM diss., University of Otago, 1972), 3.

49 YCAA 1048/17, folio 294, #4790, R1481809 (ANZ AR).

50 AG-447-6/01 Ashburn Hall, Case book, 1901–1907, folio 124, 126, #317 (HC). Information also from Papers Past and Ancestry.com. Elspeth Knewstubb, 'Influences on Medical Practice at Ashburn Hall, Dunedin, 1882–1910,' *NZJH* 46, no. 1 (2012): 19, fn. 59, points out that the word 'voluntary' is misleading. Many 'voluntary boarders' did not seek treatment but were admitted by family. Those admitted did not meet the statutory requirements for certification, or their families did not wish to have them certified.

51 AG-447-6/01, folio 131.

52 Incipient Melancholia,' *AS*, 30 May 1898, 3, https://paperspast.natlib.govt.nz/newspapers/AS18980530.2.14

53 Weaver, *Sorrows of a Century*, 177.

54 'Suicide at Coromandel — Inquest on the Body,' *DSC*, 24 December 1862, 3, https://paperspast.natlib.govt.nz/newspapers/DSC18621224.2.14

55 'Suicide at Auckland. Mental Depression the Cause,' *Wairarapa Daily Times*, 14 July 1896, 3, https://paperspast.natlib.govt.nz/newspapers/WDT18960714.2.44

56 'Outrages, Suicides and Murders,' *NZH*, 2 February 1869, 5, https://paperspast.natlib.govt.nz/newspapers/NZH18690202.2.28

57 'The Execution of Harper,' *DSC*, 23 September 1863, 3, https://paperspast.natlib.govt.nz/newspapers/DSC18630923.2.14

58 'Suicide of a Clergyman,' *Manawatu Times*, 26 November 1883, 3, https://paperspast.natlib.govt.nz/newspapers/MT18831126.2.15

59 'Obituary Notices,' *AS*, 8 December 1883, https://paperspast.natlib.govt.nz/newspapers/AS18831208.2.57

60 A newspaper report, 'Suicide of a Clergyman', states the asylum as Waipukurau, and Napier.

61 CBDB 23547, #4613 (118), R22857980 (ANZ CR).

62 YCAA 1026, #4769, R25296744 (ANZ AR).

63 Weaver, *Sorrows of a Century*, 172.

64 I. M. Allen, 'Neurasthenia with Depression,' 125–26.

65 'Drawing-room Alcoholism,' *NEM*, 5 April 1871, 3, https://paperspast.natlib.govt.nz/newspapers/NEM18710405.2.16

66 James Mark Baldwin, *Dictionary of Philosophy and Psychology* (New York, London: Macmillan, 1901), https://psychclassics.yorku.ca/Baldwin/Dictionary/defs/M2defs.htm

67 Kerrin M. Christie, 'A First Assessment of the Costs and Benefits Associated with Drug Usage in New Zealand Mental Hospitals' (Wellington: Contract Research Unit, New Zealand Institute of Economic Research, 1968), 20.

68 ACGS 16231, COR1928/1447, R23714644 (ANZ WR). Widely reported in the media.

69 'Jumped From Mast,' *EP*, 22 December 1928, 11, https://paperspast.natlib.govt.nz/newspapers/EP19281222.2.119; ACGS 16231, COR1928/1482 R23714679 (ANZ WR).

70 Fowler, 'A Study of Depression'.

71 Confidential source.

72 ACGS 16231, COR1958/931, R23880668 (ANZ WR).

73 Weaver, *Sorrows of a Century*, 192; J. M. Aubrey, 'Patient Views of Depression in a General Practice' (PM diss., University of Otago, 1973), 5. On the questioning of these distinctions, see Sadowsky, *The Empire of Depression*, 76, 197, n.20; Allan V. Horwitz and Jerome C. Wakefield, *The Loss of Sadness: How Psychiatry Transformed Normal Sorrow into Depressive Disorder* (Oxford: Oxford University Press, 2007).

74 'The Blues,' *Bruce Herald*, 1 September 1876, 3, https://paperspast.natlib.govt.nz/newspapers/BH18760901.2.5

75 'Outrages, Suicides and Murders,' *NZH*, 2 February 1869, 5, https://paperspast.natlib.govt.nz/newspapers/NZH18690202.2.28

76 *Temuka Leader*, 24 September 1898, 4, https://paperspast.natlib.govt.nz/newspapers/TEML18980924.2.30.4

77 YCAA 1048/12, folio 139, #4234; folio 341 R1481806 (ANZ AR).

78 Edward Tregear, 'Inaugural Address,' *Transactions and Proceedings of the Royal Society of New Zealand* 31 (1898): 622.

79 'Notes on Electric Lighting,' *Progress*, 1 October 1916, 747, https://paperspast.natlib.govt.nz/periodicals/P19161001.2.16

80 *ODT*, 28 July 1923, 16, https://paperspast.natlib.govt.nz/newspapers/ODT19230728.2.140

81 ACGS 16231, COR1928/570, R23713769 (ANZ WR).

82 'The Late Mr. J. W. Diddams,' *DSC*, 5 December 1872, 3, https://paperspast.natlib.govt.nz/newspapers/DSC18721205.2.22

83 DAHI 19850/30, #3407, R25259353 (ANZ DR).

84 DAHI 19956/74, #5526, R6670184 (ANZ DR).

85 DAHI 19956/75, #5589, R6670185 (ANZ DR). The death was reported in the media, but this reference is withheld as it did not disclose that he was a patient at Seacliff.

86 Maree Dawson, 'National Fitness or Failure? Heredity, Vice and Racial Decline in New Zealand Psychiatry: A Case Study of the Auckland Mental Hospital, 1868–99' (PhD thesis, University of Waikato, 2013), 109, https://hdl.handle.net/10289/7521. Dawson cites Ann Goldberg, *Sex, Religion, and the Making of Modern Madness: The Eberach Asylum and German Society, 1815–1849* (New York: Oxford University Press, 1999), 89, and discusses similar medical discourse about masturbation and madness.

87 CAHW 27346/88, #424, R18946511 (ANZ CR); COR1934/817, R23860375 (ANZ WR).

88 AG-447-6/02, Ashburn Hall, Case book, 1908–1927, #98 (HC).

89 ACGS 16231, COR1928/339 R23713539 (ANZ WR).

90 e.g., DAHI 19850/30, #3435 (R25259378) (ANZ DR).

91 YCAA 1048/12, folio 141, #4236, R1481806; R25296269 (ANZ AR).

92 YCAA 1048/12, folio 304, #4399 R1481806 (ANZ AR).

93 See Hilary Marland, '"Destined to a Perfect Recovery": The Confinement of Puerperal Insanity in the Nineteenth Century,' in *Insanity, Institutions and Society, 1800–1914: A Social History of Madness in Comparative Perspective*, eds Joseph Melling and Bill Forsythe (London: Routledge, 1999), 141–44; Hilary Marland, *Dangerous Motherhood: Insanity and Childbirth in Victorian England* (Basingstoke: Palgrave Macmillan, 2004). For Aotearoa, see V. J. Carlton, 'A Study of Postpartum Psychosis and Depression' (PM diss., University of Otago, 1974); Eric Arnold Espiner, 'Mental Illness Following Childbirth' (PM diss., University of Otago, 1956).

94 CAUY 12251, #4745, R20127941; CBDB 23547/8; #413, R22857968 (ANZ CR); DAHI 19850/44, #4881, R25260416 (ANZ DR).

95 For example, YCAA 1048/9, #2511, R1481802 (ANZ AR), who lived to 73.

96 CAUY 12251/18, #1734, R20127929 (ANZ CR).

97 YCAA 1048/17, folio 294, #4790, R1481809 (ANZ AR).

98 AG-447-6/01, folio 132, #322.

99 Name and title of dissertation withheld.

100 Patricia M. Buckfield, 'Therapeutic Forces in a Mental Hospital: A Survey of the Therapeutic Forces at Work on the Female Side of the Seacliff Mental Hospital' (PM diss., University of Otago, 1957).

101 National Advisory Committee on Health and Disability, *Guideline for the Treatment and Management of Depression by Primary Healthcare Professionals* (Wellington: Ministry of Health, 1996), www.moh.govt.nz/notebook/nbbooks.nsf/0/B78AC66F-92C61AF84C2565D700188F23/$file/depression-guideline.pdf

102 Mark A. Oakley Browne, Elisabeth Wells and K. M. Scott, eds, *Te Rau Hinengaro: The New Zealand Mental Health Survey* (Wellington: Ministry of Health, 2006), 255–56.

103 Mason Durie, *Mauri Ora: The Dynamics of Māori Health* (Auckland: Oxford University Press, 2001), 113.

2. Rāwakiwaki

1 Waata Kūkūtai at Taupari, Letter from Waata Kūkūtai at Taupari, 3 December 1866. University of Waikato (accessed 30 July 2023), https://waikato.recollect.co.nz/nodes/view/434. For an insightful discussion of grief and suicide among Māori, see Michael P. J. Reilly, 'Grief, Loss and Violence in Ancient Mangaia, Aotearoa and Te Waipounamu,' *The Journal of Pacific History* 47, no. 2 (2012): 145–61.

2 Gary Scott, 'Kūkūtai, Waata Pihikete,' *Dictionary of New Zealand Biography* (1990), *Te Ara — the Encyclopedia of New Zealand* (accessed 19 April 2023); 'Death of Waata Kukutai', *NZH*, 11 January 1867, 5.

3 'Wairarapa. A Visit to Wi Waka's Hiding Place,' *Lyttelton Times*, 13 April 1866, 2.

4 Mason Durie, 'Mental Health Patterns for New Zealand Maori,' in *Te Aro Kawa Whakaruruhau: Cultural Safety in Health* (Auckland: Mental Health Foundation of New Zealand, 1998), 53–67; Durie, *Mauri Ora*.

5 Tamāti Kruger et al., Transforming Whānau Violence — A Conceptual Framework (Wellington: Second Māori Taskforce on Whānau Violence, 2004), https://nzfvc.org.nz/sites/default/files/transforming_whanau_violence.pdf

6 Hirini Moko Mead, *Tikanga Māori: Living by Māori Values* (Wellington: Huia, 2003), 58. See also, for example, Moana Jackson, 'The Mentally Ill Offender: A Māori Perspective,' *Community Mental Health in New Zealand* 4, no. 1 (June 1988): 49–50; Te Kani Kingi et al., *Maea Te Toi Ora: Māori Health Transformations* (Wellington: Huia, 2018).

7 Durie, 'Mental Health Patterns for New Zealand Maori,' 56.

8 Durie, *Mauri Ora*, 35.

9 Leonie Pihama and Paul Reynolds, *Kia Mārama: Tane Māori and Depression: A Scoping Report* (Auckland: Hāpai Te Hauora Tapui Ltd and Mental Health Foundation, 2007), 134.

10 Durie, *Mauri Ora*, 115.

11 Ibid.

12 Peter H. Buck, (Te Rangi Hīroa), 'Medicine Amongst the Maoris in Ancient and Modern Times' (MD thesis, University of New Zealand, 1910), 103–4, http://hdl.handle.net/10523/10413

13 Durie, 'Mental Health Patterns for New Zealand Maori,' 56. See also S. Percy Smith, 'The Evils of *Makutu*, or Witchcraft', *JPS* 30, no. 119 (1921): 172–84. Lachy Paterson, 'Government, Church and Māori Responses to *Mākutu* (Sorcery) in the Nineteenth and Early Twentieth Centuries,' *Cultural and Social History* 8, no. 2 (2015): 175–94 discusses changing attitudes to mākutu among Māori, and the role of Māori reformers during the late nineteenth and early twentieth centuries.

14 Edward Shortland, *Maori Religion and Mythology* (London: Longmans Green, 1882), 32–33.

15 Personal communication, Maata Wharehoka, 23 March 2023. See also Geoffrey Blake-Palmer, 'Beliefs and Practices of the Present Day Maori', *JPS* 63, no. 2 (June 1954): 147–63.

16 Laurie Kalman Gluckman, 'Makutu: A Study in the Ethnopsychiatry of the Maori, Past and Present' (MD diss., University of Otago, 1962). Gluckman wrote several publications on New Zealand's medical history, including *Tangiwai: Medical History of New Zealand Prior to 1860* (Auckland: L. Gluckman, 1976).

17 'Makutu,' ibid., 95–100. Keira is a pseudonym.

18 Ibid., 140–421.

19 Ibid., 107–8. Gluckman reported that ECT helped the patient, whose mother had been similarly treated.

20 Ibid., 184–90. Eliza is a pseudonym.

21 Confidential source.

22 Personal communication, Wharehoka.

23 Bradford Haami, *Dr. Golan Maaka: Māori Doctor* (Auckland: Tandem Press, 1995), 141–42.

24 https://depression.org.nz/get-better/your-identity/maori/ (accessed 11 March 2021). See Joan Metge, *In and Out of Touch: Whakamaa in Cross-Cultural Context* (Wellington: Victoria University Press, 1986), especially 146–48.

25 Iwa Stewart, 'Surviving Chronic Whakamaa,' *Mental Health Quarterly* (June 1998): 10.

26 'Further Papers Relative to Native Affairs,' *AJHR*, 1860 Session I, E-01a, 8.

27 George Pitt-Rivers, 'Visit to a Maori Village. Being some Observations on the Passing of the Maori Race and the Decay of Maori Culture,' *JPS* 33, no. 129 (1924): 58. Pitt-Rivers, who was extremely wealthy, endorsed eugenics, and later was a supporter of the British fascist Oswald Mosley.

28 Personal communication, Wharehoka.

29 For example: Durie, 'Mental Health Patterns for New Zealand Maori'; Tamāti Kruger et al., 'Transforming Whānau Violence.'

30 Frederick Cooper and Ann Laura Stoler, 'Introduction. Tensions of Empire: Colonial Control and Visions of Rule,' *American Ethnologist* 16 (1989): 618.

31 See Jacqueline Leckie, 'Pacific Bodies and Personal Space Redefined, 1850–1950,' in *The Cambridge History of the Pacific Ocean. Volume II: The Pacific Ocean Since 1800*, eds Anne Perez Hattori and Jane Samson (Cambridge: Cambridge University Press, 2022), 490–513.

32 Claudia Orange, 'Te Tiriti o Waitangi — the Treaty of Waitangi,' *Te Ara — the Encyclopedia of New Zealand*, (2012, revised 2023), www.TeAra.govt.nz/en/te-tiriti-o-waitangi-the-treaty-of-waitangi (accessed 15 June 2023).

33 Jim McAloon, 'Land ownership,' *Te Ara — the Encyclopedia of New Zealand* (2008), www.TeAra.govt.nz/en/land-ownership (accessed 15 June 2023).

34 Cook drew on mainly coastal estimates, and debates persist among demographers about these numbers. There is also debate about the role of psychological malaise in depopulation. See Ian Pool, 'Death Rates and Life Expectancy — Effects of Colonisation on Māori,' *Te Ara — the Encyclopedia of New Zealand* (2011, revised 2019), www.teara.govt.nz/en/death-rates-and-life-expectancy/page-4 (accessed 15 June 2023)

35 'Future of Maoris,' *NZH*, 30 June 1934, 15, https://paperspast.natlib.govt.nz/newspapers/NZH19340630.2.140. Sutherland's own experience with depression is taken up in chapter 5.

36 Rebecca Wirihana et al., 'Māori Indigenous Healing Practices in Aotearoa (New Zealand),' in *The Routledge International Handbook of Race, Culture and Mental Health* eds Roy Moodley and Eunjung Lee (Milton: Taylor and Francis, 2020), 532–33.

37 YCAA 1048, Box 7, Case Continuation Book 1896–1898, folio 144, #2245, R1481801 (ANZ AR).

38 YCAA 1048, Box 17, folio 351, #4847, R1481809 (ANZ AR).

39 YCAA 1048/1, folio 151, R1481795 (ANZ AR).

40 Derek A. Dow, '"Pruned of Its Dangers": The Tohunga Suppression Act 1907,' *Health and History* 3, no. 1 (2001): 41–64.

41 See Paterson, 'Government, Church and Māori Responses to *Mākutu*.'

42 Shortland, *Maori Religion and Mythology*, 32–33. See also W. H. Goldie, *Maori Medical Lore: Notes on the Causes of Disease and Treatment of the Sick Among the Maori People of New Zealand, reprinted from Transactions of the New Zealand Institute, 1904* (Nelson: Southern Reprints, 1998).

43 Durie, *Mauri Ora*, 115–16.

44 Pip M. E. Williams, *Te Rongoā Māori: Māori Medicine 1904–1997* (Auckland: Raupo, 2008).

45 Laurie K. Gluckman, 'The Staff of Asklepios: A Theory of Origin Supported by Clinical Ethnopsychiatry,' *NZMJ* 65, no. 402 (February 1966): 115.

46 *Colonist*, 13 August 1858, 2, https://paperspast.natlib.govt.nz/newspapers/TC18580813.2.6. She died two days later.

47 See Berrios, *The History of Mental Symptoms*, 425–26.

48 *Nelson Examiner and New Zealand Chronicle*, 14 August 1858, 2, https://paperspast.natlib.govt.nz/newspapers/NENZC18580814.2.8

49 YCAA 1048, box 9, folio 43, #2537, R1481803 (ANZ AR).

50 YCAA 1048, box 9, folio 343, #2476, R1481802 (ANZ AR).

51 YCAA 1048, box 15, #5138, R1481810 (ANZ AR).

52 YCAA 1048, box 12, folio 70, #4165, R1481806 (ANZ AR).

53 YCAA 1048, R148180, folio 138, #5034; folio 394, #5290, R1481810 (ANZ AR).

54 See Jacqueline Leckie, 'Insanity in a Sea of Islands: Mobility and Mental Health in Aotearoa New Zealand's Pacific Sphere,' *The Journal of New Zealand Studies* NS32 (2021): 168–69.

55 YCAA 1026, R25296428, #446 (ANZ AR); 'A Wandering Maori. Found in the Bush,' *Waikato Independent*, 14 May 1912, 6, https://paperspast.natlib.govt.nz/newspapers/WAIKIN19120514.2.32

56 YCAA 1048, box 9, folio 321, R1481802 (ANZ AR).

57 YCAA 1048, box 17, R1481809, folio 155, #4651; 1026, R25296630 (ANZ AR).

58 The impact of these patterns on Māori women's mental health is captured in Patricia Grace's novel *Cousins* (Auckland: Penguin, 1992) and in the 2021 movie of the same name. See, also, the research project, Te Hau Kāinga (the Māori Home Front), led by Angela Wanhalla, Lachy Paterson and Sarah Christie, www.maorihomefront.nz

59 Jackson, 'The Mentally Ill Offender,' 49.

60 Pihama and Reynolds, *Kia Mārama*.

61 Manuka Henare, 'Te Tiriti Te Tangata Te Whānau: The Treaty, The Human Person, The Family,' in *Te Aro Whānau: Family A Cornerstone of Māori Mental Well-being* (Auckland: Mental Health Foundation of New Zealand, 1997) 26–34.

62 Felicity Goodyear-Smith et al., 'Ethnic Differences in Mental Health and Lifestyle Issues: Results from Multi-Item General Practice Screening,' *NZMJ* 118, no. 1212 (2005): 6.

63 Brent Bezo and Stefania Maggi, 'Intergenerational Perceptions of Mass Trauma's Impact on Physical Health and Well-Being,' *Psychological Trauma: Theory, Research, Practice, and Policy* 10, no.1 (2018): 87–94; Leonie Pihama et al., 'Positioning Historical Trauma Theory,' *AlterNATIVE: An International Journal of Indigenous Peoples* 10, no. 3 (2014): 248–63.

64 Karina L. Walters et al., 'Bodies Don't Just Tell Stories, They Tell Histories: Embodiment of Historical Trauma Among American Indians and Alaska Natives,' *Du Bois Review* 8, no. 1 (2011): 179–89.

65 Keri Lawson-Te Aho, *A Review of Evidence: A Background Document to Support Kia Piki te Ora o te Taitamariki* (Wellington: Te Puni Kōkiri, 1998), 16.

66 See Tākirirangi Smith, *He Ara Uru Ora: Traditional Māori Understandings of Trauma and Well-being* (Whanganui: Te Atawhai o Te Ao: Independent Māori Institute for Environment and Health, 2019), https://teatawhai.maori.nz/wp-content/uploads/2020/04/He-Ara-Uru-Ora.pdf

67 Daniel H. Tuke, *Insanity in Ancient and Modern Life with Chapters on Its Prevention* (London: Macmillan, 1878), 94. See Caitlin Murray, 'The "Colouring of the Psychosis": Interpreting Insanity in the Primitive Mind,' *Health and History* 9, no. 2 (2007): 7–21.

68 Edward Jarvis, 'On the Supposed Increase in Insanity,' *American Journal of Insanity* 8, no. 4 (1852): 363.

69 William Mathews, 'Civilization and Suicide,' *The North American Review* 152, no. 413 (April, 1891): 470–84; this article was widely reported in New Zealand during the 1890s.

70 Buck, 'Medicine Amongst the Maoris,' 77.

71 *Colonist*, 13 August 1858.

72 YCAA 1048, folio 351, #4446, R1481806 (ANZ AR).

73 Ibid., folio 303, #4398.

74 Durie, 'Mental Health Patterns for New Zealand Maori,' 63; Lorelle Barry and Catharine Coleborne, 'Insanity and Ethnicity in New Zealand: Māori Encounters with the Auckland Mental Hospital, 1860–1900,' *History of Psychiatry* 22, no. 3 (2011): 295; Lorelle Burke, '"The Voices Caused Him to Become Porangi": Maori Patients in the Auckland Lunatic Asylum, 1860–1900' (MA thesis, University of Waikato, 2006), https://hdl.handle.net/10289/12621. Similar cultural withdrawal is noted among Chinese patients in chapter 6.

75 Depression Helpline, www.depression.org.nz/get-better/your-identity/maori

76 Durie, *Mauri Ora*, 99.

77 'Maori Woman's Death', *NZH*, 13 December 1917, 4, https://paperspast.natlib.govt.nz/newspapers/NZH19171213.2.29

78 *EP*, 22 December 1942; ACGS 16231, COR1942/1630, R23744963 (ANZ WR).

79 See Reilly, 'Grief, Loss and Violence.'

80 John Weaver and Doug Munro, 'The Historical Contingency of Suicide: A Case-Based Comparison of Suicides in New Zealand in the 1930s and 1980s,' *New Zealand Sociology* 25, no. 1 (2010): 117.

81 For example, *The Gisborne Herald*, 6 June 1942, 2, https://paperspast.natlib.govt.nz/newspapers/GISH19420606.2.10; *The Waihi Daily Telegraph*, 15 May 1919, 3, https://paperspast.natlib.govt.nz/newspapers/WHDT19190515.2.26

82 *The Gisborne Herald*, ibid.; COR1942/777, R23744113 (ANZ WR).

83 These were possibly 19 pages of handwritten minutes of meetings of the Nelson Division of the British Medical Association between May and October 1936 concerning the dispute between Bydder and Potaka. Information about Potaka comes from Gerard Hindmarsh, *Nelson Mail*, 22 August 2020. Information also from ACGS 16231, COR1936/1244, R23862334 (ANZ WR); Bruce Young, 'Dr Louis Hauiti Potaka of New Zealand: A Biographical Essay,' (Waterloo: Department of Geography and Environmental Studies, Wilfrid Laurier University, 1999, revised, 2005), https://kb.osu.edu/bitstream/handle/1811/5984/potaka.pdf

84 *The Horowhenua Chronicle*, 6 August 1931, 2.

85 Different reports stated Rameka's age in 1931 as 31, 36 and 39.

86 'Murder Charge,' *AS*, 5 August 1931, 8, https://paperspast.natlib.govt.nz/newspapers/AS19310805.2.80. See also Martin Johnson, 'The H-Files: Crimes of Passion in Old Auckland,' *NZH*, 14 January 2019, www.nzherald.co.nz/nz/the-h-files-crimes-of-passion-in-old-auckland/QEDMJUJSTKSORRORFPCAGRVW7A

87 'Murder Charge.'

88 For a literature overview of Māori mental health before the 1980s, see Timothy Gassin, *Māori Mental Health: A Report Commissioned by the Waitangi Tribunal for the Wai 2575 Health Services and Outcomes Kaupapa Inquiry* (Wellington: Waitangi Tribunal, 2019), 3–9, https://forms.justice.govt.nz/search/Documents/WT/wt_DOC_153087514/Wai%202575%2C%20B026.pdf

89 'Evidence to Select Committee on the General Lunatic Asylum,' 26 May 1858, AEBE 18507, box 16, #18584, R17684412 (ANZ WR).

90 Frank Harty Foster, *Maori Patients in Mental Hospitals*. Special Report no. 8, Medical Statistics Branch, Department of Health (Wellington: Government Printer, 1962).

91 Durie, *Mauri Ora*, 117.

92 Nicole Coupe, 'Whakamomori: Māori Suicide Prevention' (PhD thesis, Massey University, 2005), 48, http://hdl.handle.net/10179/1695

93 Weaver, *Sorrows of a Century*, 42.

94 Barry and Coleborne, 'Insanity and Ethnicity in New Zealand,' 288.

95 Ernest Beaglehole, 'Culture and Psychosis in New Zealand,' *JPS* 48, no. 191 (1939): 144–55.

96 K. M. Mayo, 'A Survey of Maori and Dalmation Mental Patients Living in the Auckland and Kingseat Mental Hospitals in February, 1952' (PM diss., University of Otago, 1952).

97 Durie, *Mauri Ora*, 112. On the lack of data on the history of Māori and mental health, see Te Kani Kingi, 'Introduction', in *Maea Te Toi Ora*, 7–18.

98 Pihama and Reynolds, *Kia Mārama*.

99 Ibid.

100 Alan Duff, *Once Were Warriors* (Auckland: Tandem Press, 1990).

101 For example, Arroll Bruce et al., 'The Prevalence of Depression among Maori Patients in Auckland General Practice,' *Journal of Primary Health Care* 1 (March 2009): 26–29. See also Mason Durie, 'Mental Health and Maori Development,' *ANZJP* 33 (1999): 5–12; L. K. Edmonds et al., 'Trends in Maori Mental Health in Otago,' *ANZJP* 34, no. 4 (2000): 677–83.

102 MaGPIe Research Group, 'Mental Disorders Among Māori Attending Their General Practitioner,' *ANZJP* 39 (2005): 401–6.

103 David Thomas et al., 'General Practitioners' Views about Diagnosing and Treating Depression in Maori and Non-Maori Patients,' *Journal of Primary Health Care* 2 (2010): 208–16.

104 Mason Durie, 'Puahou: A Five-Point Plan for Improving Maori Mental Health' [paper presented to Summit] (Auckland: Maori Mental Health Summit, 1997), cited in Felicity Goodyear-Smith et al., 'Ethnic Differences in Mental Health and Lifestyle Issues,' 6.

105 Manatū Hauora Ministry of Health, 'Mental Health,' www.health.govt.nz/our-work/populations/maori-health/tatau-kahukura-maori-health-statistics/nga-mana-hauora-tutohu-health-status-indicators/mental-health (accessed 1 March 2023).

106 Discussed further in the epilogue. Mason Durie, 'Mauri Ora Practice and Mauri Ora Practitioners,' in Kingi et al., *Maea Te Toi Ora*, 92.

3. The lonely land

1 Dr Morgan Stanislaus Grace, 'Report of the Joint Committee on Lunatic Asylums, 1871' *AJHR*, 1871, Session I, H-10, appendix, 10.

2 'A Peculiar Case,' *ES*, 15 September 1877, 2, https://paperspast.natlib.govt.nz/newspapers/ESD18770915.2.11; *The Marlborough Press*, 5 October 1877, 4, https://paperspast.natlib.govt.nz/newspapers/MPRESS18771005.2.19. The name was also spelt as 'Rowen'.

3 New Zealand passenger lists, 1839–1973, available at FamilySearch, https://familysearch.org/ark:/61903/3:1:S3HT-62H9-N4X?cc=1609792&wc=MP7K-NQP%3A119260101%2C119112001%2C119319701. Derived from ANZ WR. Julia and her infant daughter were listed as Jude.

4 *ES*, 15 September 1877, 2.

5 DAHI 19956/38, folio 65, #968 R6670148; 19850/6, R25257131 (ANZ DR).

6 *ES*, 15 September 1877.

7 DAHI 19850/5, #1058, R25257216 (ANZ DR).

8 See Jock Phillips, 'History of Immigration,' *Te Ara — the Encyclopedia of New Zealand* (2005, revised 2015), www.teara.govt.nz/en/history-of-immigration (accessed 12 July 2023).

9 DAHI 19956/45 #2651 R6670155 (ANZ DR).

10 Jenny Robin Jones, *Writers in Residence: A Journey with Pioneer New Zealand Writers* (Auckland: Auckland University Press, 2004), 67–72.

11 Miles Fairburn, 'Wakefield, Edward Gibbon,' *Dictionary of New Zealand Biography, Te Ara — the Encyclopedia of New Zealand* (1990), https://teara.govt.nz/en/biographies/1w4/wakefield-edward-gibbon (accessed 31 July 2023).

12 Reeves, *The Long White Cloud.*

13 Keith Sinclair, *William Pember Reeves: New Zealand Fabian* (Oxford: Clarendon Press, 1965), 27.

14 Reeves MSS, small clipping book, 110–111, cited ibid., 26.

15 Reeves to Miss G. Colborne Veel, 25 April 1924, cited ibid., 341.

16 Sinclair, *William Pember Reeves*, 39.

17 Reeves MSS, cited ibid., 41.

18 Angela McCarthy, *Migration, Ethnicity and Madness: New Zealand, 1860–1910* (Dunedin: Otago University Press, 2015), 80–106. See also David Hastings, *Over the Mountains of the Sea: Life on the Migrant Ships 1870–1885* (Auckland: Auckland University Press, 2013).

19 Jennifer Kain, *Insanity and Immigration Control in New Zealand and Australia, 1860–1930* (Cham: Palgrave MacMillan, 2019), 61. Vogel, who had been premier of New Zealand between 1873 and 1875, and again in 1876, became New Zealand's agent-general in London between 1876 and 1880, representing New Zealand's diplomatic, legal and commercial interests in Britain.

20 Full details of Jane's voyage are in McCarthy, *Migration, Ethnicity and Madness*, 83–85.

21 'Correspondence re Miss Chapman passenger on Wave Queen; Letter from Constabulary Office to Superintendent of Auckland, 9 February 1874,' AP2 14 C 95 483, Record Number 532/74, (ANZ AR), cited in Kain, *Insanity and Immigration*, 50.

22 Oppenheim, *Shattered Nerves*, 129.

23 Sources include: *ES*, 31 May 1884; *NZT*, 10 June 1884, 2. There are several newspaper entries on Papers Past for Edgar. Information also sourced from Ancestry.com

24 See Leckie, 'Insanity in a Sea of Islands,' 170–71.

25 YCAA 1017/1, #36, R283406; 1026/1 R25295711, A914 (ANZ AR).

26 'Reports on Lunatic Asylums in New Zealand,' *AJHR*, 1870, D-29, 6.

27 DAHI 19850/1, #87, R25256271 (ANZ DR).

28 DAHI 19850/1, #270, R25256450 (ANZ DR).

29 'Attempted Suicide,' *ES*, 31 January 1877, 2, https://paperspast.natlib.govt.nz/newspapers/ESD18770131.2.10; DAHI 19956/38, folio 137, #1004 R6670148; 19850/6, #1004, R25257165; AAAR, 25135/244, #11, R13286391 (ANZ DR).

30 For example, John Mulgan, *Man Alone* (London: Selwyn and Blount, 1939); Jock Phillips, *A Man's Country? The Image of the Pakeha Male, A History* (Auckland: Penguin, 1987), 27.

31 Catharine Coleborne, *Insanity, Identity and Empire: Immigrants and Institutional Confinement in Australia and New Zealand, 1873–1910* (Manchester: Manchester University Press, 2015); McCarthy, *Migration, Ethnicity, Madness.*

32 See Warwick Brunton, 'A Choice of Difficulties: National Mental Health Policy in New Zealand, 1840–1947' (PhD thesis, University of Otago, 2001), 45–46, http://hdl.handle.net/10523/383

33 For example, Judith Holloway, '"Unfortunate Folk": A Study of the Social Context of Committal to Seacliff 1928–1937,' in *'Unfortunate Folk': Essays on Mental Health Treatment 1863–1992*, eds Barbara Brookes and Jane Thomson (Dunedin: Otago University Press, 2001), 160–62; Barbara Brookes, 'Women and Madness: A Case-study of the Seacliff Asylum, 1890–1920,' in *Women in History 2: Essays on Women in New Zealand*, eds Barbara Brookes, Charlotte Macdonald and Margaret Tennant (Wellington: Bridget Williams Books, 1992), 135; Bronwyn Labrum, 'Looking Beyond the Asylum: Gender and the Process of Committal to Auckland, 1870–1919,' *NZJH* 26 (1992): 125–44; Coleborne, *Insanity, Identity and Empire.* Angela McCarthy, 'Ethnicity, Migration and the Lunatic Asylum in Early Twentieth-Century Auckland, New Zealand,' *Social History of Medicine* 21, no. 1 (2008): 52, shows that men from Ireland and Scotland were more likely to be unmarried than those from England.

34 'Report of the Joint Committee on Lunatic Asylums, 1871', 11.

35 McCarthy, *Migration, Ethnicity and Madness*, 111–40. See also, for example, Catharine Coleborne, *Madness in the Family: Insanity and Institutions in the Australasian Colonial World, 1860–1914* (Houndmills: Palgrave Macmillan, 2010); Stevan Eldred-Grigg, *Diggers, Hatters and Whores: The Story of the New Zealand Gold Rushes* (Auckland: Random House, 2008), 247–54. Such studies are part of the historiography that challenged Fairburn's earlier thesis of an atomised society within colonial New Zealand. See Miles Fairburn, *The Ideal Society and Its Enemies: The Foundations of Modern New Zealand Society, 1850–1900* (Auckland: Auckland University Press, 1989).

36 'Despatches from the Governor of New Zealand to the Secretary of State,' *AJHR*, 1873, Session I, A-01 Enclosure No. 23, 30.

37 See Eric Pawson and Tom Brooking, *Making a New Land: Environmental Histories of New Zealand* (Dunedin: Otago University Press, 2013).

38 *Bruce Herald*, 14 September 1886, 3, https://paperspast.natlib.govt.nz/newspapers/BH18860914.2.7; DAHI 19956/40, folio 191, #2038, R6670150 (ANZ DR).

39 DAHI 19956/38, folio 103 #988 R6670148; 19850/6 #988, R25257149 (ANZ DR).

40 DAHI 19956/52, #3352, R6670162 (ANZ DR).

41 It is unclear what locked gloves referred to. These were probably stiff leather mittens, but with no separate finger or thumb compartments, with a lock to prevent the gloves being removed.

42 Susanne Hill and John Hill, *Richard Henry of Resolution Island* (Dunedin: Te Ara, 1987), 127.

43 Melland Papers: Letters from Richard Henry at Auckland Hospital and Dusky Sound, 5 October 1893, MS-0705-B (HC); *AS*, 3 October 1893, 8; *NZH*, 4 October 1893, 5.

44 'In Sanctuary,' *EP*, 11 May 1911, 2, https://paperspast.natlib.govt.nz/newspapers/EP19110511.2.6

45 'Biography of Richard Henry — Bird Conservationist (1845–1929),' https://collections.tepapa.govt.nz/topic/1473

46 CAHW 27346, folio 359–360, #441, R18946511 (ANZ CR); Ancestry.com

47 'Report of the Joint Committee on Lunatic Asylums, 1871,' 10.

48 'Year to 31 March 1872,' *AJHR*, 17.

49 YCAA 1048/1, folio 219, R1481795 (ANZ AR).

50 Eleanor Catton, *The Luminaries* (Wellington: Victoria University Press, 2013). Catton was inspired by Colin Townsend, *Misery Hill, Seaview Terrace, Hokitika, 1866–1909: The Home of the Dead, the Mad and the Bad: A Personal Cameo History of the Upper Gaol, Seaview Terrace, Hokitika and Some of Its Inmates* (Christchurch: Leon G. Morel, 1998); Eldred-Grigg, *Diggers, Hatters and Whores.*

51 'Reports on Lunatic Asylums in New Zealand,' *AJHR*, 1872, G-27, 22.

52 CAHW 27346, folio 120, R18946513 (ANZ CR); *The West Coast Times*, 18 May 1872, 2, https://paperspast.natlib.govt.nz/newspapers/WCT18720518.2.10

53 *Lyttelton Times*, 18 March 1880, 3, https://paperspast.natlib.govt.nz/newspapers/LT18800318.2.5

54 *ODT*, 30 April 1863, 4, https://paperspast.natlib.govt.nz/newspapers/ODT18630430.2.10

55 DAHI 19850/1, folio 147, #147, R25256331 (ANZ DR).

56 The term originates from the eighteenth and nineteenth centuries when workers in the felt-hat-making industry were exposed to mercury nitrate, which could cause tremors and other nervous symptoms.

57 *The Western Star*, 9 September 1876, 3, https://paperspast.natlib.govt.nz/newspapers/WSTAR18760909.2.4

58 DAHI 19956/52, #3366, R6670162; 19850/29, R25259318 (ANZ DR).

59 *ODT*, 9 May 1871, 2, https://paperspast.natlib.govt.nz/newspapers/ODT18710509.2.10. A lunatic asylum opened in Fiji in 1884. See Jacqueline Leckie, *Colonizing Madness: Asylum and Community in Fiji* (Honolulu: University of Hawai'i Press, 2020).

60 *NEM*, 23 July 1872, 2, https://paperspast.natlib.govt.nz/newspapers/NEM18720723.2.7

61 See Richard S. Hill, *Policing the Colonial Frontier: The Theory and Practice of Coercive Social and Racial Control in New Zealand, 1767–1867* (Wellington: Historical Publications Branch, Department of Internal Affairs, 1986), 556.

62 *ODT*, 28 December 1864, 5, https://paperspast.natlib.govt.nz/newspapers/ODT18641228.2.16

63 *NEM*, 23 July 1872, 2, https://paperspast.natlib.govt.nz/newspapers/NEM18720723.2.7

64 YCAA 1048/1, folio 193; R1481795; A914/2, 130, R25295789 (ANZ ARO); Rex E. Wright-St Clair, 'J. Rutherford Ryley: Pioneer of Antisepsis in New Zealand,' *Journal of Medical Biography* 7, no. 1 (1999): 32–34.

65 DAAC 20681, D140, #389, R8668764 (ANZ DR).

66 'Report of Inquest. J. R. Ryley,' *The Sydney Morning Herald*, 15 March 1884, 6; 12.

67 http://otagotaphophile.blogspot.com/2021/06

68 DAHI 19850/1, #36, R25256220 (ANZ DR).

69 YCAA 1048/1, folio 238, R1481795 (ANZ AR); *The Thames Guardian and Mining Record*, 26 June 1872, https://paperspast.natlib.govt.nz/newspapers/TGMR18720626.2.14; Gabrielle A. Fortune, 'Hugh Coolahan and the Prosperous Irish: Auckland, 1840–1870' (MA thesis, University of Auckland, 1997).

70 CAHW 27346, #834, R18946513 (ANZ CR).

71 YCAA 1048/9, #2554, R1481803 (ANZ AR).

72 *NZH*, 7 December 1883, 4, https://paperspast.natlib.govt.nz/newspapers/NZH18831207.2.21

73 www.geni.com/projects/Royal-New-Zealand-Fencibles-1847-1852/33912

74 *NZH*, July 7, 1883, 1 (*Supplement*), https://paperspast.natlib.govt.nz/newspapers/NZH18830707.2.52. The Fencibles website confirms that George Feltus died at sea. Ancestry.com has Richard's birth as January 1844. I could not ascertain what happened to Richard's mother.

75 *NZH*, 6 March 1866, 5, https://paperspast.natlib.govt.nz/newspapers/NZH18660306.2.20

76 *NZH*, 3 September 1891, https://paperspast.natlib.govt.nz/newspapers/NZH18910903.2.15

77 'Report of the Joint Committee on Lunatic Asylums, 1871,' 10.

78 *DSC*, 13 January 1871, 2, https://paperspast.natlib.govt.nz/newspapers/DSC18710113.2.14

79 Coleborne, *Insanity, Identity and Empire*, 39, drew my attention to Stuckenberg. See John Kousgård Sørensen, 'Ingeborg Stuckenberg in New Zealand,' in *Danish Emigration to New Zealand*, eds Henning Bender and Birgit Larsen, trans. Karen Veien (Danes Worldwide Archives, 1990), 46–59. Stuckenberg's letters from Aotearoa to Denmark were later published in Danish, translated as *Long Letters from a Short Voyage*. Quotations cited here are from Tina White, 'Many Early Settlers Found Life Too Tough to Bear,' *Stuff*, 10 August 2019, www.stuff.co.nz/dominion-post/114772868/flashback-many-early-settlers-found-live-too-tough-to-bear

80 *AS*, 28 December 1911, 5, https://paperspast.natlib.govt.nz/newspapers/WT19360127.2.18

81 ACGS 16231, COR1926/740, R23840070 (ANZ WR).

82 ACGS 16231, COR1928/764, R23713961 (ANZ WR).

83 ACGS 16231, COR1928/792, R23713989 (ANZ WR).

84 DAHI 19850/1, #346, R25256524 (ANZ DR).

85 YCAA 1048/17 #4697, R1481809 (ANZ AR).

86 See, for example, Coleborne, *Insanity, Identity and Empire*, 114–63; Bronwyn Labrum, 'The Boundaries of Femininity: Madness and Gender in New Zealand, 1870–1910,' in *Women, Madness and the Law: A Feminist*

Reader, eds Wendy Chan, Dorothy E. Chunn and Robert Menzies (London: The GlassHouse Press, 2005), 69.

87 Labrum, 'The Boundaries of Femininity,' 61.

88 See Angela Middleton, *Pēwhairangi: Bay of Islands Missions and Maōri, 1814 to 1845* (Dunedin: Otago University Press, 2019), 58.

89 Ibid., 128.

90 Cited in Frances Porter, Charlotte Macdonald with Tui MacDonald, eds, *My Hand Will Write What My Heart Dictates: The Unsettled Lives of Women in Nineteenth-Century New Zealand as Revealed to Sisters, Family and Friends* (Auckland: Auckland University Press, 1996), 83.

91 Margaret Bilton, 'Some of My Experiences in Backblocks Nursing,' *Kai Tiaki: The Journal of the Nurses of New Zealand* 6, no. 1 (1 January 1913): 9.

92 CAHW 27346, R18946510, folio 142 (ANZ CR).

93 Ibid.

94 See Labrum, 'The Boundaries of Femininity,' 76–77.

95 YCAA 1048/1, folio 51, R1481795 (ANZ AR).

96 DAHI 19850, #3401, R25259348 (ANZ DR).

97 YCAA 1048, box 13, #4788, R1481807 (ANZ AR).

98 YCAA 1026/1, #60, R25295734 (ANZ AR).

99 *DSC*, 3 February 1868, 3, https://paperspast.natlib.govt.nz/newspapers/DSC18680203.2.23

100 DAHI 19956/38, folio 151, #1011, R6670148; 19850/6, R25257172 (ANZ DR).

101 *ES*, 10 March 1877, 2, https://paperspast.natlib.govt.nz/newspapers/ESD18770310.2.9. The newspaper report cites the children as being charged as neglected children.

102 YCAA 1048/17, # 4523, R1481809 (ANZ ARO). It is not clear where they emigrated from.

103 CAHW, 27346, #655, R18946514 (ANZ CR).

104 YCAA,1048, box 1, folio #13, R1481795; 1026, A914, R23545527 (ANZ AR); Reported *DSC*, 21 June 1870, 3.

105 YCAA 1048/ 1, folio #47, R1481795 (ANZ AR).

106 YCAA 1048/15, #5069, R1481810 (ANZ AR). Out of respect to the family, I have given her a fictitious name and do not cite details of the tragedy, which were reported in the media.

107 It is unclear why puerperal was listed as a cause, because it had been a long time since Sara had given birth. It is possible that she had suffered post-partum depression before, but there is no evidence of this.

108 Guthrie, 'A Study of Twelve Patients with Depression.'

109 Jane's story is compiled from personal correspondence, Trevor Agnew; interview, Pinky Agnew, Wellington, 28 April 2021; Norman Agnew's diary.

110 '*Ionic*'s Draft. A Shipload of Soldiers' Wives,' *The Dominion*, 27 October 1919, 4, https://paperspast.natlib.govt.nz/newspapers/DOM19191027.2.14

4. Enduring darkness

1 ACGS 16231, COR1945/96, R23868832 (ANZ WR); Regimental No 50365. 'Trevor' is a pseudonym.

2 For example, John Horrocks, 'The Limits of Endurance: Shell Shock and Dissent in World War One,' *The Journal of New Zealand Studies* NS27 (2018): 35–49; Gwen A. Parsons, 'The Construction of Shell Shock in New Zealand, 1919–1939: A Reassessment,' *Social History of Medicine: The Journal of the Society for the Social History of*

Medicine 26, no. 1 (2013): 56–73; John Weaver and David Wright, 'Shell Shock and the Politics of Asylum Committal in New Zealand, 1916–22,' *Health and History* 7, no. 1 (2005): 17–40.

3 Peter Leese, 'Essay Review: Making Shell-shock,' *British Journal of Psychology* 92 (2001): 411–15; Harold Merskey, 'Shell-shock,' in *150 Years of British Psychiatry, 1841–1991*, eds German E. Berrios and H. Freeman (London: Gaskell, 1991), 245–67.

4 YCAA, 1026/3 #163, R25295815 (ANZ AR).

5 YCAA 1048/1, folio 53, R1481795 (ANZ AR).

6 Archives New Zealand, Research guides, 'World War One 1914–1918'; 'World War Two 1939–45', www.archives.govt.nz/research-guidance/research-guides/war-records/world-war-one-1914-1918#:~:text=In%20the%20First%20World%20War,a%20very%20high%20casualty%20rate; www.archives.govt.nz/research-guidance/research-guides/war-records/world-war-two#:~:text=A%20total%20of%20about%20105%2C000,16%2C000%20were%20wounded%20as%20well (accessed 15 September 2023).

7 'Health of the troops in New Zealand for the year 1917,' *AJHR*, 1918, Session I–II, H-19b.

8 Millais Culpin, *Recent Advances in the Study of the Psychoneuroses* (London: J. & A. Churchill, 1931), 120. See, also, Edward F. C. Hefford, 'War Neurosis. An Aspect of Psychological Medicine and Its Relation to the Maintenance of Health' (PM diss., University of Otago, and for Director General, Medical Services, 1946).

9 Allen, 'Neurasthenia with Depression.'

10 For example: Ben Shephard, *A War of Nerves. Soldiers and Psychiatrists 1914–1994* (London: Pimlico Books, 2002); Peter Leese, *Shell Shock: Traumatic Neurosis and the British Soldiers of the First World War* (Houndmills: Palgrave, 2002), 227; Anthony Babington, *Shell Shock: A History of the Changing Attitudes to War Neurosis* (London: Leo Cooper, 1997).

11 C. S. Myers, 'A Contribution to the Study of Shell Shock: Being an Account of Three Cases of Loss of Memory, Vision, Smell, and Taste, Admitted into the Duchess of Westminster's War Hospital, Le Touquet,' *The Lancet* 185 (1915): 316–320.

12 Eric T. Dean Jr., *Shook Over Hell: Post-Traumatic Stress, Vietnam, and the Civil War* (Cambridge, MA: Harvard University Press, 1999), 30.

13 Michael B. Tyquin, *Madness and the Military: Australia's Experience of the Great War* (Loftus: Australian Military History Publications, 2006), 41.

14 *The Gisborne Times*, 15 May 1915, 6, https://paperspast.natlib.govt.nz/newspapers/GIST19150515.2.36

15 CAUY 12251, #4811; #4810, R20127942 (ANZ CR). Some details are from their military records, but I have not cited these for reasons of privacy.

16 Hefford, 'War Neurosis,' 37.

17 Captain A. G. Clouston, 'War Neuroses and the General Medical Practitioner,' *NZMJ* 41, no. 221 (1942): 6–13. See Tiffany Jenks and Angela Wanhalla, 'Psychological Casualties: War Neurosis, Rehabilitation, and the Family in Post-World War II New Zealand,' *Health and History* 22, no. 2 (2020): 1–25; Paul A. H. Morris, '"Their Nerves were Shot to Shreds — Our Own Weren't too Steady Either": Attitudes Towards Psychological Casualties in the 2nd New Zealand Expeditionary Force, 1939 to 1945' (MA thesis, University of Canterbury, 2013),

70, http://hdl.handle.net/10092/8035; A. D. Macleod, 'Psychiatric Casualties of World War II,' *NZMJ* 113, no. 1112 (23 June 2000): 248–50.

18 'Brigadier J. M. Twhigg — Papers and Files — Neuropsychiatry,' Director General of Health, M. K. Watt to Brigadier I.S. Wilson, Acting Director General, Medical Services, NZ Army, 15 February 1944, CAJM 22899, R21387211 (ANZ WR) used 'psychoneurosis' in a formal reference to the treatment of repatriated psychological casualties. See M. H. Aiken, 'Psychoneuroses in the Second New Zealand Expeditionary Force,' *NZMJ* 40, no. 220 (December 1941): 345.

19 M. H. Aiken, 'Psychiatric Casualties Among New Zealand Troops in Italy,' *NZMJ* 45 (June 1946): 157.

20 Editorial, 'Wartime Psychiatric Problems in New Zealand,' *NZMJ* 41, no. 221 (1942): 1–2.

21 Harold Palmer, 'The Problem of Neurosis in Ex-Soldiers,' *NZMJ* 47, no. 258 (April 1948): 129–38.

22 Dean, *Shook Over Hell*, 195.

23 Alison Parr, *'Silent Casualties': New Zealand's Unspoken Legacy of the Second World War* (Auckland: Tandem Press, 1995), 15–16.

24 Nigel Long et al., 'Prevalence of Posttraumatic Stress Disorder, Depression and Anxiety in a Community Sample of New Zealand Vietnam War Veterans,' *ANZJP* 30, no. 2 (1996): 253–56.

25 'Report of the Commissioner of Pensions, G. C. Fache,' *AJHR*, HIB 1925, 8.

26 Peter Boston, 'The Bacillus of Work: Masculinity and the Rehabilitation of Disabled Soldiers in Dunedin 1919 to 1939' (BA Hons Long Essay, University of Otago, 1993), 4.

27 *The Manawatu Standard*, 14 October 1919, 5, https://paperspast.natlib.govt.nz/newspapers/MS19191014.2.18

28 'A Note on the Work of the Department with respect to Soldier Patients from the Beginning of the War to the 4th August, 1919,' Mental Hospitals of the Dominion (report on) for 1918, *AJHR*, 1919 Session I, H-7, 27.

29 Boston, 'The Bacillus of Work,' 17.

30 DAHI 19956, #5496, R6670184 (ANZ DR); YCAA 1026, #5375, R25297338 (ANZ AR).

31 DAHI 19956, #5673, R6670185 (ANZ DR).

32 Ibid., #5693.

33 Morris, '"Their Nerves were Shot to Shreds",' 52. Today the Maudsley is the largest mental health training institution in the United Kingdom. It was the vision of psychiatrist Henry Maudsley, and was already treating war veterans before it opened in 1915.

34 Ibid., 70; Susan Fennell, 'Psychiatry in New Zealand, 1912–1948,' in *'Unfortunate Folk': Essays on Mental Health Treatment, 1863–1992*, eds Barbara Brookes and Jane Thompson (Dunedin: Otago University Press, 2002), 145.

35 P. Chisholm and S. D. Rhind, 'Some Aspects of Post-War Psycho-Neuroses, and Their Treatment at the Queen Mary Hospital Hanmer Springs,' *NZMJ* 19 (1920): 227. See also Weaver and Wright, 'Shell Shock and the Politics of Asylum Committal in New Zealand.'

36 Russell Clarke, 'Not Mad, But Very Ill: The Treatment of New Zealand's Shell Shocked Soldiers 1914 to 1939' (MA thesis, University of Auckland, 1991), also found that psychoanalysis was a failure in the treatment of war neuroses.

37 Chisholm and Rhind, 'Some Aspects of Post-War Psycho-Neuroses,' 225–6.

38 Ibid., 224; E. W. Giesen, 'Discussion of Neurasthenia,' *NZMJ* 16, no. 74 (1917): 135–42.

39 Michael Roche, 'Failure Deconstructed: Histories and Geographies of Soldier Settlement in New Zealand Circa 1917–39,' *New Zealand Geographer* 64, no. 1 (2008): 46–56, questions whether the schemes were the utter failures, so commonly depicted in historical narratives. He also points out that there was a tendency to place blame on the veterans' own personal failings.

40 'Soldier Settlers,' *NEM*, 14 March 1929, 5, https://paperspast.natlib.govt.nz/newspapers/NEM19290314.2.48

41 John C. Weaver and Doug Munro, 'Country Living, Country Dying: Rural Suicides in New Zealand, 1900–1950,' *Journal of Social History* 42, no. 4 (2009): 946.

42 'Few Soldiers Suffer from War Neurosis,' *NZ Truth*, 29 August 1945, 10.

43 See Tiffany Jenks, '"They hold us responsible for their welfare": War Neurosis, World War Two Veterans, Families and the New Zealand Returned Servicemen's Association' (BA Hons diss., University of Otago, 2016); Ref MS-2755, Dunedin Returned Servicemen's Association, Welfare Claims Files (WCF) #1201–1270 (HC).

44 Oliver Sutherland, *Paikea: The Life of I. L. G. Sutherland* (Christchurch: Canterbury University Press, 2013), 377.

45 Ruth Manchester, *The New Zealand Association of Psychotherapists, Te Roopu Whakaora Hinengaro: Notes Towards a History: A Chronology of the First Fifty Years, 1947–1997* (Wellington: The Association, 1996), 12.

46 Term used in 'Psychological Casualties,' *The Press*, 31 July 1944, 4, https://paperspast.natlib.govt.nz/newspapers/CHP19440731.2.38. See also Weaver and Wright, 'Shell Shock and the Politics of Asylum Committal in New Zealand,' 28.

47 Cited in J. O. Melling, 'The New Zealand Returned Soldiers' Association, 1916–1923' (MA thesis, Victoria University of Wellington, 1952), 74, http://restrictedarchive.vuw.ac.nz/handle/123456789/6674

48 Stephen Clarke, *After the War: The RSA in New Zealand* (Auckland: Penguin Random House, 2016), points out that the RSA's clubs established during the First World War were initially 'dry' from alcohol, although at various reunions and events this was not always the practice.

49 'Returned Soldier's Death. Mental Depression due to War Experience,' *The Dominion*, 31 October 1918, 4, https://paperspast.natlib.govt.nz/newspapers/DOM19181031.2.24

50 ACGS 16231, COR1928/716, R23713913 (ANZ, WR). Information also from the roll of the New Zealand Expeditionary Force.

51 *NZH*, 18 February 1921, 7, https://paperspast.natlib.govt.nz/newspapers/NZH19210218.2.104

52 '"Shell Shock" Defence,' *The Waikato Times*, 12 December 1919, 2, https://paperspast.natlib.govt.nz/newspapers/WT19191212.2.4

53 'Imposter Gaoled,' *The Sun* (Auckland), 23 May 1930, 12, https://paperspast.natlib.govt.nz/newspapers/SUNAK19300523.2.140

54 *Wanganui Chronicle*, 24 May 1930, 16, https://paperspast.natlib.govt.nz/newspapers/WC19300524.2.137

55 MS-2755/006, WCF #371 (HC): Online Cenotaph.

56 ACGS 16231, COR1960/142, R23881241 (ANZ WR).

57 Robert J. Ursano, 'Prisoners of War: Long-term Health Outcomes,' *The Lancet* 362, Supplement, Extreme Medicine (December 2003): s22–s23, www.thelancet.com/pdfs/journals/lancet/PIIS0140673603150623.pdf

58 Confidential source.

59 MS-2755 /013, WCF, #729, (HC). John is a pseudonym.

60 Jenks and Wanhalla, 'Psychological Casualties,' 4. The welfare claims of the Dunedin branch of the RSA are available at MS-2755/002, WCF, 1940–1989, SER-09548, (HC). For the aftermath of the First World War, see Elizabeth Walker, '"The Living Death": The Repatriation Experience of New Zealand's Disabled Great War Servicemen' (MA thesis, Victoria University of Wellington, 2013), http://hdl.handle.net/10063/2641

61 Parr, *Silent Casualties*, 144.

62 Ibid., 120–22.

63 Ibid., 16.

64 Ibid., 144.

65 'Tenth Re-inforcements,' *ODT*, 19 November 1915, 3, https://paperspast.natlib.govt.nz/newspapers/ODT19151119.2.10

66 DAHI 19956, #5686, R6670185; DAHI 19851, #5639, R25677018 (ANZ DR); AABK, 18805, WW1 8/3913 — Army, R16792224 (ANZ WR).

67 'Soldier Admits Desertion,' *The Press*, 4 July 1941, 6, https://paperspast.natlib.govt.nz/newspapers/CHP19410704.2.37

68 Ibid.

69 Weaver, *Sorrows of a Century*, 162.

70 Aiken, 'A Review of Psychiatric Casualties,' 169.

71 Ibid., 168.

72 Hefford, 'War Neurosis.'

73 Weaver, *Sorrows of a Century*, 154–55. The sample covered suicides for the even years of the twentieth century.

74 'Soldier's Death,' *NEM*, 25 July 1917, 3, https://paperspast.natlib.govt.nz/newspapers/NEM19170725.2.14.2; ACGS 16231, COR1917/826, R23704628, (ANZ WR); 'Soldier's Suicide. Sequel to Depression,' *The Ashburton Guardian*, 15 November 1918, 4, https://paperspast.natlib.govt.nz/newspapers/AG19181115.2.14; ACGS 16231, R23728328, COR 1918/1244 (ANZ WR).

75 *The Thames Star*, 16 May 1930, 5, https://paperspast.natlib.govt.nz/newspapers/THS19300516.2.30

76 'Sad Sequel to Shell Shock,' *The Horowhenua Chronicle*, 4 February 1925, 3, https://paperspast.natlib.govt.nz/newspapers/HC19250204.2.41

77 'Shooting Fatality,' *The Poverty Bay Herald*, 1 August 1932, 6, https://paperspast.natlib.govt.nz/newspapers/PBH19320801.2.86

78 Donald McKenzie, 'Prefrontal Leucotomy,' *NZMJ* 47, no. 257 (1948): 38–9. This report did not state the patient's condition after returning home.

79 ACGS 16231, COR1938/1824, R23901781; AABK 18805, WW1 23/2538, #0023386R, R21892880 (ANZ WR).

80 ACGS 16231, COR1938/1351, R23901307 (ANZ WR).

81 Confidential source.

82 ACGS 16231, COR1943/126, R23766709 (ANZ WR).

83 CBDB 23547/8; #4743, R20127941 (ANZ CR).

84 Weaver and Munro, 'Country Living, Country Dying,' 953.

85 ACGS 16231, COR1924/367, R23798548 (ANZ WR).

86 ACGS 16231, COR1944/757, R23829093 (ANZ WR).

87 Weaver, *Sorrows of a Century*, 164.

88 'Death of Young Man,' *The Poverty Bay Herald*, 7 September 1921, 6, https://paperspast.natlib.govt.nz/newspapers/PBH19210907.2.60

89 AG-447-6/03 Ashburn Hall, Case book, 1927–1947, folio 261, #204 (HC).

90 ACGS 16231, COR1940/1259, R23865229 (ANZ WR).

91 ACGS 16231, COR1940/1605, R23865575 (ANZ WR).

92 ACGS 16231, COR1942/482, R23743818 (ANZ WR).

5. Living with, and denying, the dark cloud

1 Meg Campbell, Typescript draft of 'Arlin' (1999) an autobiography, MS-Papers-11519-64 (ATL). 'Arlin' was written with Margaret Blair's assistance, as an internal dialogue between Meg and Arlin, as well as a conversation with others. Quotes from Meg in this chapter are from 'Arlin' unless indicated otherwise.

2 Alistair's letters to mostly Meg part 1, 10 September 1960, 91-046-1/05 (ATL).

3 See Joy Mackenzie, '"My way is to be with you": Meg and Alistair Te Ariki Campbell,' in *Between the Lives: Partners in Art*, ed. Deborah Shepard (Auckland: Auckland University Press, 2005), 187–209.

4 Interview with Alistair and Meg Campbell, 27 February 2004, OHInt-0734-05 (ATL).

5 Memoirs of his parents and his early life are retold in Alistair Campbell, *Island to Island* (Christchurch: Whitcoulls, 1984).

6 See Antonella Sarti, *Spiritcarvers: Interviews with Eighteen Writers from New Zealand* (Amsterdam: Rodopi, 1998), 14. See also Seri Inthava Kau'ikealaula Luangphinith, 'Tropical Fevers: "Madness" and Colonialism in Pacific Literature,' *The Contemporary Pacific* 16, no. 1 (Spring 2004): 71–75.

7 Nelson Wattie, *Scribbling in the Dark: Alistair Te Ariki Campbell* (Wellington: Steele Roberts Aotearoa, 2011), 29–30. 'The Return' was first published in Alistair Campbell, *Mine Eyes Dazzle: Poems 1947–9* (Christchurch: Pegasus Press, 1950).

8 Alistair Campbell, *Sanctuary of Spirits* (Wellington: Wai-Te-Ata Press, 1963); *The Frigate Bird* (Auckland: Heinemann Reed, 1989).

9 Sarti, *Spiritcarvers*, 17.

10 Meg Campbell, 'Heredity,' in *The Way Back: Poems* (Pukerua Bay: Te Kotare Press, 1981), 11.

11 Meg Campbell, 'Arlin,' 18.

12 Ibid., 159.

13 Ibid., 152–56.

14 Published in *The Listener*, 14 April 1979; Campbell, *The Way Back*, 18.

15 Janet Frame, *An Angel At My Table* (London: Virago, 2010). This edition contains all three volumes of Frame's autobiography, and is introduced by Jane Campion.

16 As there is extensive literature about Janet Frame's life, I do not repeat this. See, for example, Michael King, *Wrestling with the Angel: A Life of Janet Frame* (Auckland: Viking, 2000).

17 Alistair Fox, *Jane Campion: Authorship and Personal Cinema* (Bloomington, IN: Indiana University Press, 2011).

18 Frank Sargeson, 'Review,' *Landfall* 125 (1978): 90; Edith Campion, *A Place to Pass Through and Other Stories* (Wellington: Reed, 1977).

19 Sue Williams, 'A Light on the Dark Secrets of Depression,' in *Jane Campion: Interviews*, ed. Virginia Wright Wexman (Jackson, MS: University Press of Mississippi, 1999), 175–76.

20 Fox, *Jane Campion*, 130.

21 Alison Hunt, 'Lotus-Eating in Avondale: Tennyson in Robin Hyde's Poetry and 1934 Autobiography,' *Ka mate ka ora: A New Zealand Journal of Poetry and Poetics* 1, (2005): 47.

22 Psychiatric Clinic Case Notes for Iris G. Wilkinson, June 1933, by Henry Buchanan. YCAA 1090/7 (ANZ AR), cited in Alison Hunt, '"The Cage with the Open Door": Autobiography and Psychiatry in the Life and Works of Robin Hyde' (PhD thesis, University of Auckland, 2008), 24. Due to archival access restrictions, I was unable to consult Hyde's case notes. See also Derek Challis and Gloria Rawlinson, *The Book of Iris: A Life of Robin Hyde* (Auckland: Auckland University Press, 2002).

23 Cited in Mary Edmond-Paul, ed., *Your Unselfish Kindness: Robin Hyde's Autobiographical Writings* (Dunedin, Otago University Press, 2011), 173. See also Alison Hunt, 'Angel-Guarded Liar in a Pleasant, Quiet Room: Robin Hyde's Experiences in the New Zealand Mental Health System of the 1930s,' in *Lighted Windows: Critical Essays on Robin Hyde*, eds Mary Paul and Susan Ash (Dunedin: Otago University Press, 2008), 143–50.

24 Alison Hunt, 'The Unhappy Present Recites the Past: Autobiography as Psychiatric Treatment in the 1930s Case of Robin Hyde,' in *Telling Lives: Essays in Biography and History*, eds Catharine Coleborne, Mark Houlahan and Hugh Douglas Morrison (Hamilton: University of Waikato, Departments of History and Humanities, 2006), 105–29; Edmond-Paul, *Your Unselfish Kindness*.

25 See Alison Hunt, 'A Bibliography of the Published Works of Robin Hyde (Iris G. Wilkinson, 1906–1939)' (Auckland: New Zealand Electronic Poetry Centre, University of Auckland), 22 March 2004), www.nzepc.auckland.ac.nz/authors/hyde/index.asp

26 Hunt, '"The Cage with the Open Door",' 2.

27 Robin Hyde, *The Godwits Fly* (London: Hurst & Blackett, 1938); Robin Hyde, *Wednesday's Children: A Novel* (London: Hurst & Blackett, 1937); Robin Hyde, with an introduction by Derek Challis, *A Home in this World* (Auckland: Longman Paul, 1984).

28 For details of this part of Hyde's life, see Challis and Rawlinson, *The Book of Iris*, 629–56.

29 Jacqueline Matthews, 'Hyde, Robin,' *Dictionary of New Zealand Biography* (1998), *Te Ara — the Encyclopedia of New Zealand*, https://teara.govt.nz/en/biographies/4h41/hyde-robin

30 Rosaleen Macbrayne, 'Shock therapy "changed" artist Rita Angus', *NZH*, n.d., www.nzherald.co.nz/lifestyle/shock-thera-py-changed-artist-rita-angus/XBAWSIGYJJ6YQYKZ2R3E6ITOGM. See Vita Cochran et al., *Rita Angus: Live to Paint and Paint to Live* (Auckland: Random House in association with City Gallery Wellington and Hocken Library, Dunedin, 2001).

31 James Courage, *Diaries*, ed. Chris Brickell (Dunedin: Otago University Press, 2021).

32 Ibid., 38.

33 Ibid., 8 September 1960, 37. Courage died in 1963 from a cardiac arrest.

34 Sutherland, *Paikea*, 400.

35 Ernest Beaglehole, 'Some Sociological Aspects of Race Relations in New Zealand,' *International Social Science Bulletin* 3, no.2 (1951): 253–58.

36 Cited in James Ritchie, 'Sutherland, Ivan Lorin George,' *Dictionary of New Zealand Biography* (1998, updated 2020 by Oliver Sutherland), *Te Ara — the Encyclopedia of New Zealand*, https://teara.govt.nz/en/biographies/4s57/sutherland-ivan-lorin-george (accessed 4 July 2023).

37 Sutherland, *Paikea*, 401.

38 Nancy Sutherland, cited in ibid.

39 J. C. B., A. E. C., R. M. C. and J. M. McE. 'I. L. G. Sutherland 1897–1952,' JPS 61, no. 1/2 (1952): 122–24. These initials are those of John Beaglehole, Arnold Campbell, Richard Campbell and Jock McEwan.

40 Ibid., 120.

41 Alistair Fox, *The Ship of Dreams: Masculinity in Contemporary New Zealand Fiction* (Dunedin: Otago University Press, 2008), 15.

42 Parr, *'Silent Casualties'*, 140.

43 ACGS 16231, COR1949/118, R23874607 (ANZ WR). An obituary was published in *The British Medical Journal* and in the media, but there was no public mention of suicide, so I have not disclosed his name, or the precise details of where he served.

44 Confidential source.

45 'Incipient Melancholia,' *AS*, 30 May 1898, 3, https://paperspast.natlib.govt.nz/newspapers/AS18980530.2.14

46 Hugh Freeman, 'When the Mood Swings Crazily,' *N.Z. Family Doctor*, April 1964, 22.

47 H. M. Horton, 'Attempted Suicide and Severe Depression' (PM diss., University of Otago, 1967), 26–27.

48 Allan Horwitz and Jerome Wakefield, *The Loss of Sadness: How Psychiatry Transformed Normal Sorrow into Depressive Disorder* (Oxford: Oxford University Press, 2007).

49 Francis O'Gorman, *Worrying: A Literary and Cultural History* (London: Bloomsbury, 2015), 1.

50 Derek Summerfield, 'Afterword: Against "Global Mental Health",' *Transcultural Psychiatry* 49, no. 3–4 (2012): 520.

51 Alain Ehrenberg, *The Weariness of the Self: Diagnosing the History of Depression in the Contemporary Age* (Chicago, IL: McGill Queen's University Press, 2009), 3. Originally published in French in 1998.

52 Sadowsky, 'Before and After Prozac,' 491.

53 Weaver, *Sorrows of a Century*, 169. See the table on p. 23.

54 Ibid., 176.

55 Ibid., 177.

56 Conan Fowler, 'A Study of Depression in Middle-aged Housewives' (PM diss., University of Otago, 1972), 3–4.

57 DAHI, 19956, D264; # 5598, R66070185 (ANZ DR).

58 J. M. Aubrey, 'Patient Views of Depression in a General Practice' (PM diss., University of Otago, 1973), 17.

59 Horton, 'Attempted Suicide and Severe Depression.'

60 CAHW 27346, #1170, R18946513 (ANZ CR).

61 *The Grey River Argus*, 5 April 1923, 4, https://paperspast.natlib.govt.nz/newspapers/GRA19230405.2.19

62 DAHI 19956, #5524, R6670183 (ANZ DR).

63 Horton, 'Attempted Suicide and Severe Depression'; S. D. R. Lang, 'Attempted Suicide by Overdose' (PM diss., University of Otago, 1967), R. T. Lienert, 'Aspects of Suicide and Attempted Suicide' (PM diss., University of Otago, 1967).

64 Horton, 'Attempted Suicide and Severe Depression.'

65 Weaver and Munro, 'Country Living, Country Dying,' 955.

66 Ibid., 939.

67 ACGS 16231, COR1946/800, R23873801 (ANZ WR).

68 Weaver and Munro, 'Country Living, Country Dying,' 933–61; Annette L. Beautrais, 'Farm Suicides in New Zealand, 2007–2015: A Review of Coroners' Records,' *ANZJP* 52, no.1 (2017): 78–86.

69 ACGS 16231, COR1945/44, R23868780 (ANZ WR).

70 ACGS 16231, COR1959/15, R23853530 (ANZ WR).

71 YCAA 1048/15, #5000, R1481810 (ANZ AR).

72 DAHI 19956, #5548, R6670184; 19851, R25676945 (ANZ DR).

73 DAHI, 19956, #5549, R6670184 (ANZ DR).

74 Reported in Papers Past. I have withheld details for reasons of confidentiality.

75 AG-447-6/01, folio 138, #32 (HC).

76 'The Treatment,' *The Press*, 24 May 1977, 19, https://paperspast.natlib.govt.nz/newspapers/CHP19770524.2.139

77 Alistair Campbell and Meg Campbell, *It's Love, Isn't It? The Love Poems* (Wellington: HeadworX, 2008).

6. Depression, ethnicity and culture

1 Letters on R25297075, 5 February 1916, 13 April 1916 (ANZ AR).

2 YCAA 1026/43, #5102, R25297075 (ANZ AR), where he is called Taru Singh. On the Indian diaspora to Aotearoa, see Jacqueline Leckie, *Indian Settlers: The Story of a New Zealand South Asian Community* (Dunedin: Otago University Press, 2007).

3 Ibid. Letter from J. Whittaker to medical superintendent, Avondale Mental Hospital, 18 March 1915.

4 W. H. McLeod, *A List of Punjabi Immigrants in New Zealand, 1890–1939* (Hamilton: Country Section of the Central Indian Association, 1984), 18, notes a Kahan Singh. Pheru Singh is not mentioned in McLeod's records, but McLeod provides the background Singh came from.

5 'Mental Hospitals of the Dominion (Report On) for 1916,' *AJHR*, 1917, Session I, H-07.

6 Barbara Brookes, 'Pictures of People, Pictures of Places: Photography and the Asylum,' in *Exhibiting Madness in Museums: Remembering Psychiatry through Collections and Display*, eds Catharine Coleborne and Dolly MacKinnon (New York, London: Routledge, 2011), 40–57, discusses how asylum patients sometimes performed stereotypes of madness when photographed.

7 It is quite unlikely that he would have been stoned because his hair was cut.

8 This does not deny that many earlier refugees in Aotearoa experienced depression. See Ann Beaglehole, *Refuge New Zealand: A Nation's Response to Refugees and Asylum Seekers* (Dunedin: Otago University Press, 2013), 30–42.

9 On the neglect of ethnicity in historical studies of mental health in Aotearoa, see Coleborne, *Insanity, Identity and Empire*, 9–10; Angela McCarthy and Catharine Coleborne, 'Introduction: Mental Health, Migration and Ethnicity,' in *Migration, Ethnicity, and Mental Health: International Perspectives, 1840–2010*, eds Angela McCarthy and Catharine Coleborne (New York and Abingdon: Routledge, 2012), 1–14; McCarthy, *Migration, Ethnicity and Madness*, 169–200.

10 DAHI 19850/38, #4159, R25259945 (ANZ DR).

11 Sadowsky, *The Empire of Depression*; Sadowsky, 'Before and After Prozac,' 483.

12 For example, Arthur Kleinman and Byron Good, eds, *Culture and Depression: Studies in the Anthropology and Cross-Psychiatry of Affect and Disorder* (Berkeley, CA: University of California Press, 1985).

13 Elsie Seckyee Ho, 'Mental Health of Asian Immigrants in New Zealand: A Review of Key Issues,' *Asian and Pacific Migration Journal* 13, no. 1 (March

2004): 39–60; Carol H. J. Lee et al., 'Ethnic Inequality in Diagnosis with Depression and Anxiety Disorders,' *NZMJ* 130, no. 1454 (2017): 10–20; Francis Agnew et al., 'Pacific Models of Mental Health Service Delivery in New Zealand ('PMMHSD') Project' (Auckland: Health Research Council of New Zealand, 2004), www.leva.co.nz/uploads/files/resources/Pacific-Models-of-Mental-Health-Service-Delivery-in-New-Zealand-PMMHSD-Project.pdf

14 For example, Anthony J. Marsella et al., 'Cross-Cultural Studies of Depressive Disorders: An Overview,' in *Culture and Depression: Studies in the Anthropology and Cross-Psychiatry of Affect and Disorder*, eds Arthur Kleinman and Byron Good (Berkeley, CA: University of California Press, 1985), 299-324; Arthur Kleinman and Joan Kleinman, 'Somatization: The Interconnections in Chinese Society among Culture, Depressive Experiences, and the Meanings of Pain, in *Culture and Depression*, eds Kleinman and Good, 370–429; Eng-Seong Tan, 'The Presentation of Affective Symptoms in Non-Western Countries,' in *Handbook of Studies on Depression*, ed. Graham D. Burrows (Amsterdam: Excerpta Medica, 1977), 121–33; Claire E. Edington, *Beyond the Asylum: Mental Illness in French Colonial Vietnam* (Ithaca, NY: Cornell University Press, 2019); Junko Kitanaka, *Depression in Japan: Psychiatric Cures for a Society in Distress* (Princeton, NJ: Princeton University Press, 2012).

15 Sally Swartz, 'Changing Diagnoses in Valkenberg Asylum, Cape Colony, 1891–1920: A Longitudinal View,' *History of Psychiatry* 5 (1995): 431–51; Jonathan Sadowsky, *Imperial Bedlam: Institutions of Madness in Colonial Southwest Nigeria* (Berkeley, CA: University of California Press, 1999), 108; Leckie, *Colonizing Madness*, 132–33; Tan, 'The Presentation of Affective Symptoms in Non-Western Countries,' 123.

16 Studies are cited in Sadowsky, *The Empire of Depression*, 89–90.

17 H. B. M. Murphy and R. Narayan, 'Mental Hospitalisation in Fiji,' *Fiji Medical Journal* 7, no. 1 (1979): 4–11.

18 B. G. Burton-Bradley, *Stone Age Crisis: A Psychiatric Appraisal* (Nashville, TN: Vanderbilt University Press, 1975). By 1998 Attah reported that depressive disorders were as common in Papua New Guinea as in other cultures globally. Felix Y. Attah, 'Depressive Disorders: Diagnosis, Recognition and Management of Depressive Disorders in General Medical Practice in the Pacific,' *Fiji General Practitioner* 5, no. 1 (1998): 300–5.

19 For example: Gananath Obeyesekere, 'Depression, Buddhism and the Work of Culture in Sri Lanka,' in Kleinman and Good, *Culture and Depression*, 134–52; Catherine Lutz, 'Depression and the Translation of Emotional Worlds,' in Kleinman and Good, *Culture and Depression*, 63–100.

20 DAHI 19956, #3413, R6670162 (ANZ DR).

21 James Ng, *Windows on a Chinese Past* (Dunedin: Otago Heritage Books, 4 vols, 1993–1999): vol. 3, 103, identified him as Chan Tsaan Yam (in vol. 1, 201, the name is Chan Tsaam Yam). Ng says that Chan was in and out of Seacliff, where he died in 1906. On Alexander Don's *Roll of Chinese in New Zealand 1883–1913*, (reproduced in Ng, *Windows on a Chinese Past*, 1993, vol. 4, 904), the name is Cham Jarn Yum (No. 906). I could not find any of these names in the Seacliff archive.

22 *N.Z. Presbyterian*, 1 October 1886, 62.

23 *The Outlook*, 23 March 1901, 2.

24 Ng, *Windows on a Chinese Past*, vol. 1, 333, n.58.

25 For example: Manying Ip, 'Chinese,' *Te Ara — the Encyclopedia of New Zealand* (2005, updated 2015), www.teara.govt.nz/en/chinese; Ng, *Windows on a Chinese Past.*

26 *North Otago Times*, 17 January 1868, 2, https://paperspast.natlib.govt.nz/newspapers/NOT18680117.2.10

27 'Outrages upon the Chinese,' *ODT*, 3 February 1868, 5, https://paperspast.natlib.govt.nz/newspapers/ODT18680203.2.21

28 *Otago Witness*, 13 March 1880, 9, https://paperspast.natlib.govt.nz/newspapers/OW18800313.2.23.3. See Ng, *Windows on a Chinese Past*, vol. 2, 292–325, on opium and the Chinese in Aotearoa.

29 DAHI 19956/40, #2128, R6670150; DAHI 19850/17, R25258220 (ANZ DR).

30 CAHW 27346, folio 89, #1024, R18946513 (ANZ CR).

31 *Hawera and Normanby Star*, 9 July 1909, 8, https://paperspast.natlib.govt.nz/newspapers/HNS19090709.2.63

32 ACGS 16231, COR1940/1095, R23865067 (ANZ WR); 'Death of Chinese,' *EP*, 22 August 1940, 17, https://paperspast.natlib.govt.nz/newspapers/EP19400822.2.161

33 'Chinamen,' *The Cromwell Argus*, 2 September 1873, 7, https://paperspast.natlib.govt.nz/newspapers/CROMARG18730902.2.21; *Mount Ida Chronicle*, 5 September 1873, 7, https://paperspast.natlib.govt.nz/newspapers/MIC18730905.2.24

34 DAHI 19956/40, #2128, R6670150 (ANZ DR).

35 DAHI 19956, #2643, R6670155 (ANZ DR).

36 CAHW 27346, folio 347, R18946511 (ANZ CR).

37 CAHW 27346, folio 42, #685, R18946514 (ANZ CR).

38 DAHI 19956, folio 341, R6670150 (ANZ DR).

39 Ng, *Windows on a Chinese Past*, vol. 1, 200–1; vol. 2, 44–46.

40 Chinese NZ Oral History Foundation, www.facebook.com/CNZOHF/posts/wallingford-william-chan-ting-ming-usually-known-as-wallingford-chan-was-born-in/163716344304543

41 See, for example, Jenny Agnew and Trevor Agnew, *Merchant, Miner, Mandarin: The Life and Times of the Remarkable Choie Sew Hoy* (Christchurch: Canterbury University Press, 2020).

42 DAHI 19956, #5417, R6670184 (ANZ DR).

43 See 'Scattered Seeds,' https://dunedin.recollect.co.nz/nodes/view/199784

44 After 1929 Dalmatia became part of Yugoslavia, and today Dalmatia is part of Croatia. See Carl Walrond, 'Dalmatians,' *Te Ara — the Encyclopedia of New Zealand* (2005, updated 2015), www.teara.govt.nz/en/dalmatians/print (accessed 30 June 2023).

45 YCAA 1048/12, folio 139, #4234; folio 341, #4485, R1481806 (ANZ AR).

46 YCAA 1048/8, folio 311, #2460, R1481802 (ANZ AR).

47 YCAA 1048/12, #4377, R1481806 (ANZ AR).

48 YCAA 1048/12, #4485 (ANZ AR).

49 Such as in Polynesia and Micronesia, according to Alan Howard, 'Polynesia and Micronesia in Psychiatric Perspective,' *Transcultural Psychiatry* 16 (1979): 132. See also Francis X. Hezel, 'In Search of the Social Roots of Mental Pathology in Micronesia,' in *Contemporary Issues in Mental Health Research in the Pacific Islands*, eds Albert B. Robillard and Anthony J. Marsella (Honolulu: University of Hawai'i Press, 1987): 12–31.

50 Ng, *Windows on a Chinese Past*, 291, note 185.

51 DAHI 19956/38, #963, R6670148; DAHI 19850/6, R25257126 (ANZ DR); *Lake County Press*, 12 July 1876, 2, https://paperspast.natlib.govt.nz/newspapers/LCP18760712.2.5

52 CAHW 3358, folio 187, R18946497 (ANZ CR).

53 'Determined Suicide,' *The Western Star*, 15 August 1883, 2, https://paperspast.natlib.govt.nz/newspapers/WSTAR18830815.2.9

54 'New Zealand Disasters and Tragedies. Otago Miners Inquests from The Otago Police Gazettes,' *Otago Police Gazette* (1872), http://free's.genealogy.rootsweb.ancestry.com/~sooty/otagoinquests1868.html

55 'Inquest,' *ES*, 1 September 1885, 3, https://paperspast.natlib.govt.nz/newspapers/ESD18850901.2.19; *Otago Witness*, 5 September 1885, 10, https://paperspast.natlib.govt.nz/newspapers/OW18850905.2.15

56 Daniel Davy, *Gold Rush Societies and Migrant Networks in the Tasman World* (Edinburgh: Edinburgh University Press, 2021), 189.

57 ACGS 16231, COR1938/420, R23900377 (ANZ WR).

58 This section is based on confidential sources. See also Jacqueline Leckie, 'Gumboots and Saris: Engendering Indian Settlers' History in Aotearoa,' in *Asia in the Making of New Zealand*, eds Henry Johnson and Brian Moloughney (Auckland: Auckland University Press: 2006), 76–93.

59 Siale Foliaki et al., 'Pacific People,' in *Te Rau Hinengaro: The New Zealand Mental Health Survey*, eds M. A. Oakley Browne and J. E. Wells (Wellington: Ministry of Health, 2006), 178–208, www.health.govt.nz/system/files/documents/publications/mental-health-survey-2006-pacific-people.pdf

60 See Damon I. Salesa, 'New Zealand's Pacific,' in *The New Oxford History of New Zealand*, ed. Giselle Byrnes (Melbourne: Oxford University Press, 2009), 149–72. New Zealand was also a co-trustee of Nauru, along with Australia and Britain when Nauru was a League of Nations mandate, and a United Nations trust territory.

61 Indira Stewart, 'Older Pasifika Migrants More Resilient to Mental Illness,' *RNZ*, 13 December 2018, www.rnz.co.nz/international/pacific-news/378200/older-pasifika-migrants-more-re-silient-to-mental-illness; Joanna Ataera-Minster and Holly Trowland, *Te Kaveinga — Mental Health and Wellbeing of Pacific Peoples* (Wellington: Health Promotion Agency, 2018) 10, www.hpa.org.nz/research-library/research-publications/te-kaveinga-mental-health-and-wellbe-ing-of-pacific-peoples

62 Ministry for Pacific Peoples, *Pacific Aotearoa Status Report. A Snapshot, 2020* (Wellington: Ministry for Pacific Peoples, 2021), 14, www.mpp.govt.nz/assets/Reports/Pacific-Peo-ples-in-Aotearoa-Report.pdf

63 See, for example, Leckie, *Colonizing Madness*; Jacqueline Leckie and Frances Hughes, 'Mental Health in the Smaller Pacific States,' in *Mental Health in Asia and the Pacific: Historical and Comparative Perspectives*, eds Harry Minas and Milton Lewis (New York: Springer, 2017), 253–72.

64 Stewart, 'Older Pasifika Migrants More Resilient to Mental Illness.'

65 Iain Loan et al., 'Understanding Depression in Tokelauan People in New Zealand,' *Journal of Primary Health Care* 8 (2016): 70.

66 For Samoan terms, see Dorothy C. Clement, 'Samoan Folk Knowledge of Mental Disorders,' in *Cultural Conceptions of Mental Health and Therapy*, eds Anthony J. Marsella and Geoffrey M. White (Dordecht: D. Reidel Publishing, 1974), 193–213; George Bertram Milner, *Samoan Dictionary* (London: Oxford University Press, 1966); George Pratt, *Pratt's Grammar and Dictionary of the Language* (Apia: The Malua Printing Press, 1862). For Rarotongan, see: Josephine Baddeley, 'Traditional Healing Practices,' in *Healing Practices in the South Pacific*, ed. Claire D. F. Parsons (Laie, HI: Institute for Polynesian Studies, Brigham Young University, 1985), 129–43; W. Arthur Whistler, 'Traditional and Herbal Medicine in the Cook Islands,' *Journal of Ethnopharmacology* 13 (1985): 239–80; Marsa Dodson, pers. comm. For Niuean, Wolfgang B. Sperlich, *Tohi Vagahau Niue = Niue Language Dictionary: Niuean–English, with English–Niuean Finderlist* (Honolulu, HI: Government of Niue in association with Department of Linguistics, University of Hawai'i, 1997). For Tokelauan, Office of Tokelau Affairs, *Tokelau Dictionary* (Apia: Office of Tokelau Affairs, 1986). For Fijian, Arthur Capell, The Fijian Dictionary (Suva: Government Printers, 1941); David Hazlewood, *A Fijian and English and an English and Fijian Dictionary: With Examples of Common and Peculiar Modes of Expression and Uses of Words, also, Containing Brief Hints on Native Customs, Proverbs, the Native Names of Natural Productions, and Notices of the Islands of Fiji, and a Grammar of the Language, with Examples of Native Idioms*, ed. James Calvert (London: S. Low, Marston, 1872). For Tongan: Clerk Maxwell Churchward, *Tongan Dictionary: Tongan–English and English–Tongan* (Nuku'alofa: Government of Tonga, 1959); Wendy E. Cowling, 'Eclectic Elements in Tongan Folk Belief and Healing Practice,' in *Tongan Culture and History*, eds Phyllis Herda, Jennifer Terrell and Niel Gunson (Canberra: Department of Pacific and South Asian History, Australian National University, 1990), 72–92. For ni-Vanuatu: Christopher R. Brown and Jimmy Obed, 'The State of Psychology and Mental Health Services in Vanuatu,' in *Psychology in Oceania and the Caribbean*, eds Grant J. Rich and Neeta A. Ramkumar (Cham: Springer International Publishing, 2022), 37.

67 Kiwi Tamasese et al., 'Ole Taeao Afua, the New Morning: A Qualitative Investigation into Samoan Perspectives on Mental Health and Culturally Appropriate Services,' *Australasian Psychiatry: Bulletin of the Royal Australian and New Zealand College of Psychiatrists* 39, no. 4 (2005): 300–9.

68 Ibid., 304.

69 Laurie Kalman Gluckman, 'Drau Ni Kau: The Ethnopsychiatry of Fiji in Historical and Clinical Perspective,' *ANZJP* 3 (1969): 152–58.

70 Cowling, 'Eclectic Elements in Tongan Folk Belief.'

71 WITN0452001, 18 May 2021, Royal Commission of Inquiry into Abuse In Care, Witness Statement of Rachael Lemali Umaga, www.abuseincare.org.nz/assets/Uploads/Witness-Statement-of-Rachael-Umaga-for-Tulou-Our-Pacific-Voices-Tatala-e-Pulonga.pdf

72 See Loan et al., 'Understanding Depression in Tokelauan people in New Zealand,' 69.

73 On the rich literature on humour within Pacific cultures, see, for example, Niko Besnier, 'Humour and Humility: Narratives of Modernity on Nukulaelae Atoll,' *Etnofoor* 28, no. 1 (2016): 75–95; Elisabeth Betz and Toon van Meijl, 'Humour in the Negotiations

of Social Identity in the Tongan Diaspora,' *Etnofoor* 28, no. 1 (2016): 111–25.

74 Anna Carlson, talanoa with Jacqueline Leckie, Wellington, February 1992; August 1995.

75 Jacqueline Leckie, 'Silent Immigrants? Gender, Immigration and Ethnicity in New Zealand,' in *Immigration and National Identity in New Zealand: One People, Two Peoples, Many Peoples?* ed. Stuart Greif (Palmerston North: Dunmore Press, 1995), 60–61.

76 R. Cooper, 'Unrecognized Losses in Child Adoption,' in *Disenfranchised Grief: New Directions, Challenges, and Strategies for Practice*, ed. Kenneth J. Doka (Champaign: Research Press, 2002), 265–74; Marsa Dodson, 'Practising *Tamariki 'Āngai*: Mangaia's Informal Island Adoption' (PhD thesis, University of Otago, 2009), 43–46, http://hdl.handle.net/10523/4084

77 Tamasese et al., 'Ole Taeao Afua,' 304. See Ministry for Culture and Heritage, 'The Dawn Raids: Causes, Impacts and Legacy' (updated 12 June 2023), https://nzhistory.govt.nz/culture/dawn-raids. In fact the largest number of immigration overstayers were from Europe and North America.

78 Confidential sources.

79 Confidential source.

80 Carol H. J. Lee et al., 'Ethnic Inequality in Diagnosis with Depression and Anxiety Disorders,' *NZMJ* 130, no. 1454 (2017): 10.

81 'Nightmare for Patients,' *Mana* 1, no. 7 (29 September 1977): 1, https://paperspast.natlib.govt.nz/newspapers/MANAK19770929.2.6

7. 'Quacks', shocks, docs and drugs

1 'Reports on Lunatic Asylums in New Zealand,' *AJHR*, 1873, D-29, 6.

2 *NZH*, 13 February 1904, 5, https://paperspast.natlib.govt.nz/newspapers/NZH19040213.2.54.55

3 'Lecture Delivered to Auckland Trained Nurses,' *Kai Tiaki: The Journal of the Nurses of New Zealand* 5, no. 1 (1 January 1912): 6.

4 Oppenheim, *Shattered Nerves*, 112; 110–40.

5 *South Canterbury Times*, 18 March 1885, 2, https://paperspast.natlib.govt.nz/newspapers/SCANT18850318.2.5 2

6 *EP*, 21 March 1885, 2, https://paperspast.natlib.govt.nz/newspapers/EP18850321.2.11

7 *NZT*, 14 April 1883, 4, https://paperspast.natlib.govt.nz/newspapers/NZTIM18830414.2.27.1

8 See 'Humoral Theory,' Curiosity Collections, Harvard Library, https://curiosity.lib.harvard.edu/contagion/feature/humoral-theory (accessed 2 July 2023).

9 *ES*, 8 October 1903, 2, https://paperspast.natlib.govt.nz/newspapers/ESD19031008.2.12.2; advertised 1903–1910.

10 *AS*, 26 May 1913, 11, https://paperspast.natlib.govt.nz/newspapers/AS19130526.2.124.1

11 *The Poverty Bay Herald*, 28 July 1932, 12, https://paperspast.natlib.govt.nz/newspapers/PBH19320728.2.125.3

12 *The Press*, 28 October 1936, 11, https://paperspast.natlib.govt.nz/newspapers/CHP19361028.2.92.2

13 *The Ashburton Guardian*, 15 July 1895, 1, https://paperspast.natlib.govt.nz/newspapers/AG18950715.2.2.5

14 *ES*, 13 December 1906, 3, https://paperspast.natlib.govt.nz/newspapers/ESD19061213.2.19.2

15 For example, *The Manawatu Standard*, 17 October 1901, 2, https://

paperspast.natlib.govt.nz/newspapers/MS19011017.2.5

16 Alternative healing practitioners reject the term 'quacks' as derogatory. See also Athol Maurice Abrahams, 'Quackery: Or a Study of Unorthodox Medical Practitioners in Auckland' (PM diss., University of Otago, 1955), 48.

17 Kate Duke, 'A Century of CAM in New Zealand: A Struggle for Recognition,' *Complementary Therapies in Clinical Practice* 11, no. 1 (2005): 11–16.

18 *The Timaru Herald*, 31 May 1911, 1, https://paperspast.natlib.govt.nz/newspapers/THD19110531.2.2.4

19 *ODT*, 20 February 1906, 6, https://paperspast.natlib.govt.nz/newspapers/ODT19060220.2.63.5; *The Southland Times*, 10 February 1911, 6, https://paperspast.natlib.govt.nz/newspapers/ST19110210.2.51.6

20 Oppenheim, *Shattered Nerves*, 121.

21 *NZT*, 3 June 1905, 13, https://paperspast.natlib.govt.nz/newspapers/NZTIM19050603.2.86.1

22 *NZT*, 17 August 1907, 7, https://paperspast.natlib.govt.nz/newspapers/NZTIM19070817.2.52.6

23 DAHI 19956/73, #5555, R6670183 (ANZ DR).

24 *ES*, 26 April 1938, 16, https://paperspast.natlib.govt.nz/newspapers/ESD19380426.2.148

25 *The Thames Star*, 4 November 1897, 2, https://paperspast.natlib.govt.nz/newspapers/THS18971104.2.8

26 See Mathew Thomson, 'Practical Psychology,' in *Psychological Subjects: Identity, Culture, and Health in Twentieth-Century Britain*, ed. Mathew Thomson (Oxford: Oxford University Press, 2006), 17–53.

27 *ES*, 26 April 1938, 16, https://paperspast.natlib.govt.nz/newspapers/ESD19380426.2.148

28 E. Stolkind, 'A Case of Acute Fatal Medinal Poisoning, with Notes on the Ill-Effects of the Medinal Habit,' *The Lancet* 207 (1926): 391–92.

29 Robin Hyde, 'The Veronal Menace,' *The New Zealand Observer*, 28 July 1932. See also Redmar Yska, 'Veronal; Who Remembers Veronal?', *Matters of Substance*, 1 August 2016, www.drugfoundation.org.nz/matters-of-substance/archive/august-2016/veronal-who-remembers-veronal

30 Hunt, 'The Cage with the Open Door,' 23; Challis and Rawlinson, *The Book of Iris*, 219, 238, 244, 307–8.

31 ACGS 16231, COR1936/395, R23861489 (ANZ WR).

32 John King, inspector of asylums, 'Reports on Lunatic Asylums in New Zealand', *AJHR*, 1870, D-29, 5.

33 'Special Wards Urged. Treating of Melancholia,' *NZH*, 9 October 1937, 14, https://paperspast.natlib.govt.nz/newspapers/NZH19371009.2.111

34 See Edmond-Paul, *Your Unselfish Kindness*, 34–35.

35 'Mental hospitals of the Dominion (report on) for 1935.'

36 Ibid.

37 Jeff Kavanagh, 'Cherry Farm 1952–1992. Social and Economic Forces in the Evolution of Mental Health Care in Otago,' in *'Unfortunate Folk': Essays on Mental Health Treatment, 1863–1992*, eds Barbara Brookes and Jane Thomson (Dunedin: Otago University Press, 2001), 168–82. The villa or outdoor system was established at Tokanui in 1912, with patients housed in separate units according to their mental condition.

38 See Warwick Brunton, 'The Origins of Deinstitutionalisation in New Zealand,' *Health and History* 5, no. 2 (2003): 75–103.

39 Wendy Hunter Williams, *Out of Sight Out of Mind: The Story of Porirua Hospital* (Wellington: Porirua Hospital, 1987), 273–77. Meg's name was not published, but this interview is similar to parts of 'Arlin', and Meg and Alistair Campbell's interview, 27 February 2004, Porirua Oral History (ATL).

40 Campbell, 'Arlin,' 156–57.

41 CAHW 27346, #840, R1894651 (ANZ CR).

42 DAHI 19956/73, #5439, R6670183; DAHI 19851/58, R25676882 (ANZ DR).

43 Alan Somerville, 'Ashburn Hall and its Place in Society, 1882–1904' (MA thesis, University of Otago, 1996), 38; Cameron Duder, *The Ashburn Clinic: The Place and the People* (Dunedin: Ashburn Clinic, 2007). Ashburn Hall was renamed as Ashburn Clinic in 2001.

44 Warwick Brunton, 'Mental Health Services — Psychiatric Hospitals, 1940s to 1960s,' *Te Ara — the Encyclopedia of New Zealand* (2011, revised 2022), www.teara.govt.nz/en/mental-health-services/page-4 (accessed 13 July 2023). We need more historical research on patient and family pressures and their subjective reasons for agreeing to voluntary admission in mental institutions. Unfortunately, the inaccessibility of case records inhibits such research.

45 AG-447-6/04 Ashburn Hall, Case book, folio 74, #46, vol. 1, 1882–1890 (HC); DAHI 19956/40, folio 387, R6670150 (ANZ DR).

46 DAHI 19956/73, #5437, R6670183 (ANZ DR).

47 *The Ashburton Guardian*, 28 April 1921, 5.

48 AG-447-6/05 Ashburn Hall, Case book vol. 3, 1895–1898, folio 32, #202; AG-447-6/01, folio 139 #32; (HC); DAAC, D140/269, #L73 R22355984; DAHI 19850/44, #4835 R25260386 (ANZ DR); CAUY 12251/26, #3603, R20127937 (ANZ CR).

49 Sadowsky, 'Before and After Prozac,' 487.

50 'Mental Hospitals of the Dominion (Report On) for 1924,' *AJHR* 1925, Session I, H-07, 3; 7.

51 'Modern Treatments at Sunnyside Hospital,' *The Press*, 3 June 1961, 14, https://paperspast.natlib.govt.nz/newspapers/CHP19610603.2.163

52 Chisholm and Rind, 'Some Aspects of Post-War Psycho-Neuroses,' 224; E. W. Giesen, 'Discussion of Neurasthenia,' *NZMJ* 16, no. 74 (1917): 135–42.

53 Stuart Moore, 'Psychotherapy,' *NZMJ* 12, no. 47 (1913): 514–38.

54 Allen, 'Neurasthenia with Depression'; Charles Burns and W. Ironside, 'Obituary: Kathleen Mary Todd,' *NZMJ* 68, no. 436 (1968): 193; 'Obituary, Dr. C. M. Bevan-Brown,' *The Press*, 28 February 1967. Peter S. Cook, 'The Early History of the New Zealand Association of Psychotherapists and the Related Movement for Primary Prevention in Mental Health: Some Recollections,' *ANZJP* 30, no. 3 (June 1996): 405–9.

55 Cook, ibid., 405. See also Manchester, *The New Zealand Association of Psychotherapists.*

56 J. C. McKenzie, 'Maurice Bevan-Brown and His Influence on Thinking and Practice at Timaru Hospital,' Memorial Lecture, 22 August 1967, cited, ibid.

57 'Electrotherapy For Mental Illness,' *The Press*, 7 December 1957, 10, https://paperspast.natlib.govt.nz/newspapers/CHP19571207.2.49

58 See John Spencer Bonar Lindsay, 'The Affect in Prefrontal Leucotomy' (MD thesis, University of New Zealand, 1952); Paula Frances Rathbone, 'The Psychological Effects of Prefrontal Leucotomy: A Review of the Literature and Observations of Some Cases Studied' (MA thesis, University of New Zealand, 1948); Perminder Sachdev

and Jagdeep Sachdev, 'Sixty Years of Psychosurgery: Its Present Status and its Future,' *ANZJP* 31, no. 4 (1997): 457–64.

59 'New Treatments,' *NEM*, 20 October 1943, 3, https://paperspast.natlib.govt.nz/newspapers/NEM19431020.2.35

60 Reginald W. Medlicott, 'Prefrontal Leucotomy,' *NZMJ* 42, (1943): 113–20.

61 Ibid., 116–17.

62 Reginald W. Medlicott, 'Psychiatric Treatments,' *The New Zealand Nursing Journal* 38, no. 2 (1945): 31.

63 Medlicott, 'Prefrontal Leucotomy,' 120.

64 'Doubts Claims of Los Angeles Doctor', *The Northern Advocate*, 23 April 1946, 3, https://paperspast.natlib.govt.nz/newspapers/NA19460423.2.25

65 D. G. McLachlan and M. A. Falconer, 'Prefrontal Leucotomy (Lobotomy): A Report on 65 Cases,' *NZMJ* 49, no. 273 (1950): 522–30. The file 'Leucotomy and lobotomy', 1947–1960, ADCB 16173, #4/7/12, R16195661 (ANZ WR) contains details of patients who were melancholic or depressive and had leucotomies.

66 McLachlan and Falconer, ibid., 524.

67 'Mental Hospitals of the Dominion (Report On) for 1945,' *AJHR*, 1946 Session I, H–07.

68 K. R. Stallworthy, 'Clinical Findings Following Leucotomy,' *NZMJ* 52, no. 291 (1953): 405–12. See also Memo from medical superintendent, Auckland Mental Hospital to Director, Division of Mental Hygiene, 1 June 1955, R16195661 (ANZ WR).

69 'Doubts Claims of Los Angeles Doctor.'

70 Weaver, *Sorrows of a Century*, 205.

71 See Jacqueline Leckie, 'Infrastructure and "Magic Bullets" in Mental Health in the Colonial Pacific,' *Health and History* 23, no. 2 (2021): 29–50.

72 Reginald W. Medlicott, 'The Place of Electronarcosis in Psychiatric Treatment. A Clinical Assessment Based on the Treatment of Four Hundred Patients,' *NZMJ* 53, no. 294 (1954): 136; Duder, *The Ashburn Clinic*, 46, cites Medlicott's, First Decennial Report, 1957, 4.

73 *Ellesmere Guardian*, 31 October 1941, 5, https://paperspast.natlib.govt.nz/newspapers/EG19411028.2.32.1

74 Medlicott, 'Psychiatric Treatments.' See Edward Shorter and David Healy, *Shock Therapy: A History of Electroconvulsive Treatment in Mental Illness* (New Brunswick, NJ: Rutgers University Press, 2007), 11–21. Schizophrenia was a serious and complex mental disorder. It has undergone several diagnostic shifts and descriptions of causes and symptoms. Contrary to popular discourse, schizophrenia does not mean that a person has a 'split personality'. It is often, but not always, associated with psychosis (delusions, hallucinations) and confusion. Many people diagnosed with schizophrenia also suffer from depression. See, for example, Kieran McNally, *A Critical History of Schizophrenia* (London: Palgrave Macmillan, 2016).

75 'Shock Treatment,' *ES*, 12 April 1938, 16, https://paperspast.natlib.govt.nz/newspapers/ESD19380412.2.143

76 Fennell, 'Psychiatry in New Zealand,' 146; 'New Methods on Trial in New Zealand,' *The Press*, 23 November 1938, 9, https://paperspast.natlib.govt.nz/newspapers/CHP19381123.2.44

77 *AJHR*, 1961 (1962), H 31.

78 Harold Bourne, 'The Insulin Myth,' *The Lancet* 262 (7 November 1953): 964–68.

79 *NEM*, 20 October 1943.

80 Kenneth Stallworthy, 'Melancholia Treated with Cardiazol,' *NZMJ* 42, no. 232 (December 1943): 268.

81 Medlicott, 'Psychiatric Treatments,' 30.

82 Lothar B. Kalinowsky. 'Convulsive Shock Treatment,' in *American Handbook of Psychiatry*, vol. 2, ed. Silvano Arieti (New York: Basic Books, 1959), 1500; 'Mental Hospitals of the Dominion (report on) for 1948,' *AJHR*, 1949, H-07, 13.

83 'Electric Shock Treatments,' *The Press*, 7 June 1944, 2, https://paperspast.natlib.govt.nz/newspapers/CHP19440607.2.22

84 Alexander McKinnon, *Come Back to Mona Vale: Life and Death in a Christchurch Mansion* (Dunedin: Otago University Press, 2021), 238–82.

85 'Mental Hospitals of the Dominion (report on) for 1946,' 9, 12.

86 'Mental Hospitals of the Dominion (report on) for 1945,' 4.

87 Medlicott, 'Psychiatric Treatments.'

88 Interview, Meg and Alistair Campbell.

89 Medlicott, 'Psychiatric Treatments.'

90 Reginald W. Medlicott, 'Convulsive Therapy: Results and Complications in Four Hundred Cases,' *NZMJ* 47 (1948): 340.

91 'Mental Hospitals of the Dominion (report on) for 1948,' *AJHR*, 1949, H-07, 13.

92 Duder, *The Ashburn Clinic*, 35, citing Medlicott's Collected Publications, Dunedin, 1978, n.p. Dr Hart in 'Mental Hospitals of the Dominion (report on) for 1946,' *AJHR*, 1947 Session I, H-07, 9, qualifies Medlicott's claim to say that this was the first time that electronarcosis was applied in the Southern Hemisphere. See Medlicott, 'The Place of Electronarcosis.'

93 Reginald W. Medlicott, 'Brief Stimuli Electroconvulsive Therapy,' *NZMJ* 47 (February 1948): 29–37.

94 Rina Moore, 'Therapeutic Dissociation by Electro-Convulsive Therapy,' *NZMJ* 57, no. 320 (August 1958): 361.

95 Ibid., 363.

96 'Interview with Peter Sanders, 13 July 1989' (by Margaret Whineray), OHInt-0139/1, Psychiatric Nurses Oral History Project (ATL); D. J. Sage, 'Depression (As it Occurs in General Practice)' (PM diss., University of Otago, 1973).

97 Brian Barraclough, *Sunnyside Up* (Auckland: Brian Barraclough, 2017), 10.

98 'Modern Treatments at Sunnyside Hospital.'

99 Jennifer Hamilton, 'Wide Divergence of Opinion About the Treatment,' *The Press*, 25 May 1977, 21, https://paperspast.natlib.govt.nz/newspapers/CHP19770525.2.151

100 'The Treatment,' *The Press*, 24 May 1977, 19, https://paperspast.natlib.govt.nz/newspapers/CHP19770524.2.139

101 Ibid.

102 R. Presland and H. Palmer, 'The Comparative Value of Curarizing Agents with Special Reference to Convulsion Therapy,' *NZMJ* 49, no. 271 (1950): 263.

103 See Jonathan Sadowsky, *Electroconvulsive Therapy in America: The Anatomy of a Medical Controversy* (New York: Routledge, 2016).

104 Sylvie Gambaudo, 'Melancholia in Janet Frame's *Faces in the Water*.' *Literature and Medicine* 30, no. 1 (2012): 47.

105 Frame, *An Angel at My Table*, 252.

106 Interview with Estelle McInnes, 1 July 1993 (by R. MacBeth), OHInt-0067/010, Women in a Mining Town, Waihi 1883–1993, Oral History Project, (ATL).

107 'U.S. Psychiatrist on New Zealand Methods,' *The Press*, 20 January 1958, 10, https://paperspast.natlib.govt.nz/newspapers/CHP19580120.2.116

108 'Interview with Peter Sanders.'

109 'N.Z. Mental Hospitals Defended by Director,' *The Press*, 24 January 1958, 16, https://paperspast.natlib.govt.nz/newspapers/CHP19580124.2.171

110 ABQU 632/139, 'Mental Health — Treatments — Electro-Convulsant Therapy,' box 139, R16648103 (ANZ WR).

111 Ibid. Letter to Minister of Health, 24 October 1985. It is unclear which years she is referring to.

112 'Abuse in Care Royal Commission of Inquiry,' www.abuseincare.org.nz; David Williams, 'Our Terrifying "Treatment" of Mental Illness,' *Newsroom*, 15 August 2022, www.newsroom.co.nz/our-terrifying-treatment-of-mental-illness

113 Interview, Meg and Alistair Campbell.

114 Campbell, 'Arlin,' 145.

115 'The Treatment', *The Press*, 24 May 1977.

116 Medlicott, 'The Place of Electronarcosis,' 134.

117 Guthrie, 'A Study of Twelve Patients,' 13.

118 Ibid.

119 Mental Hospitals of the Dominion (report on) for 1946, 5.

120 *The Timaru Herald*, 29 December 1945, 8, https://paperspast.natlib.govt.nz/newspapers/THD19451229.2.108.2

121 See also the Royal Australian and New Zealand College of Psychiatrists, 'Deep Sleep Therapy,' February 2018, www.ranzcp.org/news-policy/policy-and-advocacy/position-statements/deep-sleep-therapy

122 Graham Mellsop and Michael Radford, *Report of Graham Mellsop and Michael Radford as Sought by the Department of Health on the Use of 'Deep Sleep Therapy'* (Wellington: Department of Health, 1991), 6, www.moh.govt.nz/notebook/nbbooks.nsf/0/D542CD5D4F91E-DEA4C2565D7000DEE5E/$file/REport_deep_sleep-therapy_1991.pdf

123 Fran O'Sullivan, 'Questionable "Medical" Practices not Confined to Overseas Horror Stories,' *NZH*, 4 April 2015.

124 Mellsop and Radford, 'Report,' 10.

125 S. S. Tafuna'i, 'The Efficacy of Modified Narcosis Therapy' (DPM thesis, University of Otago, November 1977). I could not locate this.

126 Mellsop and Radford, 'Report,' 12. These drugs included Valium, Serepax, chlordiazepoxide (Librium), and Halcion.

127 See also Williams, 'Our Terrifying "Treatment"; Confidential Forum for Former In-patients of Psychiatric Hospitals, *Te Āiotanga: Report of the Confidential Forum for Former In-Patients of Psychiatric Hospitals* (Wellington: Department of Internal Affairs, 2007), https://d3n8a8pro7vhmx.cloudfront.net/nzhrc/pages/174/attachments/original/1487714414/Report_of_the_Confidential_Forum_for_Former_In-Patients_of_Psychiatric_Hospitals.pdf?1487714414

128 'Modern Treatments at Sunnyside Hospital.'

129 The brand names (usually in parentheses) are those commonly prescribed in New Zealand.

130 Sage, 'Depression.'

131 Earlier sources for this data include Aubrey, 'Patient Views'; Guthrie, 'A Study of Twelve Patients with Depression'; Herd, 'Assessment of Patients'; Sage, 'Depression.'

132 Aubrey, 'Patient Views'; Sage, 'Depression'; Herd, 'Assessment of Patients.'

133 Sage, 'Depression.'

134 See full details on the Mayo Clinic's website: www.mayoclinic.org/diseas-

es-conditions/depression/in-depth/maois/art-20043992

135 See, for example, Moncrieff et al., 'The Serotonin Theory of Depression: A Systematic Umbrella Review of the Evidence,' *Molecular Psychiatry* (2022), https://doi.org/10.1038/s41380-022-01661-0

136 Sutherland, *Paikea*, 403–4.

137 Ronald Valentine Trubohovich, 'Letter: Tricyclic Antidepressants: Dangers with Overdosage,' *NZMJ* 78, no. 504 (12 December 1973): 502–3.

138 Confidential source.

139 Lang, 'Attempted Suicide by Overdose,' 31.

140 Peter Dunn, 'A Six Month Follow up Study of a Group of Psychiatric Patients' (PM diss., University of Otago, 1968), 6–9; Guthrie, 'A Study of Twelve Patients with Depression,' 18; Judy C. Herd, 'Assessment of Patients and Choice of Tranquillising and Antidepressant Drugs in General Practice' (PM diss., University of Otago, 1969), 41.

141 J. M. Berryman, 'Depressive Illness in Housewives' (PM diss., University of Otago, 1971), 27–28. See also Horton, 'Attempted Suicide.'

142 See J. C. Lopdell, 'Some Psychiatric Responsibilities in General Practice,' *NZMJ* 54, no. 300 (1955): 180–83.

143 See, for example, Wallace Ironside, 'Feelings that Disturb Our Peace of Mind,' *N.Z. Family Doctor*, May 1958, 30–1, 56; K. R. Stallworthy, 'In the Depths of Depression,' *N.Z. Family Doctor*, February 1962, 44–45; Hugh Freeman, 'You Can't Live with Your Nerves,' *N.Z. Family Doctor*, November 1962, 14–16; Hugh Freeman, 'When the Mood Swings Crazily,' *N.Z. Family Doctor*, April 1964, 22–24. Freeman wrote, 'Depression, for instance, is one of the most treatable of illnesses.' Hugh Freeman, 'Time to Consult a Psychiatrist,' *N.Z. Family Doctor*, August 1966, 14–16; 'Kind of "Blue" Feeling,' *N.Z. Family Doctor*, January 1969, 16–17, 40 (post-partum depression); Eva Le Fevre, 'Something On Your Mind,' *N.Z. Family Doctor*, November 1968, 8–10 (neurosis and psychotherapy).

144 J. M. Aubrey, 'Patient Views of Depression in a General Practice' (PM diss., University of Otago, 1973). See also Sage, 'Depression'; Berryman, 'Depressive Illness in Housewives'; Penelope Cook, 'Mental Illness Associated with Childbirth' (PM diss., University of Otago, 1967).

145 Dunn, 'A Six Month Follow up Study,' 61.

146 Confidential information from a person with lived experience of bipolar disorder and several mental health hospitalisations.

Epilogue: Bursting the black cloud?

1 'Our purpose,' Like Minds, Like Mine, www.likeminds.org.nz (accessed 23 August 2010), cited in Warwick Brunton, 'Mental Health Services — Contemporary Issues,' *Te Ara — the Encyclopedia of New Zealand* (2011, revised 2022), 7, www.teara.govt.nz/en/mental-health-services/page-7 (accessed 21 July 2023).

2 Ibid.

3 Ken H. Mason, *Report of the Ministerial Inquiry [In Respect of Certain Mental Health Services] to the Minister of Health Hon Jenny Shipley* (Wellington: Ministry of Health, 1996), 164, www.moh.govt.nz/notebook/nbbooks.nsf/0/70FC4C46F-860CFEE4C2565D70018A26A/%24file/Inquiry%20under%20section%2047%20of%20the%20health%20and%20disability%20services%20act%201993%20in%20respect%20of%20certain%20mental%20

health%20services.pdf

4 https://thenuttersclub.co.nz; Mike King with David Codyre, *The Nutters Club: Helping Nutters from the Inside Out* (Auckland: Random House, 2011). *The Nutters Club* was a long-running series on Newstalk radio, Māori Television and Facebook.

5 Brunton, 'Mental Health Services.'

6 John Kirwan with Margie Thomson, *All Blacks Don't Cry: A Story of Hope* (Auckland: Penguin, 2010), 11.

7 John Kirwan with Elliot Bell, Kirsty Louden-Bell and Margie Thomson, *Stand By Me: Helping Your Teen Through Tough Times* (Auckland: Penguin, 2014).

8 https://jkfoundation.org.nz (accessed 21 July 2023).

9 On research and proposals see, for example, 2014-029-089, Mental Health Foundation of New Zealand, 'Reports of Think Tank Meetings on Depression, Anxiety and Mental Distress Campaign, 2003–2004; Review of Depression Resources and Proposal for the Research and Design of a National Depression Awareness Initiative, November 2004' (ATL). The website is https://mentalhealth.org.nz/about

10 'Media release: Launch of Major New Depression Awareness Campaign "Out of the Blue / Kia Marama",' 23 May 2005 (Auckland: Mental Health Foundation of New Zealand); A. Woodley, *Evaluation of the Out of the Blue / Kia Marama Campaign* (Auckland: Point Research, 2007).

11 Weaver, *Sorrows of a Century*, 19, 254–91.

12 Ibid., 24.

13 Although focused on Māori, Gassin, 'Māori Mental Health,' 103–34, provides an excellent overview of the barriers to accessing mental health services in Aotearoa.

14 See Nicky Pellegrino, 'High Anxiety,' *New Zealand Listener*, 12–19 December 2020: 16–19.

15 T. P. Oei and L. M. Sullivan, 'Cognitive Changes Following Recovery from Depression in a Group Cognitive-Behaviour Therapy Program,' *ANZJP* 33, no. 3 (1999): 407–15. See also Simon T. Bennett et al., 'Considerations for Culturally Responsive Cognitive-Behavioural Therapy for Māori With Depression,' *Journal of Pacific Rim Psychology* 10 (2016): article e8, doi:10.1017/prp.2016.5

16 See Pamela Melding, 'Electroconvulsive Therapy in New Zealand: Terrifying or Electrifying?' *NZMJ* (Online) 119, no. 1237 (2006): U2051.

17 Ken H. Mason, *Report of the Committee of Inquiry into Procedures Used in Certain Psychiatric Hospitals in Relation to Admission, Discharge or Release on Leave of Certain Classes of Patients* (Wellington: Department of Health, 1988), www.moh.govt.nz/NoteBook/nbbooks.nsf/0/2DC94A246D93272C-4C2565D7000DDA26/%24file/Mason%20Report.pdf; Mason, Report of the Ministerial Inquiry (1996), www.moh.govt.nz/notebook/nbbooks.nsf/0/70FC4C46F860CFEE4C-2565D70018A26A/%24file/Inquiry%20under%20section%2047%20of%20the%20health%20and%20disability%20services%20act%201993%20in%20respect%20of%20certain%20mental%20health%20-services.pdf

18 Mental Health Commission, *Te Haererenga mo te Whakaòranga 1996–2006: The Journey of Recovery for the New Zealand Mental Health Sector* (Wellington: Mental Health Commission, 2007), 4–6, www.moh.govt.nz/notebook/nbbooks.nsf/0/12912EA93B-0B85EFCC2573C90068845D/$file/

te_haererenga%20%201996-2006.pdf

19 *Te Āiotanga: Report of the Confidential Forum for Former In-Patients of Psychiatric Hospitals* (Wellington: Department of Internal Affairs, 2007), https://d3n8a8pro7vhmx.cloudfront.net/nzhrc/pages/174/attachments/original/1487714414/Report_of_the_Confidential_Forum_for_Former_In-Patients_of_Psychiatric_Hospitals.pdf?1487714414

20 Oakley Browne et al., *Te Rau Hinengaro*; Te Whatu Ora Health New Zealand, 'Our Surveys,' www.hpa.org.nz/our-work/research/our-surveys

21 Ron Paterson et al., *He Ara Oranga. Report of the Government Inquiry into Mental Health and Addiction* (Wellington: Department of Internal Affairs, 2018), 11, https://mentalhealth.inquiry.govt.nz/inquiry-report/he-ara-oranga

22 New Zealand Mental Health and Wellbeing Commission, *Te Huringa: Change and Transformation. Mental Health Service and Addiction Service Monitoring* (Wellington: New Zealand Mental Health and Wellbeing Commission, 2022), www.mhwc.govt.nz/assets/Te-Huringa/FINAL-MHWC-Te-Huringa-Service-Monitoring-Report.pdf. See also Manatū Hauora Ministry of Health, *Kia Manawanui Aotearoa: Long-term Pathway to Mental Wellbeing* (Wellington: Ministry of Health; 2021).

23 Manatū Hauora Ministry of Health. *Te Puāwaitanga: Māori Mental Health National Strategic Framework* (Wellington: Ministry of Health, 2002), www.health.govt.nz/system/files/documents/publications/maorimentalhealthnationalstrategicframework.pdf

24 Mental Health Commission, *Blueprint II: Improving Mental Health and Wellbeing for All New Zealanders* (Wellington: Mental Health Commission, 2012), www.hdc.org.nz/media/1075/blueprint-ii-how-things-need-to-be.pdf

25 Gassin, *Māori Mental Health*, 167.

26 Wirihana et al., 'Māori Indigenous Healing Practices in Aotearoa (New Zealand)', 536–37.

27 Wikaire et al., *Nōku te Ao*.

28 Pounamu Jade Aikman, *Ka mua, ka muri: Nōku te Ao Like Minds Whakapapa and Procurement Approaches* (Wellington: Te Whatu Ora, 2022), 9, www.hpa.org.nz/our-work/research/publications

29 Wikaire et al., *Nōku te Ao*, 48.

30 2014-029-089, Kathryn Nemec, 'Review of Depression Resources, Report for the Mental Health Foundation', 21 August 2006 (ATL).

31 Susan Tutty, and Felicity Goodyear-Smith, 'Eighteen Months of Depression: Examining the Chronic Care Management of Depression with Particular Reference to Pacific People,' *Journal of Primary Health Care* 6, (2014): 31–39. Reasons for these cultural differences were not evident.

32 Joanne Baxter et al., for the New Zealand Mental Health Survey Research Team, 'Ethnic Comparisons of the 12 Month Prevalence of Mental Disorders and Treatment Contact in Te Rau Hinengaro: The New Zealand Mental Health Survey,' *ANZJP* 4010 (2006): 905–13. See also Phillipa Gaines et al., *New Zealand Mental Health Classification and Outcomes Study: Final Report* (Auckland: Health Research Council of New Zealand, 2003), www.moh.govt.nz/notebook/nbbooks.nsf/0/0384022B008C9AD5C-C256FBA0003906F/$file/mental%20health%20classification%20outcomes%20study.pdf

33 See, for example, McDaid et al., 'Antenatal Depression Symptoms in Pacific Women: Evidence from Growing Up in New Zealand,' *Journal of Primary Health Care* 11, no. 2 (2019): 96–108.

34 Ataera-Minster and Trowland, *Te Kaveinga.*

35 Le Va's website has translated the depression factsheet into Samoan and Tongan.

36 See Karlo Mila-Schaaf, 'Not Another New Zealand-Born Identity Crisis: Well-Being and the Politics of Belonging,' in *Pacific Identities and Well-being: Cross-cultural Perspectives,* eds Margaret Nelson Agee, Tracey McIntosh, Philip Culbertson and Cabrini 'Ofa Makasiale (New York, London: Routledge, 2013), 27–45.

37 Statement No: Witn0452001 Exhibits: Witn0452002 Dated:18.05.2021, Royal Commission of Inquiry into Abuse in Care.

38 2014-029-089, 21 August 2006, 'Review of Depression Resources' (ATL).

39 Sally F. Wong, *Asian Public Health in Aotearoa New Zealand* (Auckland: The Asian Network, 2021), 3–4.

40 Elsie Seckyee Ho, 'Mental Health of Asian Immigrants in New Zealand: A Review of Key Issues,' *Asian and Pacific Migration Journal* 13, no. 1 (March 2004): 39–60.

41 For example, Max Abbott et al., 'Depression in Older Chinese Migrants to Auckland,' *ANZJP* 37, no. 4, (2003): 445–51.

42 Confidential source.

43 See: Jacqueline Leckie, *Invisible: New Zealand's History of Excluding Kiwi-Indians* (Auckland: Massey University Press, 2021); Angela McCarthy, ed., *Narratives of Migrant and Refugee Discrimination in Aotearoa New Zealand* (London: Routledge, 2022).

44 Although, see Te Pou (Mental Health Programmes Limited), *Talking Therapies for Asian People: Best and Promising Practice Guide for Mental Health and Addiction Services* (Auckland: Te Pou o te Whakaaro Nui, 2010), www.tepou.co.nz/resources/talking-therapies-for-asian-people

45 Stats NZ, '2018 Census Ethnic Groups Dataset,' (June 2020), www.stats.govt.nz/information-releases/2018-census-ethnic-groups-dataset; Stats NZ, 'Population Projected to Become More Ethnically Diverse,' (28 May 2021), www.stats.govt.nz/news/population- projected-to-be-come-more-ethnically-diverse

46 Andrew Zhu, *New Zealand Asian Mental Health and Wellbeing Report 2020: A Snapshot Survey* (Auckland: Asian Family Services, 2020), www.asianfamilyservices.nz/resources/resource-items/nz-asian-mental-health-wellbeing-report-2020; Rex Liao, 'In the Shadow of Exclusion: The State of New Zealand Asian Health,' *New Zealand Medical Student Journal* 29 (2019): 32–36.

47 For example, Asian Family Services, www.asianfamilyservices.nz, offers a helpline in Mandarin, Cantonese, Korean, Vietnamese, Thai, Japanese, Hindi and English, with more specialised services. It was established in 1998 to address problem gambling, and then included mental health issues. Asian Mental Health Service caters to people in Waitematā, (asianhealthservices.co.nz), and some other regions offer similar services. Several ethnic associations now have support groups for older members, such as Shanti Niwas (www.shantiniwas.org.nz). Gender and sexuality issues that may be associated with depression and suicide are also addressed through non-governmental

organisations; for example, Shakti (for Asian, African and Middle Eastern women, children and youth; https://shaktiinternational.org/shakati-new-zealand) and Indian Origin Pride New Zealand (https://iopnz.org).

48 Lee et al., 'Ethnic Inequality in Diagnosis with Depression and Anxiety Disorders.'

49 Videos and blogs are available at www.tepapa.govt.nz/discover-collections/read-watch-play/asian-mental-health. The zine can be downloaded at www.tepapa.govt.nz/sites/default/files/asian-mental-health-zine.pdf

50 Mehwish Mughal, 'Why Asian Mental Health Matters in Aotearoa,' 28 September 2022, https://blog.tepapa.govt.nz/2022/09/28/why-asian-mental-health-matters-in-aotearoa

51 Te Pou offers several resources, working alongside mental health and addiction services, and disability organisations.

52 For example, 'A Solution to Declining Mental Health in Teens?' *RNZ*, 5 April 2023. Interview with Zach Rausch by Jesse Mulligan.

53 Earlier research that identified depression among Indo-Chinese refugees in Aotearoa included: Max Abbot, 'Refugees and Immigrants,' in *Mental Health in New Zealand from a Public Health Perspective*, eds Pete M. Ellis and Sunny C. D. Collings (Wellington: Ministry of Health, 1997), 250–64; Peter Cheung, 'Somatisation as a Presentation in Depression and Post-Traumatic Stress Disorder Among Cambodian Refugees,' *ANZJP* 27 (1993): 422–28; Hean Tan, 'Indo-Chinese Refugees' Well-Being from the Sponsors' Perspective' (MA thesis, University of Auckland, 1995); Ho, 'Mental Health of Asian Immigrants in New Zealand,' 44–50.

54 'Cultural Safety in Our Mental Health System is a Collective Responsibility,' interview of Maria Milmine by Grace Gassin, 16 March 2023, https://blog.tepapa.govt.nz/2023/03/16/cultural-safety-in-our-mental-health-system-is-a-collective-responsibility

Bibliography

Newspapers and other media sources

Most newspapers below are available online covering limited periods at Papers Past, National Library of New Zealand Te Puna Mātauranga o Aotearoa, https://paperspast.natlib.govt.nz/newspapers

Ashburton Guardian
Auckland Star
Bruce Herald
Canterbury Times
The Colonist
Daily Southern Cross
The Dominion (now *The Post*)
Ellesmere Guardian
Evening Post
Evening Star
Gisborne Herald
Gisborne Times
Grey River Argus
Horowhenua Chronicle
Lyttelton Times
Manawatu Standard (now *Manawatū Standard*)
Marlborough Press
Nelson Evening Mail
Nelson Examiner and New Zealand Chronicle
Nelson Mail
Newshub
New Zealand Herald
New Zealand Times
NZ Truth
Otago Daily Times
Otago Witness
Poverty Bay Herald
The Press (Christchurch)
Progress
Radio New Zealand (*RNZ*)
Southland Times
Stuff
The Sun (Auckland)
Temuka Leader
Thames Guardian and Mining Record
Timaru Herald
Waikato Independent
Waikato Times
Wairarapa Daily Times
Wanganui Chronicle (now *Whanganui Chronicle*)
West Coast Times
Western Star

Publications

Abbot, Max. 'Refugees and Immigrants.' In *Mental Health in New Zealand from a Public Health Perspective*, edited by Pete M. Ellis and Sunny C. D. Collings, 250–64. Wellington: Ministry of Health, 1997.

Abbott, Max W., Sai Wong, Lynne C. Giles, Sue Wong, Wilson Young, and Ming Au. 'Depression in Older Chinese Migrants to Auckland.' *Australian and New Zealand Journal of Psychiatry* 37, no. 4 (2003): 445–51.

Abrahams, Athol Maurice. 'Quackery: Or a Study of Unorthodox Medical Practitioners in Auckland.' PM diss., University of Otago, 1955.

Agnew, Francis, Fuimaono Karl Pulotu-Endemann, Gail Robinson, and Helen Schmidt-Sopoaga. 'Pacific Models of Mental Health Service Delivery in New Zealand ("PMMHSD") Project.' Auckland: Health Research Council of New Zealand, 2004. www.leva.co.nz/uploads/files/resources/Pacific-Models-of-Mental-Health-Service-Delivery-in-New-Zealand-PMMHSD-Project.pdf

Agnew, Jenny, and Trevor Agnew. *Merchant, Miner, Mandarin: The Life and Times of the Remarkable Choie Sew Hoy*. Christchurch: Canterbury University Press, 2020.

Aiken, M. H. 'Psychoneuroses in the Second New Zealand Expeditionary Force.' *The New Zealand Medical Journal* 40, no. 220 (December 1941): 345–58.

Aiken, M. H. 'Psychiatric Casualties among New Zealand Troops in Italy.' *The New Zealand Medical Journal* 45 (June 1946): 155–69.

Aikman, Pounamu Jade. *Ka mua, ka muri: Nōku te Ao Like Minds' Whakapapa and Procurement Approaches*. Wellington: Te Whatu Ora, 2022. www.hpa.org.nz/our-work/research/publications

Allen, I. M. 'Neurasthenia with Depression.' *The New Zealand Medical Journal* 13 (1933): 122–33.

Andreasen, Nancy C. *The Broken Brain: The Biological Revolution in Psychiatry*. New York: Harper and Row, 1984.

Appendix to the Journal of the House of Representatives, 1858–1961. (Until 1950, available at https://paperspast.natlib.govt.nz/parliamentary/appendix-to-the-journals-of-the-house-of-representatives)

Arroll, Bruce, Felicity Goodyear-Smith, Ngaire Kerse, Melanie Hwang, Susan Crengle, Jane Gunn, Tana Fishman, Simon Hatcher, Sanat Pradhan, and Karishma Sidhu. 'The Prevalence of Depression Among Maori Patients in Auckland General Practice.' *Journal of Primary Health Care* 1, no. 1 (March 2009): 26–29.

Ataera-Minster, Joanna, and Holly Trowland. *Te Kaveinga — Mental Health and Wellbeing of Pacific Peoples*. Wellington: Health Promotion Agency, 2018. www.hpa.org.nz/research-library/research-publications/te-kaveinga-mental-health-and-wellbeing-of-pacific-peoples

Attah, Felix Y. 'Depressive Disorders: Diagnosis, Recognition and Management of Depressive Disorders in General Medical Practice in the Pacific.' *Fiji General Practitioner* 5, no. 1 (1998): 300–5.

Aubrey, J. M. 'Patient Views of Depression in a General Practice.' PM diss., University of Otago, 1973.

Babington, Anthony. *Shell Shock: A History of the Changing Attitudes to War Neurosis.* London: Leo Cooper, 1997.

Baddeley, Josephine. 'Traditional Healing Practices.' In *Healing Practices in the South Pacific*, edited by Claire D. F. Parsons, 129–43. Laie, Hawai'i: Institute for Polynesian Studies, Brigham Young University, 1985.

Barraclough, Brian. *Sunnyside Up.* Auckland: Brian Barraclough, 2017.

Barry, Lorelle, and Catharine Coleborne. 'Insanity and Ethnicity in New Zealand: Māori Encounters with the Auckland Mental Hospital, 1860–1900.' *History of Psychiatry*, 22, no. 3 (2011): 285–301.

Baxter, Joanne, Jesse Kokaua, Elisabeth Wells, Magnus A. McGee, and Mark A. Oakley Browne, for the New Zealand Mental Health Survey Research Team. 'Ethnic Comparisons of the 12 Month Prevalence of Mental Disorders and Treatment Contact in Te Rau Hinengaro: The New Zealand Mental Health Survey.' *Australian and New Zealand Journal of Psychiatry* 40, no. 10 (2006): 905–13.

Beaglehole, Ann. *Refuge New Zealand: A Nation's Response to Refugees and Asylum Seekers.* Dunedin: Otago University Press, 2013.

Beaglehole, Ernest. 'Some Sociological Aspects of Race Relations in New Zealand.' *International Social Science Bulletin* 3, no. 2 (1951): 253–58.

Beautrais, Annette L. 'Farm Suicides in New Zealand, 2007–2015: A Review of Coroners' Records.' *Australian and New Zealand Journal of Psychiatry* 52, no. 1 (2017): 78–86.

Bell, Matthew. *Melancholia: The Western Malady.* Cambridge: Cambridge University Press, 2014.

Bennett, Simon T., Ross A Flett, and Duncan R Babbage. 'Considerations for Culturally Responsive Cognitive-Behavioural Therapy for Māori With Depression.' *Journal of Pacific Rim Psychology* 10 (2016): article e8. https://doi:10.1017/prp.2016.5

Berrios, German E. 'Mood Disorders: Clinical Section.' In *A History of Clinical Psychiatry: The Origin and History of Psychiatric Disorders*, edited by German E. Berrios and Roy Porter, 384–408. New York: New York University Press, 1995.

Berrios, German E. *The History of Mental Symptoms: Descriptive Psychopathology Since the Nineteenth Century.* Cambridge: Cambridge University Press, 1996.

Berryman, J. M. 'Depressive Illness in Housewives.' PM diss., University of Otago, 1971.

Besnier, Niko. 'Humour and Humility: Narratives of Modernity on Nukulaelae Atoll.' *Etnofoor* 28, no. 1 (2016): 75–95.

Betz, Elisabeth, and Toon van Meijl. 'Humour in the Negotiations of Social Identity in the Tongan Diaspora.' *Etnofoor* 28, no. 1 (2016): 111–25.

Bezo, Brent, and Stefania Maggi. 'Intergenerational Perceptions of Mass Trauma's Impact on Physical Health and Well-Being.' *Psychological Trauma: Theory, Research, Practice, and Policy* 10, no. 1 (2018): 87–94.

Bilton, Margaret. 'Some of My Experiences in Backblocks Nursing.' *Kai Tiaki: The Journal of the Nurses of New Zealand* 6, no. 1 (1 January 1913): 9.

Blake-Palmer, Geoffrey. 'Beliefs and Practices of the Present Day Maori.' *The Journal of the Polynesian Society* 63, no. 2 (June 1954): 147–63.

Blazer, Dan G. *The Age of Melancholy: Major Depression and Its Social Origins.* New York: Routledge, 2005.

Boston, Peter. 'The Bacillus of Work: Masculinity and the Rehabilitation of Disabled Soldiers in Dunedin 1919 to 1939.' BA Hons long essay, University of Otago, 1993. http://hdl.handle.net/10523/2747

Bourne, Harold. 'The Insulin Myth.' *The Lancet* 262 (7 November 1953): 964–68.

Brasted, E. P. 'The Female Division of a Mental Hospital: Porirua Mental Hospital, Wellington.' PM diss., University of Otago, 1945.

Brookes, Barbara. 'Mental Health Records: Who Controls the Past?' *Archifacts* (April 2015): 8–16.

Brookes, Barbara. 'Pictures of People, Pictures of Places: Photography and the Asylum.' In *Exhibiting Madness in Museums: Remembering Psychiatry through Collections and Display*, edited by Catharine Coleborne and Dolly MacKinnon, 40–57. New York, London: Routledge, 2011.

Brookes, Barbara. 'Women and Madness: A Case-study of the Seacliff Asylum, 1890–1920.' In *Women in History 2: Essays on Women in New Zealand*, edited by Barbara Brookes, Charlotte Macdonald and Margaret Tennant, 129–47. Wellington: Bridget Williams Books, 1992.

Brookes, Barbara, and Jane Thomson, eds. *'Unfortunate Folk': Essays on Mental Health Treatment 1863–1992.* Dunedin: Otago University Press, 2001.

Brown, Christopher R., and Jimmy Obed. 'The State of Psychology and Mental Health Services in Vanuatu.' In *Psychology in Oceania and the Caribbean*, edited by Grant J. Rich and Neeta A. Ramkumar, 33–44. Cham: Springer International, 2022.

Brunton, Warwick. 'Mental Health Services.' *Te Ara — the Encyclopedia of New Zealand* (2011, revised 2022), https://teara.govt.nz/en/mental-health-services

Brunton, Warwick. 'The Origins of Deinstitutionalisation in New Zealand.' *Health and History* 5, no.2 (2003): 75–103.

Brunton, Warwick. 'A Choice of Difficulties: National Mental Health Policy in New Zealand, 1840–1947.' PhD thesis, University of Otago, 2001. http://hdl.handle.net/10523/383

Buck, P. H. (Te Rangi Hīroa). 'Medicine Amongst the Maoris in Ancient and Modern Times.' MD thesis, University of New Zealand, 1910. http://hdl.handle.net/10523/10413.

Buckfield, Patricia M. 'Therapeutic Forces in a Mental Hospital: A Survey of the Therapeutic Forces at Work on the Female Side of the Seacliff Mental Hospital.' PM diss., University of Otago, 1957.

Burke, Lorelle. '"The Voices Caused Him to Become Porangi": Maori Patients in the Auckland Lunatic Asylum, 1860–1900.' MA thesis, University of Waikato, 2006. https://hdl.handle.net/10289/12621

Burns, Charles, and W. Ironside, 'Obituary: Kathleen Mary Todd.' *The New Zealand Medical Journal* 68 (1968): 191–93.

Burrell, R. H. 'Depression Associated with Resperine Therapy.' *The New Zealand Medical Journal* 55, no. 307 (1956): 228–31.

Burton-Bradley, B. G. *Stone Age Crisis: A Psychiatric Appraisal.* Nashville, Tennessee: Vanderbilt University Press, 1975.

Campbell, Alistair. *Island to Island.* Christchurch: Whitcoulls, 1984.

Campbell, Alistair. *Mine Eyes Dazzle: Poems 1947–9.* Christchurch: Pegasus Press, 1950.

Campbell, Alistair. *Sanctuary of Spirits.* Wellington: Wai-Te-Ata Press, 1963.

Campbell, Alistair. *The Frigate Bird.* Auckland: Heinemann Reed, 1989.

Campbell, Alistair, and Meg Campbell, *It's Love, Isn't It? The Love Poems.* Wellington: HeadworX, 2008.

Campbell, Meg. *The Way Back: Poems.* Pukerua Bay: Te Kotare Press, 1981.

Campion, Edith. *A Place to Pass Through and Other Stories.* Wellington: Reed, 1977.

Capell, Arthur. *The Fijian Dictionary.* Suva: Government Printers, 1941.

Carlton, V. J. 'A Study of Postpartum Psychosis and Depression.' PM diss., University of Otago, 1974.

Catton, Eleanor. *The Luminaries.* Wellington: Victoria University Press, 2013.

Challis, Derek, and Gloria Rawlinson. *The Book of Iris: A Life of Robin Hyde.* Auckland: Auckland University Press, 2002.

Cheung, Peter. 'Somatisation as a Presentation in Depression and Post-Traumatic Stress Disorder Among Cambodian Refugees.' *Australian and New Zealand Journal of Psychiatry* 27 (1993): 422–28.

Chisholm, P., and S. D. Rhind. 'Some Aspects of Post-war Psycho-Neuroses, and Their Treatment at the Queen Mary Hospital, Hanmer Springs.' *The New Zealand Medical Journal* 19 (1920): 222–29.

Christie, Kerrin M. 'A First Assessment of the Costs and Benefits Associated with Drug Usage in New Zealand Mental Hospitals.' Wellington: Contract Research Unit, New Zealand Institute of Economic Research, 1968.

Churchward, Clerk Maxwell. *Tongan Dictionary: Tongan–English and English–Tongan.* Nuku'alofa: Government of Tonga, 1959.

Clarke, Russell. 'Not Mad, But Very Ill: The Treatment of New Zealand's Shell Shocked Soldiers 1914 to 1939.' MA thesis, University of Auckland, 1991.

Clarke, Stephen. *After the War: The RSA in New Zealand.* Auckland: Penguin Random House, 2016.

Clement, Dorothy C. 'Samoan Folk Knowledge of Mental Disorders.' In *Cultural Conceptions of Mental Health and Therapy*, edited by Anthony J. Marsella and Geoffrey M. White, 193–213. Dordecht: D. Reidel Publishing, 1974.

Clouston, A. G. 'War Neuroses and the General Medical Practitioner.' *The New Zealand Medical Journal* 41, no. 221 (1942): 6–13.

Cochran, Vita, Jill Trevelyan, and Rita Angus. *Rita Angus: Live to Paint & Paint to Live.* Auckland: Random House in association with City Gallery Wellington and Hocken Library, Dunedin, 2001.

Coleborne, Catharine. *Insanity, Identity and Empire: Immigrants and Institutional Confinement in Australia and New Zealand, 1873–1910.* Manchester: Manchester University Press, 2015.

Coleborne, Catharine. 'Locating Ethnicity in the Hospitals for the Insane: Revisiting Case Books as Sites of Knowledge Production about Colonial identities in Victoria, Australia, 1873–1910.' In *Migration, Ethnicity, and Mental Health: International Perspectives, 1840–2010*, edited by Angela McCarthy and Catharine Coleborne, 73–90. New York and Abingdon: Routledge, 2012.

Coleborne, Catharine. *Madness in the Family: Insanity and Institutions in the Australasian Colonial World, 1860–1914*. Houndsmills: Palgrave Macmillan, 2010.

Confidential Forum for Former In-patients of Psychiatric Hospitals. *Te Āiotanga: Report of the Confidential Forum for Former In-patients of Psychiatric Hospitals*. Wellington: Department of Internal Affairs, 2007.

Cook, Penelope. 'Mental Illness Associated with Childbirth.' PM diss., University of Otago, 1967.

Cook, Peter S. 'The Early History of the New Zealand Association of Psychotherapists and the Related Movement for Primary Prevention in Mental Health: Some Recollections.' *Australian and New Zealand Journal of Psychiatry* 30, no. 3 (June 1996): 405–9.

Cooper, Frederick, and Ann Laura Stoler. 'Introduction. Tensions of Empire: Colonial Control and Visions of Rule.' *American Ethnologist* 16 (1989): 609–21.

Cooper R. 'Unrecognized Losses in Child Adoption.' In *Disenfranchised Grief: New Directions, Challenges, and Strategies for Practice*, edited by K. J. Doka, 265–74. Champaign: Research Press, 2002.

Coupe, Nicole. 'Whakamomori: Māori Suicide Prevention.' PhD thesis, Massey University, 2005. http://hdl.handle.net/10179/1695

Courage, James. *Diaries*, edited by Chris Brickell. Dunedin: Otago University Press, 2021.

Cowling, Wendy E. 'Eclectic Elements in Tongan Folk Belief and Healing Practice.' In *Tongan Culture and History*, edited by Phyllis Herda, Jennifer Terrell and Niel Gunson, 72–92. Canberra: Department of Pacific and South Asian History, Australian National University, 1990.

Culpin, Millais. *Recent Advances in the Study of the Psychoneuroses*. London: J. & A. Churchill, 1931.

Davy, Daniel. *Gold Rush Societies and Migrant Networks in the Tasman World*. Edinburgh: Edinburgh University Press, 2021.

Dawson, Maree. 'National Fitness or Failure? Heredity, Vice and Racial Decline in New Zealand Psychiatry: A Case Study of the Auckland Mental Hospital, 1868–99.' PhD thesis, University of Waikato, 2013. https://hdl.handle.net/10289/7521

Dean Jr., Eric T. *Shook Over Hell: Post-Traumatic Stress, Vietnam, and the Civil War*. Cambridge, Massachusetts: Harvard University Press, 1999.

de Jong, Eleanor. 'Kind of Blue.' *New Zealand Listener*, 10–16 July 2021, 16–25.

Dodson, Marsa. 'Practising *Tamariki 'Āngai*: Mangaia's Informal Island Adoption.' PhD thesis, University of Otago, 2009. http://hdl.handle.net/10523/4084

Dow, Derek A. '"Pruned of Its Dangers": The Tohunga Suppression Act 1907.' *Health and History* 3, no. 1 (2001): 41–64.

Duder, Cameron. *The Ashburn Clinic: The Place and the People*. Dunedin: Ashburn Clinic, 2007.

Duff, Alan. *Once Were Warriors*. Auckland: Tandem Press, 1990.

Duke, Kate. 'A Century of CAM in New Zealand: A Struggle for Recognition.' *Complementary Therapies in Clinical Practice* 11, no. 1 (2005): 11–16.

Dunn, Peter. 'A Six Month Follow up Study of a Group of Psychiatric Patients.' PM diss., University of Otago, 1968.

Durie, Mason. 'Mauri Ora Practice and Mauri Ora Practitioners.' In *Maea Te Toi Ora: Māori Health Transformations*, edited by Te Kani Kingi, Mason Durie, Hinemoa Elder, Rees Tapsell, Mark Lawrence and Simon Bennett, 91–99. Wellington: Huia, 2018.

Durie, Mason. *Mauri Ora: The Dynamics of Māori Health*. Auckland: Oxford University Press, 2001.

Durie, Mason. 'Mental Health and Maori Development.' *Australian and New Zealand Journal of Psychiatry* 33 (1999): 5–12.

Durie, Mason. 'Mental Health Patterns for the New Zealand Maori.' In *Te Aro Kawa Whakaruruhau: Cultural Safety in Health*, 53–67. Auckland: Mental Health Foundation of New Zealand, 1998.

Edington, Claire E. *Beyond the Asylum: Mental Illness in French Colonial Vietnam*. Ithaca, New York: Cornell University Press, 2019.

Editorial. 'Wartime Psychiatric Problems in New Zealand.' *The New Zealand Medical Journal* 41, no. 221 (1942): 1–5.

Edmond-Paul, Mary, ed. *Your Unselfish Kindness: Robin Hyde's Autobiographical Writings*. Dunedin: Otago University Press, 2011.

Edmonds, L. K., S. Williams, and A. E. Walsh. 'Trends in Maori Mental Health in Otago.' *Australian and New Zealand Journal of Psychiatry* 34, no. 4 (2000): 677–83.

Ehrenberg, Alain. *The Weariness of the Self: Diagnosing the History of Depression in the Contemporary Age*. Chicago, Illinois: McGill Queen's University Press, 2009.

Eldred-Grigg, Stevan. *Diggers, Hatters and Whores: The Story of the New Zealand Gold Rushes*. Auckland: Random House, 2008.

Espiner, Eric Arnold. 'Mental Illness Following Childbirth.' PM diss., University of Otago, 1956.

Fairburn, Miles. *The Ideal Society and Its Enemies: The Foundations of Modern New Zealand Society, 1850–1900*. Auckland: Auckland University Press, 1989.

Fairburn, Miles. 'Wakefield, Edward Gibbon.' *Dictionary of New Zealand Biography, Te Ara — the Encyclopedia of New Zealand* (1990), https://teara.govt.nz/en/biographies/1w4/wakefield-edward-gibbon

Fennell, Susan. 'Psychiatry in New Zealand 1912–1948.' In *'Unfortunate Folk': Essays on Mental Health Treatment 1863–1992*, edited by Barbara Brookes and Jane Thomson, 137–52. Dunedin: Otago University Press, 2001.

Foliaki, Siale, Jesse Kokaua, David Schaaf, and Colin Tukuitonga. 'Pacific People.' In *Te Rau Hinengaro: The New Zealand Mental Health Survey*, edited by M. A. Oakley Browne, J. E. Wells and K. M. Scott, 178–208. Wellington: Ministry of Health, 2006. www.health.govt.nz/system/files/documents/publications/mental-health-survey-2006-pacific-people.pdf

Foliaki, Siale A., Jesse Kokaua, David Schaaf, and Colin Tukuitonga. 'Twelve-Month and Lifetime Prevalences of Mental Disorders and Treatment Contact Among Pacific People in Te Rau Hinengaro: The New Zealand Mental Health Survey.' *Australian and New Zealand Journal of Psychiatry* 40, no. 10 (2006): 924–34.

Fortune, Gabrielle A. 'Hugh Coolahan and the Prosperous Irish: Auckland, 1840–1870.' MA thesis, University of Auckland, 1997.

Foster, Frank Harty. *Maori Patients in Mental Hospitals.* Special Report no. 8. Medical Statistics Branch, Department of Health. Wellington: Government Printer, 1962.

Foulkes, Lucy. *Losing Our Minds, What Mental Illness Really Is — and What It Isn't.* London: The Bodley House, 2021.

Fowler, Conan. 'A Study of Depression in Middle-aged Housewives.' PM diss., University of Otago, 1972.

Fox, Alistair. *Jane Campion: Authorship and Personal Cinema.* Bloomington, Indiana: Indiana University Press, 2011.

Fox, Alistair. *The Ship of Dreams: Masculinity in Contemporary New Zealand Fiction.* Dunedin: Otago University Press, 2008.

Frame, Janet. *An Angel at My Table.* London: Virago, 2010.

Frame, Janet. *Faces in the Water.* Christchurch: Pegasus, 1961.

Frame, Janet. *Scented Gardens for the Blind.* Christchurch: Pegasus, 1963.

Freeman, Hugh. 'Kind of "Blue" Feeling.' *N.Z. Family Doctor* (January 1969): 16–17, 40.

Freeman, Hugh. 'Time to Consult a Psychiatrist.' *N.Z. Family Doctor* (August 1966): 14–16.

Gaines, Phillipa, Alison Bower, Bill Buckingham, Kathy Eagar, Philip Burgess, and Janette Green. *New Zealand Mental Health Classification and Outcomes Study: Final Report.* Auckland: Health Research Council of New Zealand, 2003, www.moh.govt.nz/notebook/nbbooks.nsf/0/0384022B008C9AD5CC256FBA0003906F/$file/mental%20health%20classification%20outcomes%20study.pdf

Gambaudo, Sylvie. 'Melancholia in Janet Frame's *Faces in the Water.' Literature and Medicine* 30, no. 1 (2012): 42–60. www.doi.org/10.1353/lm.2012.0008

Gassin, Timothy. *Māori Mental Health: A Report Commissioned by the Waitangi Tribunal for the Wai 2575 Health Services and Outcomes Kaupapa Inquiry.* Wellington: Waitangi Tribunal, 2019, https://forms.justice.govt.nz/search/Documents/WT/wt_DOC_153087514/Wai%202575%2C%20B026.pdf

Giesen, E. W. 'Discussion of Neurasthenia.' *The New Zealand Medical Journal* 16, no. 74 (1917): 135–42.

Gluckman, Laurie Kalman. 'Drau Ni Kau: The Ethnopsychiatry of Fiji in Historical and Clinical Perspective.' *Australian and New Zealand Journal of Psychiatry* 3 (1969): 152–58.

Gluckman, Laurie Kalman. 'Makutu: A Study in the Ethnopsychiatry of The Maori, Past and Present.' MD diss., University of Otago, 1962.

Gluckman, Laurie Kalman. *Tangiwai: Medical History of New Zealand Prior to 1860.* Auckland: L. Gluckman, 1976.

Gluckman, Laurie Kalman. 'The Staff of Asklepios: A Theory of Origin Supported by Clinical Ethnopsychiatry.' *The New Zealand Medical Journal* 65, no. 402 (1966): 111–18.

Goldie, W. H. *Maori Medical Lore: Notes on the Causes of Disease and Treatment of the Sick among the Maori People of New Zealand*, reprinted from *Transactions of the New Zealand Institute*, 1904. Nelson: Southern Reprints, 1998.

Goodyear-Smith, Felicity, Bruce Arroll, Nicole Coupe, and Stephen Buetow. 'Ethnic Differences in Mental Health and Lifestyle Issues: Results from Multi-Item General Practice Screening.' *The New Zealand Medical Journal* 118, no. 1212 (2005): U1374.

Greenberg, Gary. *Manufacturing Depression: The Secret History of a Modern Disease.* New York: Simon & Schuster, 2011.

Guthrie, J. J. 'A Study of Twelve Patients with Depression.' PM diss., University of Otago, 1973.

Haami, Bradford. *Dr. Golan Maaka: Māori Doctor.* Auckland: Tandem Press, 1995.

Hastings, David. *Over the Mountains of the Sea: Life on the Migrant Ships 1870–1885.* Auckland: Auckland University Press, 2013.

Hazlewood, David. *A Fijian and English and an English and Fijian Dictionary: With Examples of Common and Peculiar Modes of Expression and Uses of Words, also, Containing Brief Hints on Native Customs, Proverbs, the Native Names of Natural Productions, and Notices of the Islands of Fiji, and a Grammar of the Language, with Examples of Native Idioms*, edited by James Calvert. London: S. Low, Marston, 1872.

Healy, David. *The Anti-depressant Era.* London: Harvard University Press, 1997.

Hefford, Edward F. C. 'War Neurosis. An Aspect of Psychological Medicine and its Relation to the Maintenance of Health.' PM diss., University of Otago, and for Director General, Medical Services, 1946.

Henare, Manuka. 'Te Tiriti Te Tangata Te Whānau: The Treaty, The Human Person, The Family.' In *Te Aro Whānau: Family A Cornerstone of Māori Mental Well-being*, 26–34. Auckland: Mental Health Foundation of New Zealand, 1997.

Herd, Judy C. 'Assessment of Patients and Choice of Tranquillising and Antidepressant Drugs in General Practice.' PM diss., University of Otago, 1969.

Hezel, Francis X. 'In Search of the Social Roots of Mental Pathology in Micronesia.' In *Contemporary Issues in Mental Health Research in the Pacific Islands*, edited by Albert B. Robillard and Anthony J. Marsella, 12–31. Honolulu, Hawai'i: University of Hawai'i Press, 1987.

Hill, Richard S. *Policing the Colonial Frontier: The Theory and Practice of Coercive Social and Racial Control in New Zealand, 1767–1867.* Wellington: Historical Publications Branch, Department of Internal Affairs, 1986.

Hill, Susanne, and John Hill. *Richard Henry of Resolution Island.* Dunedin: Te Ara, 1987.

Ho, Elsie Seckyee. 'Mental Health of Asian Immigrants in New Zealand: A Review of Key Issues.' *Asian and Pacific Migration Journal* 13, no. 1 (March 2004): 39–60.

Holloway, Judith. '"Unfortunate Folk": A Study of the Social Context of Committal to Seacliff 1928–1937.' In *'Unfortunate Folk': Essays on Mental Health Treatment 1863–1992*, edited by Barbara Brookes and Jane Thomson, 153–67. Dunedin: Otago University Press, 2001.

Horrocks, John. 'The Limits of Endurance: Shell Shock and Dissent in World War One.' *The Journal of New Zealand Studies* NS27 (2018): 35–49.

Horton, H. M. 'Attempted Suicide and Severe Depression.' PM diss., University of Otago, 1967.

Horwitz, Allan, and Jerome Wakefield. *The Loss of Sadness: How Psychiatry Transformed Normal Sorrow into Depressive Disorder*. Oxford: Oxford University Press, 2007.

Howard, Alan. 'Polynesia and Micronesia in Psychiatric Perspective.' *Transcultural Psychiatry* 16 (1979): 123–45.

Hunt, Alison. 'A Bibliography of the Published Works of Robin Hyde (Iris G. Wilkinson, 1906–1939).' Auckland: New Zealand Electronic Poetry Centre, University of Auckland 22 March 2004. www.nzepc.auckland.ac.nz/authors/hyde/index.asp

Hunt, Alison. 'Angel-Guarded Liar in a Pleasant, Quiet Room: Robin Hyde's Experiences in the New Zealand Mental Health System of the 1930s.' In *Lighted Windows: Critical Essays on Robin Hyde*, edited by Mary Paul and Susan Ash, 143–50. Dunedin: Otago University Press, 2008.

Hunt, Alison. 'Lotus-Eating in Avondale: Tennyson in Robin Hyde's Poetry and 1934 Autobiography.' *Ka mate ka ora: A New Zealand Journal of Poetry and Poetics* 1 (2005): 34–66.

Hunt, Alison. '"The Cage with the Open Door": Autobiography and Psychiatry in the Life and Works of Robin Hyde.' PhD thesis, University of Auckland, 2008.

Hunt, Alison. 'The Unhappy Present Recites the Past: Autobiography as Psychiatric Treatment in the 1930s Case of Robin Hyde.' In *Telling Lives: Essays in Biography and History*, edited by Catharine Coleborne, Mark Houlahan and Hugh Douglas Morrison, 105–29. Hamilton: University of Waikato, Departments of History and Humanities, 2006.

Hunter Williams, Wendy. *Out of Sight Out of Mind: The Story of Porirua Hospital.* Wellington: Porirua Hospital, 1987.

Hyde, Robin. *The Godwits Fly*. London: Hurst & Blackett, 1938.

Hyde, Robin. *Wednesday's Children: A Novel.* London: Hurst & Blackett, 1937.

Hyde, Robin, with an introduction by Derek Challis. *A Home in This World.* Auckland: Longman Paul, 1984.

Ip, Manying. 'Chinese.' *Te Ara — the Encyclopedia of New Zealand.* www.teara.govt.nz/en/chinese (2005, revised 2015).

Ironside, Wallace. 'Feelings that Disturb our Peace of Mind.' *N.Z. Family Doctor* (May 1958): 30–31, 56.

J. C. B., A. E. C., R. M. C., and J. M. McE. 'I. L. G. SUTHERLAND 1897–1952.' *The Journal of the Polynesian Society* 61, no. 1/2 (1952): 120–29.

Jackson, Moana. 'The Mentally Ill Offender: A Māori Perspective.' *Community Mental Health in New Zealand* 4, no. 1 (June 1988): 49–50.

Jackson, Stanley W. 'A History of Melancholia and Depression.' In *History of Psychiatry and Medical Psychology*, edited by E. R. Wallace and J. Gach, 443–60. Boston, Massachusetts: Springer, 2008.

Jackson, Stanley W. *Melancholia and Depression: From Hippocratic Times to Modern Times.* New Haven, Connecticut: Yale University Press, 1985.

Jansson, Åsa. *From Melancholia to Depression: Disordered Mood in Nineteenth-Century Psychiatry*. Cham: Palgrave MacMillan, 2021.

Jarvis, Edward. 'On the Supposed Increase in Insanity.' *American Journal of Insanity* 8, no. 4 (1852): 333–64.

Jenks, Tiffany. '"They hold us responsible for their welfare": War Neurosis, World War Two Veterans, Families and the New Zealand Returned Servicemen's Association.' BA Hons diss., University of Otago, 2016.

Jenks, Tiffany, and Angela Wanhalla. 'Psychological Casualties: War Neurosis, Rehabilitation, and the Family in Post-World War II New Zealand.' *Health and History* 22, no. 2 (2020): 1–25.

Jones, Jenny Robin. *Writers in Residence: A Journey with Pioneer New Zealand Writers*. Auckland: Auckland University Press, 2004.

Kain, Jennifer. *Insanity and Immigration Control in New Zealand and Australia, 1860–1930*. Cham: Palgrave MacMillan, 2019.

Kalinowsky, Lothar B. 'Convulsive Shock Treatment.' In *American Handbook of Psychiatry*, vol. 2, edited by Silvano Arieti, 1499–520. New York: Basic Books, 1959.

Kavanagh, Jeff. 'Cherry Farm 1952–1992: Social and Economic Forces in the Evolution of Mental Health Care in Otago.' In *'Unfortunate Folk': Essays on Mental Health Treatment 1863–1992*, edited by Barbara Brookes and Jane Thomson, 168–82. Dunedin: Otago University Press, 2001.

King, Michael. *Wrestling With the Angel: A Life of Janet Frame*. Auckland: Viking, 2000.

King, Mike, with David Codyre. *The Nutters Club: Helping Nutters from the Inside Out*. Auckland: Random House, 2011.

Kingi, Te Kani. 'Introduction.' In *Maea Te Toi Ora: Māori Health Transformations*, edited by Te Kani Kingi, Mason Durie, Hinemoa Elder, Rees Tapsell, Mark Lawrence and Simon Bennett, 7–18. Wellington: Huia, 2018.

Kingi, Te Kani, Mason Durie, Hinemoa Elder, Rees Tapsell, Mark Lawrence and Simon Bennett. *Maea Te Toi Ora: Māori Health Transformations*. Wellington: Huia, 2018.

Kirwan, John, with Margie Thomson. *All Blacks Don't Cry: A Story of Hope*. Auckland: Penguin, 2010.

Kirwan, John, with Elliot Bell, Kirsty Louden-Bell, and Margie Thomson. *Stand By Me: Helping Your Teen Through Tough Times*. Auckland: Penguin, 2014.

Kitanaka, Junko. *Depression in Japan: Psychiatric Cures for a Society in Distress*. Princeton, New Jersey: Princeton University Press, 2012.

Kleinman, Arthur, and Byron Good, eds. *Culture and Depression: Studies in the Anthropology and Cross-Cultural Psychiatry of Affect and Disorder*. Berkeley, California: University of California Press, 1985.

Knewstubb, Elspeth M. 'Respectability, Religion and Psychiatry in New Zealand: A Case Study of Ashburn Hall, Dunedin, 1882–1910.' MA thesis, University of Otago, 2011, http://hdl.handle.net/10523/1734

Knewstubb, Elspeth M. 'The Models of Home? Influences on Medical Practice at Ashburn Hall, Dunedin, 1882–1910.' *The New Zealand Journal of History* 46, no. 1 (2012): 3–20.

Kruger, Tamāti, Mereana Pitman, Di Grennell, Tahuaroa McDonald, Dennis Mariu, Alva Pomare, Teina Mita, Matehaere Maihi, and Keri Lawson Te-Aho. 'Transforming Whānau Violence — A Conceptual Framework. An updated version of the report from the former Second Māori Taskforce on Whānau Violence.' Wellington: Second Māori Taskforce on Whānau Violence, 2004, https://nzfvc.org.nz/sites/default/files/transforming_whanau_violence.pdf

Labrum, Bronwyn. 'Looking Beyond the Asylum: Gender and the Process of Committal to Auckland, 1870–1919.' *The New Zealand Journal of History* 26 (1992): 125–44.

Labrum, Bronwyn. 'The Boundaries of Femininity: Madness and Gender in New Zealand, 1870–1910.' In *Women, Madness and the Law: A Feminist Reader*, edited by Wendy Chan, Dorothy E. Chunn and Robert Menzies, 59–77. London: The GlassHouse Press, 2005.

Lang, S. D. R. 'Attempted Suicide by Overdose.' PM diss., University of Otago, 1967.

Lawlor, C. *From Melancholia to Prozac: A History of Depression*. Oxford: Oxford University Press, 2012.

Leckie, Jacqueline. *Colonizing Madness: Asylum and Community in Fiji*. Honolulu, Hawai'i: University of Hawai'i Press, 2020.

Leckie, Jacqueline. 'Gumboots and Saris: Engendering Indian Settlers' History in Aotearoa.' In *Asia in the Making of New Zealand*, edited by Henry Johnson and Brian Moloughney, 76–93. Auckland: Auckland University Press, 2006.

Leckie, Jacqueline. *Indian Settlers: The Story of a New Zealand South Asian Community*. Dunedin: Otago University Press, 2007.

Leckie, Jacqueline. 'Infrastructure and "Magic Bullets" in Mental Health in the Colonial Pacific.' *Health and History* 23, no. 2 (2021): 29–50.

Leckie, Jacqueline. 'Insanity in a Sea of Islands: Mobility and Mental Health in Aotearoa New Zealand's Pacific Sphere.' *The Journal of New Zealand Studies* NS32 (2021): 166–82.

Leckie, Jacqueline. *Invisible: New Zealand's History of Excluding Kiwi-Indians*. Auckland: Massey University Press, 2021.

Leckie, Jacqueline. 'Pacific Bodies and Personal Space Redefined, 1850–1950.' In *The Cambridge History of the Pacific Ocean. Volume II: The Pacific Ocean since 1800*, edited by Anne Perez Hattori and Jane Samson, 490–513. Cambridge: Cambridge University Press, 2022.

Leckie, Jacqueline. 'Serendipity or Working with Circumstances.' In *Serendipity: Experience of Pacific Historians*, edited by Brij V. Lal, 258–77. Honolulu, Hawai'i: University of Hawai'i Press, 2024.

Leckie, Jacqueline. 'Silent Immigrants? Gender, Immigration and Ethnicity in New Zealand.' In *Immigration and National Identity in New Zealand; One People, Two Peoples, Many Peoples?* edited by Stuart Greif, 50–76. Palmerston North: Dunmore Press, 1995.

Leckie, Jacqueline, and Frances Hughes. 'Mental Health in the Smaller Pacific States.' In *Mental Health in Asia and the Pacific: Historical and Comparative Perspectives*, edited by Harry Minas and Milton Lewis, 253–72. New York: Springer, 2017.

Lee, Carol H. J., Isabelle M. Duck and Chris G. Sibley. 'Ethnic Inequality in Diagnosis with Depression and Anxiety Disorders.' *The New Zealand Medical Journal* 130, no. 1454 (2017): 10–20.

Leese, Peter. 'Essay Review: Making Shell-shock.' *British Journal of Psychology* 92 (2001): 411–15.

Leese, Peter. *Shell Shock: Traumatic Neurosis and the British Soldiers of the First World War*. Houndmills: Palgrave, 2002.

Le Fevre, Eva. 'Something on Your Mind.' *N.Z. Family Doctor* (November 1968): 8–10.

Liao, Rex. 'In the Shadow of Exclusion: The State of New Zealand Asian Health.' *New Zealand Medical Student Journal* 29 (2019): 32–36.

Lienert, R. T. 'Aspects of Suicide and Attempted Suicide.' PM diss., University of Otago, 1967.

Lindsay, John Spencer Bonar. 'The Affect in Prefrontal Leucotomy.' MD thesis, University of New Zealand, 1952.

Loan, Iain, Wayne Cunningham, and Chrystal Jaye. 'Understanding Depression in Tokelauan People in New Zealand.' *Journal of Primary Health Care* 8 (2016): 67–74.

Long, Nigel, Carol MacDonald, and Kerry Chamberlain. 'Prevalence of Posttraumatic Stress Disorder, Depression and Anxiety in a Community Sample of New Zealand Vietnam War Veterans.' *Australian and New Zealand Journal of Psychiatry* 30, no. 2 (1996): 253–56.

Lopdell, J. C. 'Some Psychiatric Responsibilities in General Practice.' *The New Zealand Medical Journal* 54, no. 300 (1955): 180–83.

Luangphinith, Seri Inthava Kau'ikealaula. 'Tropical Fevers: "Madness" and Colonialism in Pacific Literature.' *The Contemporary Pacific* 16, no. 1 (Spring 2004): 59–85.

Lutz, Catherine. 'Depression and the Translation of Emotional Worlds.' In *Culture and Depression: Studies in the Anthropology and Cross-Cultural Psychiatry of Affect and Disorder*, edited by Arthur Kleinman and Byron Good, 63–100. Berkeley, California: University of California Press, 1985.

Macbrayne, Rosaleen. 'Shock Therapy "Changed" Artist Rita Angus.' *The New Zealand Herald*, n.d., www.nzherald.co.nz/lifestyle/shock-therapy-changed-artist-rita-angus/XBAWSIGYJJ6YQYKZ2R3E6ITOGM

Mackenzie, Joy. '"My Way is to be with You": Meg and Alistair Te Ariki Campbell.' In *Between the Lives: Partners in Art*, edited by Deborah Shepard, 187–209. Auckland: Auckland University Press, 2005.

Macleod, A. D. 'Psychiatric Casualties of World War II.' *The New Zealand Medical Journal* 113, no. 1112 (23 June 2000): 248–50.

MaGPIe Research Group. 'Mental Disorders Among Māori Attending Their General Practitioner.' *Australian and New Zealand Journal of Psychiatry* 39 (2005): 401–6.

Manatū Hauora Ministry of Health. *Kia Manawanui Aotearoa: Long-term Pathway to Mental Wellbeing*. Wellington: Ministry of Health, 2021, www.health.govt.nz/publication/kia-manawanui-aotearoa-long-term-pathway-mental-wellbeing

Manatū Hauora Ministry of Health. *Te Puāwaitanga: Māori Mental Health National Strategic Framework*. Wellington: Ministry of Health, 2002, www.health.govt.nz/system/files/documents/publications/maorimentalhealthnationalstrategicframework.pdf

Manchester, Ruth. *The New Zealand Association of Psychotherapists, Te Roopu Whakaora Hinengaro: Notes Towards a History: A Chronology of the First Fifty Years, 1947–1997*. Wellington: The Association, 1996.

Marland, Hilary. '"Destined to a Perfect Recovery": The Confinement of Puerperal Insanity in the Nineteenth Century.' In *Insanity, Institutions and Society, 1800–1914: A Social History of Madness in Comparative Perspective*, edited by Joseph Melling and Bill Forsythe, 137–56. London: Routledge, 1999.

Marland, Hilary. *Dangerous Motherhood: Insanity and Childbirth in Victorian England.* Basingstoke: Palgrave Macmillan, 2004.

Marsella, Anthony J., Norman Sartorius, Assen Jablensky, and Fred R. Fenton. 'Cross-Cultural Studies of Depressive Disorders: An Overview.' In *Culture and Depression: Studies in the Anthropology and Cross-Cultural Psychiatry of Affect and Disorder*, edited by Arthur Kleinman and Byron Good, 299–324. Berkeley, California: University of California Press, 1985.

Mason, K. H. *Report of the Committee of Inquiry into Procedures Used in Certain Psychiatric Hospitals in Relation to Admission, Discharge or Release on Leave of Certain Classes of Patients.* Wellington: Department of Health, 1988, www.moh.govt.nz/NoteBook/nbbooks.nsf/0/2DC94A246D93272C4C2565D7000DDA26/%24file/Mason%20Report.pdf

Mason, K. H. *Report of the Ministerial Inquiry [In Respect of Certain Mental Health Services] to the Minister of Health Hon Jenny Shipley.* Wellington: Ministry of Health, 1996, www.moh.govt.nz/notebook/nbbooks.nsf/0/70FC4C46F860CFEE4C2565D70018A26A/%24file/Inquiry%20under%20section%2047%20of%20the%20health%20and%20disability%20services%20act%201993%20in%20respect%20of%20certain%20mental%20health%20services.pdf

Matthews, Jacqueline. 'Hyde, Robin.' *Dictionary of New Zealand Biography. Te Ara — the Encyclopedia of New Zealand* (1998), https://teara.govt.nz/en/biographies/4h41/hyde-robin

Mayo, K. M. 'A Survey of Maori and Dalmatian Mental Patients Living in the Auckland and Kingseat Mental Hospitals in February, 1952.' PM diss., University of Otago, 1952.

McAloon, Jim. 'Land Ownership.' *Te Ara — the Encyclopedia of New Zealand* (2008), www.teara.govt.nz/en/land-ownership

McCarthy, Angela. 'Ethnicity, Migration and the Lunatic Asylum in Early Twentieth-Century Auckland, New Zealand.' *Social History of Medicine* 21, no. 1 (2008): 47–65.

McCarthy, Angela. *Migration, Ethnicity and Madness. New Zealand, 1860–1910.* Dunedin: Otago University Press, 2015.

McCarthy, Angela, ed. *Narratives of Migrant and Refugee Discrimination in Aotearoa New Zealand.* London: Routledge, 2022.

McCarthy, Angela, and Catharine Coleborne. 'Introduction: Mental Health, Migration and Ethnicity.' In *Migration, Ethnicity, and Mental Health: International Perspectives, 1840–2010*, edited by Angela McCarthy and Catharine Coleborne, 1–14. New York and Abingdon: Routledge, 2012.

McDaid, Frances, Lisa Underwood, Jacinta Fa'alili-Fidow, Karen E. Waldie, Elizabeth R. Peterson, Amy Bird, and Stephanie D'Souza. 'Antenatal Depression Symptoms in Pacific Women: Evidence from Growing Up in New Zealand.' *Journal of Primary Health Care* 11, no. 2 (2019): 96–108.

McKenzie, Donald. 'Prefrontal Leucotomy.' *The New Zealand Medical Journal* 47, no. 257 (1948): 38–39.

McKinnon, Alexander. *Come Back to Mona Vale: Life and Death in a Christchurch Mansion.* Dunedin: Otago University Press, 2021.

McLachlan D. G., and M. A. Falconer. 'Prefrontal Leucotomy (Lobotomy): A Report on 65 Cases.' *The New Zealand Medical Journal* 49 (1950): 522–30.

McLeod, W. H. *A List of Punjabi Immigrants in New Zealand, 1890–1939.* Hamilton: Country Section of the Central Indian Association, 1984.

Mead, Hirini Moko. *Tikanga Māori: Living by Māori Values.* Wellington: Huia, 2003.

Medlicott, Reginald W. 'Convulsive Therapy: Results and Complications in Four Hundred Cases.' *The New Zealand Medical Journal* 47 (1948): 338–48.

Medlicott, Reginald W. 'Prefrontal Leucotomy.' *The New Zealand Medical Journal* 42 (1943): 113–20.

Medlicott, Reginald W. 'Psychiatric Treatments.' *The New Zealand Nursing Journal* 38, no. 2 (1945): 28–32.

Medlicott, Reginald W. 'The Place of Electronarcosis in Psychiatric Treatment. A Clinical Assessment based on the Treatment of Four Hundred Patients.' *The New Zealand Medical Journal* 53, no. 294 (April 1954): 128–37.

Melding, Pamela. 'Electroconvulsive Therapy in New Zealand: Terrifying or Electrifying?' *The New Zealand Medical Journal* 119, no. 1237 (2006): U2051.

Melling, J. O. 'The New Zealand Returned Soldiers' Association, 1916–1923.' MA thesis, Victoria University of Wellington, 1952, 74.

Mellsop, Graham, and Michael Radford. 'Report of Graham Mellsop and Michael Radford as Sought by the Department of Health on the Use of "Deep Sleep Therapy".' Wellington: Department of Health, 1991, www.moh.govt.nz/notebook/nbbooks.nsf/0/D542CD5D4F91EDEA4C2565D7000DEE5E/$file/REport_deep_sleep-therapy_1991.pdf

Mental Health Commission. *Blueprint for Mental Health Services in New Zealand: How Things Need to Be.* Wellington: Mental Health Commission, 1998, www.moh.govt.nz/notebook/nbbooks.nsf/0/0E6493ACAC236A394C25678D000BEC3C/%24file/Blueprint_for_mental_health_services.pdf

Mental Health Commission. *Blueprint II: Improving Mental Health and Wellbeing for all New Zealanders.* Wellington: Mental Health Commission, 2012, www.hdc.org.nz/media/1075/blueprint-ii-how-things-need-to-be.pdf

Mental Health Commission. *Te Haererenga mo te Whakōranga 1996–2006: The Journey of Recovery for the New Zealand Mental Health Sector*. Wellington, Mental Health Commission, 2007, www.moh.govt.nz/notebook/nbbooks.nsf/0/12912EA93B0B85EFCC2573C90068845D/$file/te_haererenga%20%201996-2006.pdf

Mental Health Foundation of New Zealand. *Change in Mind. Kia Puawai a Mua.* Auckland: Mental Health Foundation of New Zealand, 2008.

Merskey, Harold. 'Shell-shock.' In *150 Years of British Psychiatry 1841–1991*, edited by German E. Berrios and H. Freeman, 245–67. London: Gaskell, 1991.

Metge, Joan. *In and Out of Touch: Whakamaa in Cross-Cultural Context.* Wellington: Victoria University Press, 1986.

Middleton, Angela. *Pēwhairangi: Bay of Islands Missions and Māori 1814 to 1845.* Dunedin: Otago University Press, 2019.

Mila-Schaaf, Karlo. 'Not Another New Zealand-Born Identity Crisis: Well-being and the Politics of Belonging.' In *Pacific Identities and Well-being: Cross-cultural Perspectives,* edited by Margaret Nelson Agee, Tracey McIntosh, Philip Culbertson and Cabrini 'Ofa Makasiale, 27–45. New York, London: Routledge, 2013.

Milner, George Bertram. *Samoan Dictionary.* London: Oxford University Press, 1966.

Ministry for Pacific Peoples. *Pacific Aotearoa Status Report: A Snapshot, 2020.* Wellington: Ministry for Pacific Peoples, 2021, www.mpp.govt.nz/assets/Reports/Pacific-Peoples-in-Aotearoa-Report.pdf

Moncrieff, Joanna, Ruth E. Cooper, Tom Stockmann, Simone Amendola, Michael P. Hengartner, and Mark A. Horowitz. 'The Serotonin Theory of Depression: A Systematic Umbrella Review of the Evidence.' *Molecular Psychiatry* (2022), https://doi.org/10.1038/s41380-022-01661-0

Moore, Rina. 'Therapeutic Dissociation by Electro-Convulsive Therapy.' *The New Zealand Medical Journal* 57 (1958): 359–64.

Moore, Stuart. 'Psychotherapy.' *The New Zealand Medical Journal* 12, no. 47 (1913): 514–38.

Morris, Paul A. H. '"Their Nerves were Shot to Shreds — Our Own Weren't Too Steady Either": Attitudes Towards Psychological Casualties in the 2nd New Zealand Expeditionary Force, 1939 to 1945.' MA thesis, University of Canterbury, 2013, http://hdl.handle.net/10092/8035

Mulgan, John. *Man Alone.* London: Selwyn and Blount, 1939.

Murphy, Henry B. M., and Ram Narayan. 'Mental Hospitalisation in Fiji.' *Fiji Medical Journal* 7, no. 1 (1979): 4–11.

Murray, Caitlin. 'The "Colouring of the Psychosis": Interpreting Insanity in the Primitive Mind.' *Health and History* 9, no. 2 (2007): 7–21.

Myers, C. S. 'A Contribution to the Study of Shell Shock: Being an Account of Three Cases of Loss of Memory, Vision, Smell, and Taste, Admitted into the Duchess of Westminster's War Hospital, Le Touquet.' *The Lancet* 185 (1915): 316–20.

National Advisory Committee on Health and Disability. *Guideline for the Treatment and Management of Depression by Primary Healthcare Professionals.* Wellington: Ministry of Health, 1996, www.moh.govt.nz/notebook/nbbooks.nsf/0/B78AC66F92C61AF84C2565D700188F23/$file/depression-guideline.pdf

Nelson, T. V. 'Functional Nervous Disorder in New Zealand Forces.' PM diss., University of Otago, 1949.

Neumaier, Felix, Mario Paterno, Serdar Alpdogan, Etienne E. Tevoufouet, Toni Schneider, Jürgen Hescheler, and Walid Albanna. 'Surgical Approaches in Psychiatry: A Survey of the World Literature on Psychosurgery.' *World Neurosurgery* 97 (2016): 603–34.

New Zealand Mental Health and Wellbeing Commission. *Te Huringa: Change and Transformation. Mental Health Service and Addiction Service Monitoring.* Wellington: New Zealand Mental Health and Wellbeing Commission, 2022, www.mhwc.govt.nz/assets/Te-Huringa/FINAL-MHWC-Te-Huringa-Service-Monitoring-Report.pdf

Ng, James. *Windows on a Chinese Past* (4 vols). Dunedin: Otago Heritage Books, 1993–1999.

Obeyesekere, Gananath. 'Depression, Buddhism and the Work of Culture in Sri Lanka.' In *Culture and Depression: Studies in the Anthropology and Cross-Cultural Psychiatry of Affect and Disorder*, edited by Arthur Kleinman and Byron Good, 134–52. Berkeley, California: University of California Press, 1985.

Oei, T. P., and L. M. Sullivan. 'Cognitive Changes Following Recovery from Depression in a Group Cognitive-Behaviour Therapy Program.' *Australian and New Zealand Journal of Psychiatry* 33, no. 3 (1999): 407–15.

Office of Tokelau Affairs. *Tokelau Dictionary*. Apia: Office of Tokelau Affairs, 1986.

O'Gorman, Francis. *Worrying A Literary and Cultural History*. London: Bloomsbury, 2015.

Oppenheim, Janet. *Shattered Nerves: Doctors, Patients, and Depression in Victorian England*. New York: Oxford University Press, 1991.

Orange, Claudia. 'Te Tiriti o Waitangi — the Treaty of Waitangi.' *Te Ara — the Encyclopedia of New Zealand* (2012, revised 2023), www.teara.govt.nz/en/te-tiriti-o-waitangi-the-treaty-of-waitangi

Page, Dorothy. *Anatomy of a Medical School: A History of Medicine at the University of Otago, 1875–2000*. Dunedin: Otago University Press, 2008.

Palmer, Harold. 'The Problem of Neurosis in Ex-Soldiers.' *The New Zealand Medical Journal* 47, no. 258 (April 1948): 129–38.

Parkins, Wendy. *Every Morning, So Far, I'm Alive: A Memoir*. Dunedin: Otago University Press, 2019.

Parr, Alison. *Silent Casualties: New Zealand's Unspoken Legacy of the Second World War*. Auckland: Tandem Press, 1995.

Parsons, Gwen A. 'The Construction of Shell Shock in New Zealand, 1919–1939: A Reassessment.' *Social History of Medicine: The Journal of the Society for the Social History of Medicine* 26, no. 1 (2013): 56–73.

Paterson, Lachy. 'Government, Church and Māori Responses to *Mākutu* (Sorcery) in the Nineteenth and Early Twentieth Centuries.' *Cultural and Social History* 8, no. 2 (2015): 175–94.

Paterson, Ron, Mason Durie, Barbara Disley, Dean Rangihuna, Jemaima Tiatia-Seath and Josiah Tualamali'i. *He ara oranga: Report of the Government Inquiry into Mental Health and Addiction*. Wellington: Department of Internal Affairs, 2018, https://mentalhealth.inquiry.govt.nz/inquiry-report/he-ara-oranga

Pellegrino, Nicky. 'High Anxiety.' *New Zealand Listener*, 12–18 December 2020: 16–19.

Pawson, Eric, and Tom Brooking. *Making a New Land: Environmental Histories of New Zealand*. Dunedin: Otago University Press, 2013.

Phillips, Jock. *A Man's Country? The Image of the Pakeha Male, A History*. Auckland: Penguin, 1987.

Phillips, Jock. 'History of Immigration.' *Te Ara — the Encyclopedia of New Zealand* (2005, revised 2015), www.teara.govt.nz/en/history-of-immigration

Philp, Matthew. 'Scientific Pastors: The Professionalisation of Psychiatry in New Zealand 1877–1920.' In *'Unfortunate Folk': Essays on Mental Health Treatment 1863–1992*, edited by Barbara Brookes and Jane Thomson, 185–99. Dunedin: University of Otago Press, 2001.

Pihama, Leonie, and Paul Reynolds. *Kia Mārama: Tane Māori and Depression. A Scoping Report.* Auckland: Hāpai Te Hauora Tapui and Mental Health Foundation, 2007.

Pihama, Leonie, Paul Reynolds, C. Smith, J. Reid, Linda Tuhiwai-Smith, and R. Te Nana. 'Positioning Historical Trauma Theory.' *AlterNATIVE: An International Journal of Indigenous Peoples* 10, no. 3 (2014): 248–63.

Pitt-Rivers, George. 'Visit to a Maori Village. Being Some Observations on the Passing of the Maori Race and the Decay of Maori Culture.' *The Journal of the Polynesian Society* 33, no. 129 (1924): 48–65.

Pool, Ian. 'Death Rates and Life Expectancy — Effects of Colonisation on Māori.' *Te Ara — the Encyclopedia of New Zealand*, (2011, revised 2019), www.teara.govt.nz/en/death-rates-and-life-expectancy/page-4

Porter, Frances, Charlotte Macdonald, and Tui MacDonald. *My Hand Will Write What My Heart Dictates: The Unsettled Lives of Women in Nineteenth-Century New Zealand as Revealed to Sisters, Family and Friends.* Auckland: Auckland University Press, 1996.

Porter, Roy. 'Mood Disorders: Social Section.' In *A History of Clinical Psychiatry: The Origin and History of Psychiatric Disorders*, edited by German Berrios and Roy Porter, 409–20. New York: New York University Press, 1995.

Pratt, George. *Pratt's Grammar and Dictionary of the Language.* Apia: The Malua Printing Press, 1862.

Presland, R., and H. Palmer. 'The Comparative Value of Curarizing Agents with Special Reference to Convulsion Therapy.' *The New Zealand Medical Journal* 49, no. 271 (1950): 262–66.

Radden, Jennifer. *Moody Minds Distempered: Essays on Melancholy and Depression.* Oxford: Oxford University Press, 2009.

Rathbone, Paula Frances. 'The Psychological Effects of Prefrontal Leucotomy: A Review of the Literature and Observations of Some Cases Studied.' MA thesis, University of New Zealand, 1948.

Reeves, William Pember. *The Long White Cloud: Ao Tea Roa.* London: Horace Marshall & Son, 1898.

Reilly, Michael P. J. 'Grief, Loss and Violence in Ancient Mangaia, Aotearoa and Te Waipounamu.' *The Journal of Pacific History* 47, no. 2 (2012): 145–61.

Ritchie, James. 'Sutherland, Ivan Lorin George.' *Dictionary of New Zealand Biography, Te Ara — the Encyclopedia of New Zealand* (1998, updated 2020 by Oliver Sutherland), https://teara.govt.nz/en/biographies/4s57/sutherland-ivan-lorin-george

Roche, Michael. 'Failure Deconstructed: Histories and Geographies of Soldier Settlement in New Zealand Circa 1917–39.' *New Zealand Geographer* 64, no. 1 (2008): 46–56.

Royal Commission of Inquiry into Abuse in Care, 2023, www.abuseincare.org.nz

Sachdev, Perminder, and Jagdeep Sachdev. 'Sixty Years of Psychosurgery: Its Present Status and Its Future.' *Australian and New Zealand Journal of Psychiatry* 31, no. 4 (1997): 457–64.

Sadowsky, Jonathan. *Bedlam: Institutions of Madness in Colonial Southwest Nigeria.* Berkeley, California: University of California Press, 1999.

Sadowsky, Jonathan. 'Before and After Prozac: Psychiatry as Medicine, and the Historiography of Depression.' *Culture, Medicine and Psychiatry* 45, no. 3 (2021): 479–502.

Sadowsky, Jonathan. *Electroconvulsive Therapy in America: The Anatomy of a Medical Controversy*. New York: Routledge, 2016.

Sadowsky, Jonathan. *The Empire of Depression: A New History*. Cambridge, Massachusetts: Polity Books, 2021.

Sage, D. J. 'Depression (As it Occurs in General Practice).' PM diss., University of Otago, 1973.

Salesa, Damon I. 'New Zealand's Pacific.' In *The New Oxford History of New Zealand*, edited by Giselle Byrnes, 149–72. Melbourne: Oxford University Press, 2009.

Sargeson, Frank. 'Review.' *Landfall* 125 (1978): 90–91.

Sarti, Antonella. *Spiritcarvers: Interviews with Eighteen Writers from New Zealand*. Amsterdam: Rodopi, 1998.

Scott, Gary. 'Kūkūtai, Waata Pihikete.' *Dictionary of New Zealand Biography* (1990). *Te Ara — the Encyclopedia of New Zealand*, https://teara.govt.nz/en/biographies/1k17/kukutai-waata-pihikete

Seckyee Ho, Elsie. 'Mental Health of Asian Immigrants in New Zealand: A Review of Key Issues.' *Asian and Pacific Migration Journal* 13, no. 1 (March 2004): 39–60.

Shephard, Ben. *A War of Nerves: Soldiers and Psychiatrists 1914–1994*. London: Pimlico Books, 2002.

Short, Gordon. 'Case of Mental Depression.' *The New Zealand Medical Journal* 34, no. 83 (1935): 342–43.

Shorter, Edward, and David Healy. *Shock Therapy: A History of Electroconvulsive Treatment in Mental Illness*. New Brunswick: Rutgers University Press, 2007.

Shortland, Edward. *Maori Religion and Mythology*. London: Longmans Green, 1882.

Simcock, Keith R. 'War Neurosis with Special References to Some Hamilton Cases.' PM diss., University of Otago, 1949.

Sinclair, Keith. *William Pember Reeves: New Zealand Fabian*. Oxford: Clarendon Press, 1965.

Sinclair, Keith, and Trudie McNaughton. *A History of the University of Auckland, 1883–1983*. Auckland: Auckland University Press / Oxford University Press, 1983.

Smith, S. Percy. 'The Evils of *Makutu*, or Witchcraft.' *The Journal of the Polynesian Society* 30, no. 3 (119) (1921): 172–84.

Smith, Tākirirangi. *He Ara Uru Ora: Traditional Māori Understandings of Trauma and Well-being*. Whanganui: Te Atawhai o Te Ao: Independent Māori Institute for Environment and Health, 2019, https://teatawhai.maori.nz/wp-content/uploads/2020/04/He-Ara-Uru-Ora.pdf

Somerville, Alan. 'Ashburn Hall and Its Place in Society, 1882–1904.' MA thesis, University of Otago, 1996.

Sørensen, John Kousgård. 'Ingeborg Stuckenberg in New Zealand.' In *Danish Emigration to New Zealand*, edited by Henning Bender and Birgit Larsen, translated by Karen Veien, 46–59. Danes Worldwide Archives, 1990.

Sperlich, Wolfgang B. *Tohi Vagahau Niue = Niue Language Dictionary: Niuean–English, with English–Niuean Finderlist*. Honolulu, Hawai'i: Government of Niue in association with Department of Linguistics, University of Hawai'i, 1997.

Stallworthy, Kenneth. 'Clinical Findings Following Leucotomy.' *The New Zealand Medical Journal* 52, no. 291 (1953): 405–12.

Stallworthy, Kenneth. 'In the Depths of Depression.' *N.Z. Family Doctor* (February 1962): 44–45.

Stallworthy, Kenneth. 'Melancholia Treated with Cardiazol.' *The New Zealand Medical Journal* 42, no. 232 (December 1943): 268.

Stewart, Indira. 'Older Pasifika Migrants More Resilient to Mental Illness.' *Radio New Zealand*, 13 December 2018.

Stewart, Iwa. 'Surviving Chronic Whakamaa.' *Mental Health Quarterly* (June 1998): 10.

Stolkind, E. 'A Case of Acute Fatal Medinal Poisoning, with Notes on the Ill-Effects of the Medinal Habit.' *The Lancet* 207 (1926): 391–92.

Summerfield, Derek. 'Afterword: Against "Global Mental Health".' *Transcultural Psychiatry* 49, no. 3–4 (2012): 519–30.

Sutherland, Oliver. *Paikea: The Life of I. L. G. Sutherland.* Christchurch: Canterbury University Press, 2013.

Swartz, Sally. 'Changing Diagnoses in Valkenberg Asylum, Cape Colony, 1891–1920: A Longitudinal View.' *History of Psychiatry* 5 (1995): 431–51.

Tamasese, Kiwi, Carmel Peteru, Charles Waldegrave, and Allister Bush. 'Ole Taeao Afua, the New Morning: A Qualitative Investigation into Samoan Perspectives on Mental Health and Culturally Appropriate Services.' *Australasian Psychiatry: Bulletin of the Royal Australian and New Zealand College of Psychiatrists* 39, no. 4 (2005): 300–9.

Tan, Eng-Seong. 'The Presentation of Affective Symptoms in Non-Western Countries.' In *Handbook of Studies on Depression*, edited by Graham D. Burrows, 121–33. Amsterdam: Excerpta Medica, 1977.

Tan, Hean. 'Indo-Chinese Refugees' Well-Being from the Sponsors' Perspective.' MA thesis, University of Auckland, 1995.

Te Pou (Mental Health Programmes). *Talking Therapies for Asian People: Best and Promising Practice Guide for Mental Health and Addiction Services.* Auckland: Te Pou o te Whakaaro Nui, 2010, www.tepou.co.nz/resources/talking-therapies-for-asian-people

Thomson, Mathew. 'Practical Psychology.' In *Psychological Subjects: Identity, Culture, and Health in Twentieth-century Britain*, edited by Mathew Thomson, 17–53. Oxford: Oxford University Press, 2006.

Tod, Frank. 'Terry, Edward Lionel.' *Dictionary of New Zealand Biography* (1996). *Te Ara — the Encyclopedia of New Zealand*, https://teara.govt.nz/en/biographies/3t27/terry-edward-lionel

Townsend, Colin. *Misery Hill, Seaview Terrace, Hokitika, 1866–1909: The Home of the Dead, the Mad and the Bad: A Personal Cameo History of the Upper Gaol, Seaview Terrace, Hokitika and Some of Its Inmates.* Christchurch: Leon G. Morel, 1998.

Tregear, Edward. 'Inaugural Address.' *Transactions and Proceedings of the Royal Society of New Zealand* 31 (1898): 605–23.

Trubohovich, Ronald Valentine. 'Letter: Tricyclic Antidepressants: Dangers with Overdosage.' *The New Zealand Medical Journal* 78, no. 504 (12 December 1973): 502–3.

Tuke, Daniel Hack, ed. *A Dictionary of Psychological Medicine. Giving the Definition, Etymology and Synonyms of the Terms Used in Medical Psychology with the Symptoms, Treatment, and Pathology of Insanity and the Law of Lunacy in Great Britain and Ireland.* Philadelphia, Pennsylvania: P. Blakiston, Son & Co., 1892.

Tuke, Daniel Hack. *Insanity in Ancient and Modern Life with Chapters on its Prevention.* London: Macmillan, 1878.

Tutty, Susan, and Felicity Goodyear-Smith. 'Eighteen Months of Depression: Examining the Chronic Care Management of Depression with Particular Reference to Pacific People.' *Journal of Primary Health Care* 6, no. 1 (2014): 31–39.

Tyquin, Michael B. *Madness and the Military: Australia's Experience of the Great War.* Loftus: Australian Military History Publications, 2006.

Ursano, Robert J. 'Prisoners of War: Long-term Health Outcomes.' *The Lancet* 362, Supplement, Extreme Medicine (December 2003): s22–s23.

Walker, Elizabeth. '"The Living Death": The Repatriation Experience of New Zealand's Disabled Great War Servicemen.' MA thesis, Victoria University of Wellington, 2013, http://hdl.handle.net/10063/2641

Walrond, Carl. 'Dalmatians.' *Te Ara — the Encyclopedia of New Zealand.* (2005, revised 2015), www.TeAra.govt.nz/en/dalmatians/print

Walters, Karina L., Selina A Mohammed, Teresa Evans-Campbell, Ramona E. Beltrán, David H. Chae, and Bonnie Duran. 'Bodies Don't Just Tell Stories, They Tell Histories: Embodiment of Historical Trauma Among American Indians and Alaska Natives.' *Du Bois Review* 8, no. 1 (2011): 179–89.

Wattie, Nelson. *Scribbling in the Dark: Alistair Te Ariki Campbell.* Wellington: Steele Roberts Aotearoa, 2011.

Weaver, John C. *Sorrows of a Century: Interpreting Suicide in New Zealand, 1900–2000.* Montreal: McGill-Queen's University Press / Wellington: Bridget Williams Books, 2014.

Weaver, John C., and Doug Munro. 'Country Living, Country Dying: Suicide Inquests and Rural Hardship in New Zealand, 1900–1950.' *Journal of Social History* 42, no. 4 (2009): 933–61.

Weaver, John C., and Doug Munro. 'The Historical Contingency of Suicide: A Case-Based Comparison of Suicides in New Zealand in the 1930s and 1980s.' *New Zealand Sociology* 25, no. 1 (2010): 100–30.

Weaver, John C., and David Wright. 'Shell Shock and the Politics of Asylum Committal in New Zealand, 1916–22.' *Health and History* 7, no. 1 (2005): 17–40.

Whistler, W. Arthur. 'Traditional and Herbal Medicine in the Cook Islands.' *Journal of Ethnopharmacology* 13, no. 3 (1985): 239–80.

Wikaire, Erena, Kayla Wikaire-Mackey, Shaquille Graham, Michael Naera, and Mason Durie. *Nōku te Ao: Sovereignty of the Māori Mind.* Wellington: Te Whatu Ora, 2022, www.nokuteao.org.nz/noku-te-ao-sovereignty-of-the-maori-min

Williams, Pip M. E. *Te Rongoā Māori: Māori Medicine 1904–1997.* Auckland: Penguin, 2008.

Williams, Sue. 'A Light on the Dark Secrets of Depression.' In *Jane Campion: Interviews.* edited by Virginia Wright Wexman, 175–76. Jackson, Mississippi: University Press of Mississippi, 1999.

Wirihana, Rebecca, Cherryl Smith, and Takirirangi Smith. 'Māori Indigenous Healing Practices in Aotearoa (New Zealand).' In *The Routledge International Handbook of Race, Culture and Mental Health,* edited by Roy Moodley and Eunjung Lee, 530–40. Milton: Taylor and Francis, 2020.

Wong, Sally F. *Asian Public Health in Aotearoa New Zealand.* Auckland: The Asian Network, 2021.

Wright-St Clair, Rex E. 'J. Rutherford Ryley: Pioneer of Antisepsis in New Zealand.' *Journal of Medical Biography* 7, no. 1 (1999): 32–34.

Young, Bruce. *Dr Louis Hauiti Potaka of New Zealand: A Biographical Essay.* Waterloo: Department of Geography and Environmental Studies, Wilfrid Laurier University, 1999, revised, 2005, https://kb.osu.edu/bitstream/handle/1811/5984/potaka.pdf;jsessionid=095489F752BE246BB88169209A3E2A32?sequence=1

Zhu, Andrew. *New Zealand Asian Mental Health and Wellbeing Report 2020: A Snapshot Survey.* Auckland: Asian Family Services, 2020, www.asianfamilyservices.nz/resources/resource-items/nz-asian-mental-health-wellbeing-report-2020

Psychiatric hospitals in Aotearoa New Zealand

This list refers to names mentioned in this book. Because of slight variations between sources, dates may be approximate, and precise names sometimes varied. In 1911 the official term 'asylum' was nationally replaced by 'mental hospital' and later by 'psychiatric hospital'. It is unclear when 'psychiatric' was officially used in the terminology.

Auckland

Auckland Provincial Lunatic Asylum (also known as Avondale Lunatic Asylum), 1854–1910 (also known as 'The Whau' asylum, established 1853 in the grounds of the Auckland Hospital; moves to Point Chevalier in 1876)

Auckland Mental Hospital, 1911–1959

Oakley Hospital, 1960–1973

Carrington Hospital (also known as Avondale), 1973–1992

Kingseat Psychiatric Hospital (Karaka, South Auckland), 1932–1999

Waikato

Tokanui Psychiatric Hospital (Te Awamutu), 1912–1988

Manawatū

Lake Alice Hospital (Marton/Bulls) 1950–1999

Wellington

Karori Lunatic Asylum, 1854–1873

Mount View, 1873–1910

Porirua Lunatic Asylum Hospital, 1887–1910

Porirua Mental Hospital (usually known as Porirua Hospital), 1911–2007

Nelson

Nelson Lunatic Asylum, 1864–1911

Nelson Mental Hospital, 1912–c.1922

Ngawhatu Psychiatric Hospital (Stoke), 1922–2000

West Coast

Hokitika Lunatic Asylum (initially a lunatic ward at South Spit Hospital), 1865–1872

Seaview Asylum (also known as Seaview Hospital), 1872–1911

Seaview Psychiatric Hospital, 1911–2009

Christchurch

Sunnyside Lunatic Asylum, 1863–1911

Sunnyside Hospital, 1911–1999

Hillmorton Hospital, 2007–

Hanmer Springs

Queen Mary Hospital for Sick and Wounded Soldiers, 1916–1921

Queen Mary Hospital, 1922–2003

Otago

Dunedin Lunatic Asylum, 1863–1878

Seacliff Lunatic Asylum, 1879–1911

Seacliff Mental Hospital, 1911–1973

Cherry Farm Hospital (Some patients were also treated at Orokonui Home, Waitati), 1952–1992

Ashburn Hall, 1882–2001

Ashburn Clinic, 2001–

Glossary

Te reo Māori

hapū subtribe, kinship group sharing descent from a common ancestor

hauora to be well, healthy, in good spirits

hinengaro intellectual wellbeing

iwi extended kinship group, tribe

karakia chant, prayer

kaumātua elder

kaupapa Māori Māori approach, customary practice incorporating the attitudes, knowledge, skills and values of Māori society

kuia female elder, grandmother

kūmara sweet potato, *Ipomoea batatas*

mākutu witchcraft, sorcery

marae area in front of the wharenui (meeting house) where formal greetings and discussions take place. Often used to describe the complex of buildings nearby

mate atua illnesses with no obvious physical causes

mate Māori sickness attributed to transgressions of tapu or to mākutu

mate pāpōuri depression

mate taua physical accidents

ngākau emotional wellbeing

Pākehā New Zealander usually of European descent, non-Māori

pōkē mental depression

pōrangi madness, mad

pōuritanga depression, sadness

poururu to be darkish, gloomy, depressed

rangatira of high rank, leader, chief

raupatu conquest, confiscation

rāwakiwaki intense grief, depression, despair

rongoā indigenous medicinal plants

taipō ghost

tāngata whaiora person seeking health, including mental health

tangata whenua Indigenous people

taonga tapu sacred or restricted treasured possession

tapu sacred, prohibited, restricted

taua war party

te reo Māori Māori language

tinana physical wellbeing

tiwhatiwha to be dark, gloomy, depressed

tohunga priest, healer, expert

wairangi depression

wairua spiritual wellbeing

whakamā to be ashamed, shame

whakamomori suicide

whakapōuri depression, despair

whānau family group

whenua land

Medical

affective moods, feelings and emotions.

affective psychoses psychotic symptoms, such as hallucinations or delusions, with a mood disorder

amnesic confusional state loss of memory for certain events and confusion

anticonvulsant anti-seizure medication

antidepressant medication used to treat depressive disorders and other conditions such as anxiety disorders

antipsychotic medication used to manage psychosis

antisocial personality disorder referred to people who disregarded others and property, and the social and legal norms of right and wrong

artificial feeding tubal or intravenous feeding

automatism nonpurposeful behaviour performed mechanically without intention and without conscious awareness

bipolar disorder mental illness that causes unusual shifts in a person's mood, energy, activity levels and concentration. People with bipolar disorder often experience shifting moods, from being highly active to very depressed; at other times they may feel neither unusually high nor low, or can experience manic and depressive symptoms within the same episode

biochemical chemical processes and substances within humans

Cardiozol therapy Cardiozol was the brand name for metrazol, used in early shock therapy

cataleptic stupor extreme unresponsiveness

catamenia blood and other matter discharged from the uterus at menstruation

climacteric menopuase

clinical depression term used by a medical practitioner to diagnose depression that requires medical or other intervention

cognitive behavioural therapy (CBT) talking therapy that deals with current psychological and behavioural problems, aiming to change negative patterns to improve thinking and wellbeing

convulsion rapid, involuntary muscle contractions that cause uncontrollable shaking and limb movement

convulsive therapy electroconvulsive therapy that induces a convulsion in the brain

deep sedation and deep sleep therapy injection of drugs to induce a patient to be under prolonged or intermittent sleep, during which other drugs, and ECT, might be administered

dementia loss of cognitive functioning that interferes with a person's daily life and activities

dopamine a 'feel-good' chemical released in the brain

electroconvulsive therapy (ECT) electric stimulation to the brain that causes a brief surge of electrical activity (also known as a seizure) with the aim of relieving severe symptoms of some mental health problems

electronarcosis electrical stunning leading to sleep

endogenous depression depression considered long-term, biological and physiological

exogenous depression depression considered to be a response to life events or the environment

Freudian therapy talk therapy based on Sigmund Freud's theories of psychoanalysis, in which the therapist probes the patient to uncover past subconscious thoughts and feelings

Gestalt therapy therapy focused on the client's present, often through exploring connections between form, shapes and feelings

homoeopathy works on the belief that the body can cure itself. Tiny amounts of natural substances are used to stimulate the healing process

hydropathy 'water cure', treating illness through the use of water

hypomania considered a milder version of mania lasting for a shorter period

insulin coma psychiatric treatment in which patients are given doses of insulin in order to induce hypoglycemia (low blood glucose), coma and a shock to the brain

insulin subcoma inducing hypoglycemia that causes clouded consciousness for up to an hour, but does not induce a coma

involutional melancholia serious depression later in life (middle-aged or older), according to the definitions of age at the time

leucotomy/lobotomy operation to sever the connections in the brain's prefrontal cortex from the thalamus in order to disconnect thoughts and affect

magnetic healing use of magnets in healing

mania extremely elevated and excitable mood

manic depression earlier term for bipolar disorder

metaphysician non-medical 'doctor' who explored alternative forms of healing

metrazol generic of Cardiozol

narcoanalysis/narcohypnosis analysis or hypnosis while the patient is sleeping under the influence of drugs

neuralgia intense, sharp pain that can be caused by damage to pain-signalling nerves or to the brain

neurasthenia term for melancholia and depression

neurotic depression/neurotic depressive reaction terms for a depressed reaction to external circumstances, considered to be out of proportion to events

neurotransmitter neurons that message, regulate and modulate across a synapse, and affect mood, memory, and mental health

non-convulsive stimulatory treatment elecroconvulsion with no seizures

nosology disease classification

paresis weakness

postnatal depression depression following childbirth

post-traumatic stress disorder (PTSD) extraordinary stress during a traumatic event with long-term effects

prolonged narcosis deep sleep therapy

Prozac brand name for fluoxetine, the most well-known selective serotonin reuptake inhibitor (SSRI)

psychasthenia phobias, obsessions or compulsions that the person knows are irrational

psychoanalysis 'talking therapy' designed to uncover subconscious thoughts and repressed feelings and memories

psychotherapy client/patient and therapist work together using various techniques to explore the patient's thinking and feelings in order to seek change or accepatance

psychoneurosis mental disorders that cause a sense of distress and impair functioning. Neuroses were often considered to be out of proportion to actual life circumstances

puerperal insanity severe mental disorders associated with pregnancy, childbirth and lactation

puerperal mania pyschosis, delusions or confusion following childbirth

puerperal melancholia severe depression following childbirth

reactive depression depression considered to be a response to life events or the environment

schizophrenia mental health condition where people experience psychosis — hallucinations and delusions and unusual patterns of thinking or speaking

serotonin neurotransmitter, a natural substance in the brain that helps maintain mental balance

shell shock/war neurosis terms formerly applied to the psychological impact of trauma through war

somatic physical or bodily

SSRIs selective serotonin reuptake inhibitors, newer-generation antidepressants that increase the amount of serotonin in the brain

suicide ideation thinking about committing suicide

therapeutic dissociation where therapeutic techniques are applied to fragment and separate thoughts and experiences

Image credits

Pages 2–3: E. Mervyn Taylor, *Dark Valley*, 1937, Museum of New Zealand Te Papa Tongarewa, 1999-0035-3. Courtesy of the Taylor whānau.

Pages 12–13, clockwise from top left: Auckland Libraries Heritage Collections, 7-A10156; Hocken Collections Uare Taoka o Hākena, 26907; Museum of New Zealand Te Papa Tongarewa, C.014031; Auckland Libraries Heritage Collections, AWNS-19030806-13-02; Auckland Libraries Heritage Collections, NZG-19060721-0037-01

Page 28, clockwise from top left: Archives New Zealand, DAHI/20271/D266/520a; Alexander Turnbull Library, 1/4-020299-F; David Wiltshire, Massey University

Page 29: The New Zealand Medical Journal 23, no. 113 (February 1924): ix. Courtesy of Hocken Collections Uare Taoka o Hākena

Page 70, from top: Auckland Libraries Heritage Collections, NZG-19010323-0552-01; Alexander Turnbull Library, PA1-q-232-10-4

Page 71, clockwise from top: Golden Bay Museum; Marion Davis Library; Auckland Libraries Heritage Collections, AWNS-19310701-48-04

Page 82: State Library Victoria, 1654096

Page 83: Auckland Libraries Heritage Collections, AWNS-19190529-33-04

Pages 96–97, clockwise from top left: Museum of New Zealand Te Papa Tongarewa, C.011731; Alexander Turnbull Library, 1/2-031744-F; Hocken Collections Uare Taoka o Hākena, 694-02852; courtesy of the Agnew whānau; Alamy

Pages 124–25, clockwise from top left: Hocken Collections Uare Taoka o Hākena, 25531; photograph by Philip McManaway, courtesy of Liz Dench; Alexander Turnbull Library, A-313-1-034; Olaf Peterson, Auckland War Memorial Museum Tāmaki Paenga Hira, PH-1988-9; Hocken Collections Uare Taoka o Hākena, S12-152a

Page 143, clockwise from top left: Hocken Collections Uare Taoka o Hākena, S21-566a MS-0999-176; Alexander Turnbull Library, 1/2-043599-F; Alexander Turnbull Library, 1/1-018914-F; courtesy of Mark Pirie and the Campbell whānau

Page 149, from top: Alexander Turnbull Library, 114/109/15-G; Porirua Hospital Museum

Pages 172–73, clockwise from top left: Alexander Turnbull Library, 1/2-019164-F; New Zealand Chinese Heritage Charitable Trust; *The Press*, 9 April 1938, 9, courtesy of the Alexander Turnbull Library; courtesy of Anna Carlson; Auckland Libraries Heritage Collections, 1727-087; Auckland Libraries Heritage Collections, 1790-10

Page 189, clockwise from top left: Stratford Evening Post, 4 May 1923, 2, courtesy of the Alexander Turnbull Library; *Evening Star*, 15 November 1903, 2, courtesy of Papers Past; *Evening Star*, 15 March 1915, 3, courtesy of Papers Past

Pages 198–99, from left: The New Zealand Medical Journal (October 1955): page lv. Courtesy of Hocken Collections Uare Taoka o Hākena; *The New Zealand Medical Journal* (December 1957), colour supplement. Courtesy of Hocken Collections Uare Taoka o Hākena

Page 213, from top: Alexander Turnbull Library, 1/2-057704-F; Warwick Brunton, private collection

Page 230, from top: Daniel Crichton-Rouse, Museum of New Zealand Te Papa Tongarewa; Mark Taylor, Stuff Limited; Lawrence Gullery, Stuff Limited

Acknowledgements

Once again it has been a pleasure to work with Massey University Press, and under the direction of Nicola Legat and Emily Goldthorpe. My thanks also to editor Kate Stone, designer Sarah Elworthy and indexer Diane Lowther. A big shout out to Tracey Borgfeldt, who encouraged me in this project and with whom I initially worked. I also appreciate the care and attention from a reviewer and feedback from Maata Wharehoka and Angela Wanhalla on chapter 2.

Much of this book was written during the Covid pandemic when doing research outside the home could be a logistical nightmare. I applaud staff who responded to requests for information and access to source material during these trying years when there were many personnel shortages. Thanks to Archives New Zealand Te Rua Mahara o te Kāwanatanga; Hocken Library Collections Uare Taoka o Hākena (especially Anna Blackman and Judith Holloway); Alexander Turnbull Library and Collections; Karen Johnson at the Golden Bay Museum Te Waka Huia o Mohua; Presbyterian Archives Research Centre; Mental Health Foundation (particularly Kim Higginson); Ashburn Clinic; Dunedin Returned Services Association; Ministry of Justice Te Tāhū o te Ture; Mental Health and Addiction Services; Ministry of Health Manatu Hauora; and the former Canterbury District Health Board.

Doug Munro was a great source of advice about coronial records, as well as offering convivial company when I was researching in Wellington. I appreciated conversations, advice and support from Angela Wanhalla, Effie Karageorgos, Tiffany Jenks, Kate Hunter, Richard Hill, Chris Prentice, Christine Brett Vickers, Hilary Radner, Sue Tait, Helen Gardner, Judy Bennett, Annabel Cooper, Jenny Bryant-Tokalau and Michelle Walker. I am indebted to Jonathon Sadowsky for his early encouragement of a local history of depression. His scholarship provided me with much inspiration. I also acknowledge my sister 'pioneers' of New Zealand's mental health history, notably Cathy Coleborne, Angela McCarthy and Barbara Brookes.

Several people and organisations generously granted permission to access material, including Andrew Campbell, Estelle McInness, Chris Brickell, Warwick Brunton, Liz Dench, Helen Bichan and the Porirua Museum, the Taylor whānau and the New Zealand Nurses Organisation. Pinky Agnew and Trevor Agnew kindly shared material about their grandmother Jane and I only wish I could have been able to access her mental health records to shed light on her situation.

My warmest thanks to the friends and whānau who have hosted me. These included Carmen Marsh and Tony Richardson, Savita Kesry, Pinky Agnew and Allan Abbott, Bee Dawson and Sandy Dawson.

It cannot have been easy living with someone who is writing about what appears to be a gloomy subject that can be all consuming. My deepest love to my partner, Graham, and our daughter, Tara, for their support and patience and belief that a book about the 'old dark cloud' was worthwhile.

I am most grateful to Anna Green, Jim McAloon and Professor Brigitte Bonich-Brednich at the Stout Centre for New Zealand Studies, Victoria University of Wellington Te Herenga Waka, and Cathy Coleborne at the University of Newcastle in Australia for enabling my institutional support during the writing of this book. Financial support is also crucial for researchers and writers and my thanks to the Ministry for Culture and Heritage for a New Zealand History Research Trust Fund Award, 2020–2021, the Copyright Licensing New Zealand for a Cultural Fund Grant in 2021 and to Creative New Zealand.

About the author

Jacqueline Leckie is a researcher and writer based in Ōtepoti Dunedin. She was a former J. D. Stout research fellow and is now an adjunct research fellow with the Stout Centre for New Zealand Studies at Victoria University of Wellington Te Herenga Waka, and conjoint associate professor in the School of Creative Industries and Social Science at the University of Newcastle, Australia. She is a fellow of the New Zealand Indian Research Institute, an affiliated researcher of Centre for Global Migrations (Otago), and co-editor of the *Journal of Pacific History*. She has taught at the University of the South Pacific, Kenyatta University and the University of Otago. Her publications have covered health history, the Indian diaspora, gender, ethnicity, and work within the Asia–Pacific. Her books include *Invisible: New Zealand's History of Excluding Kiwi-Indians* (2021), *Colonizing Madness: Asylum and Community in Fiji* (2020), *Indian Settlers: The Story of a New Zealand South Asian Community* (2007), *To Labour with the State* (1997), and *A University for the Pacific: 50 Years of USP* (2018).

Index

Page numbers in **bold** refer to images

MASSEY
UNIVERSITY
PRESS

First published in 2024 by Massey University Press
Private Bag 102904, North Shore Mail Centre
Auckland 0745, New Zealand
www.masseypress.ac.nz

Design by Sarah Elworthy

Cover: Detail of E. Mervyn Taylor, *Dark Valley*, 1937, wood engraving, 255 × 189 mm. Museum of New Zealand Te Papa Tongarewa, 1999-0035-3. Courtesy of the Taylor whānau

Poems by Alistair Te Ariki Campbell and Meg Campbell on pages 139, 158 and 214 published with the kind permission of the Campbell whānau

A catalogue record for this book is available from the National Library of New Zealand

Printed and bound in Singapore by Markono Print Media Pte Ltd

ISBN: 978-1-99-101672-0
eISBN: 978-1-99-101673-7

creative nz
Arts Council of New Zealand Toi Aotearoa

COPY RIGHT LICENSING NEW ZEALAND

Manatū Taonga Ministry for Culture & Heritage

The publisher gratefully acknowledges the assistance of Creative New Zealand, Copyright Licensing New Zealand and Manatū Taonga Ministry for Culture and Heritage.